高等教育出版社　中國·北京

Higher Education Press, Beijing, China

英漢實用中醫藥大全

趙樸初題

12

GYNECOLOGY

婦科學

# THE ENGLISH-CHINESE ENCYCLOPEDIA OF PRACTICAL TRADITIONAL CHINESE MEDICINE

| | |
|---|---|
| Chief Editor | Xu Xiangcai |
| Assistants | You Ke  Kang Kai |
| | Bao Xuequan  Lu Yubin |

# 英汉实用中医药大全

主　编　　徐象才
主编助理　尤　可　　康　凯
　　　　　鲍学全　　路玉滨

Higher Education Press
高等教育出版社

# 12
# 妇 科 学

|  | 中文 | 英文 |  |  |
|---|---|---|---|---|
| 主 编 | 李竹兰 | 宣家声 |  |  |
| 副主编 | 国 培 | 张志祥 | 周令娴 | 宁 越 |
| 编 者 | 刘瑞芬 | 谢 光 | 朱 玉 | 刘艳艳 |
|  |  | 张秀娟 | 杨晓平 |  |

# GYNECOLOGY

|  | English | Chinese |
|---|---|---|
| Chief Editor | Xuan Jiasheng | Li Zhulan |
| Deputy Chief Editors | Zhang Zhixiang |  |
|  | Zhou  Lingxian | Guo Pei |
|  | Ning Yue |  |
| Editors | Xie Guang | Liu Ruifen |
|  | Zhu Yu |  |
|  | Liu Yanyan |  |
|  | Zhang Xiujuan |  |
|  | Yang Xiaoping |  |

· 2 ·

| Deputy Directors<br>副主任委员 | Zhang Zhigang,<br>张志刚 | Zhang Wengao<br>张文高 | Jiang Zhaojun,<br>姜兆俊 |
|---|---|---|---|
| | Qi Xiuheng<br>亓秀恒 | ,Xuan Jiasheng<br>宣家声 | ,Sun Xiangxie<br>孙祥燮 |
| Members<br>委员<br>(以姓氏笔划为序) | Yu Wenping<br>于文平 | ,Wang Zhengzhong,<br>王正忠 | Wang Chenying,<br>王陈应 |
| | Wang Guocai<br>王国才 | ,Fang Tingyu<br>方廷钰 | ,Fang Xuwu ,<br>方续武 |
| | Tian Jingzhen<br>田景振 | ,Bi Yongsheng<br>毕永升 | ,Liu Yutan ,<br>刘玉檀 |
| | Liu Chengcai<br>刘承才 | ,Liu Jiaqi<br>刘家起 | ,Liu Xiaojuan ,<br>刘晓娟 |
| | Zhu Zhongbao,<br>朱忠宝 | Zhu Zhenduo<br>朱振铎 | ,Xun Jianying<br>寻建英 |
| | Li Lei<br>李磊 | ,Li Zhulan<br>李竹兰 | ,Xin Shoupu ,<br>辛守璞 |
| | Shao Nianfang,<br>邵念方 | Chen Shaomin<br>陈绍民 | ,Zou Jilong ,<br>邹积隆 |
| | Zu Shengnian<br>陆胜年 | ,Zhou Xing<br>周行 | ,Zhou Ciqing ,<br>周次清 |
| | Zhang Sufang<br>张素芳 | ,Yang Chongfeng<br>杨崇峰 | ,Zhao Chunxiu ,,<br>赵纯修 |
| | Yu Changzheng<br>俞昌正 | ,Hu Zunda<br>胡遵达 | ,Xu Heying ,<br>须鹤瑛 |
| | Yuan Jiurong<br>袁久荣 | ,Huang Naijian<br>黄乃健 | ,Huang Kuiming,<br>黄奎铭 |
| | Huang Jialing<br>黄嘉陵 | ,Cao Yixun<br>曹贻训 | ,Lei Xilian<br>雷希濂 |
| | Cai Huasong<br>蔡华松 | ,Cai Jianqian<br>蔡剑前 | |

# Preface

I am delighted to learn that THE ENGLISH–CHINESE ENCYCLOPEDIA OF PRACTICAL TRADITIONAL CHINESE MEDICINE will soon come into the world.

TCM has experienced many vicissitudes of times but has remained evergreen. It has made great contributions not only to the power and prosperity of our Chinese nation but to the enrichment and improvement of world medicine. Unfortunately, differences in nations, states and languages have slowed down its spreading and flowing outside China. At present, however, an upsurge in learning, researching and applying TCM is unfolding. In order to maximize the effect of this upsurge and to lead TCM, one of the brilliant cultural heritages of the Chinese nation, to the world for it to expand and bring benefit to the people of all nations, Mr. Xu Xiangcai called intellectuals of noble aspirations and high intelligence together from Shandong and many other provinces in China and took charge of the work of both compilation and translation of THE ENGLISH–CHINESE ENCYCLOPEDIA OF PRACTICAL TRADITIONAL CHINESE MEDICINE. With great pleasure, the medical staff both at home and abroad will hail the appearance of this encyclopedia.

I believe that the day when the world's medicine is fully developed will be the day when TCM has spread throughout the world.

I have written my preface with pleasure.

By Prof. Dr. Hu ximing

Deputy ministerof The Ministry of Public Health
of the People's Republic of China,

Director general of The State Administrative Bureau of Traditional Chinese Medicine and
Pharmacology,

President of The World Federation of Acupuncture
—Moxibustion Societies,

Member of China Association of Science & Technology,

Deputy president of All—China Association of
Traditional Chinese Medicine,

President of China Acupuncture & Moxibustion
Society.

December, 1989.

# Preface

The Chinese Nation has been through a long, arduous course of struggling against diseases and has developed its own traditional medicine—Traditional Chinese Medicine and Pharmacology (TCMP). TCMP has a unique, comprehensive, scientific system including both theories and clinical practice. Some thousand years since its beginnings, not only has it been well preserved but also continuously developed. It has special advantages, such as remarkable curative effects and few side effects. Hence it is an effective means by which people prevent and treat diseases and keep themselves strong and healthy.

All achievements attained by any nation in the development of medicine are the public wealth of all mankind. They should not be confined within a single country. What is more, the need to set them free to flow throughout the world as quickly and precisely as possible is greater than that of any other kind of science. During my more than thirty years of being engaged in Traditional Chinese Medicine(TCM), I have been looking forward to the day when TCMP will have spread all over the world and made its contributions to the elimination of diseases of all mankind. However it is to be deeply regretted that the pace of TCMP in extending outside China has been unsatisfactory due to the major difficulties in expressing its concepts in foreign languages.

Mr. Xu Xiangcai, a teacher of Shandong College of TCM, has sponsored and taken charge of the work of compilation and translation of The English—Chinese Encyclopedia of Practical Traditional Chinese Medicine—an extensive series. This work is a great project, a large—scale scientific research, a courageous effort and a novel creation. I deeply esteem Mr. Xu Xiangcai and his compilers and translators for their hard labor, working day and night for such a long time, for their firm and indomitable will displayed in overcoming one difficulty after another, and for their great success achieved in this way. As a leader in the circles of TCM, I am duty—bound to do my best to support them.

I believe this encyclopedia will be certain to find its position both in the history of Chinese medicine and in the history of world science and technology.

By Mr. Zhang Qiwen
Member of The Standing Committee of
All—China Association of TCM,
Deputy head of The Health Department of
Shandong Province.
March, 1990.

# Publisher's Preface

Traditional Chinese Medicine(TCM) is one of China's great cultural heritages,. Since the founding of the People's Republic of China in 1949, guided by the farsighted TCM policy of the Chinese Communist Party and the Chinese government, the treasure house of the theories of TCM has been continuously explored and the plentiful literature researched and compiled. As a result, great success has been achieved. Today there has appeared a world—wide upsurge in the studying and researching of TCM. To promote even more vigorous development of this trend in order that TCM may better serve all mankind, efforts are required to further it throughout the world. To bring this about, the language barriers must be overcome as soon as possible in order that TCM can be accurately expressed in foreign languages.

Thus the compilation and translation of a series of Chinese —English books of basic knowledge of TCM has become of great urgency to serve the needs of medical and educational circles both inside and outside China.

In recent years, at the request of the health departments, satisfactory achievements have been made in researching the expression of TCM in English. Based on the investigation into the history and current state of the research work mentioned above, The English—Chinese Encyclopedia of Practical TCM has been published to meet the needs of extending the knowledge of TCM around the world.

The encyclopedia consists of twenty—one volumes, each dealing with a particular branch of TCM. In the process of compilation, the distinguishing features of TCM have been given close attention and great efforts have been made to ensure that the content is scientific, practical, comprehensive and concise. The chief writers of the Chinese manuscripts include professors or associate professors with at least twenty years of practical clinical and / or teaching experience in TCM. The Chinese manuscript of each volume has been checked and approved by a specialist of the relevant branch of TCM. The team of the translators and revisers of the English versions consists of TCM specialists with a good command of English, professional medical translators, and teachers of English from TCM colleges or universities. At a symposium to standardize the English versions, scholars from twenty—two colleges or universities, research institutes of TCM or other health institutes probed the questions of how to express TCM in English more comprehensively; systematically and accurately, and discussed and deliberated in detail the English versions of some volumes in order to upgrade the English versions of the whole series. The English version of each volume has been re—examined and then given a final checking.

Obviously this encyclopedia will provide extensive reading material of TCM English for senior students in colleges of TCM in China and will also greatly benefit foreigners studying TCM.

The assiduous efforts of compiling and translating this encyclopedia have been supported by the responsible leaders of the State Education Commission of the People's Republic of China, the State Administrative Bureau of TCM and Pharmacy, the Education Commission and Health Department of Shandong Province. Under the direction of the Higher Education Department of the State Education Commission, the leading board of compilation and translation of this encyclopedia was set up. The leaders of many colleges of TCM and pharmaceutical factories of TCM have also given assitance.

We hope that this encyclopedia will bring about a good effect on enhancing the teaching of TCM English at the colleges of TCM in China, on cultivating skills in medical circles in exchanging ideas of TCM with patients in English, and on giving an impetus to the study of TCM outside China.

Higher Education Press

March, 1990.

# Foreword

The English—Chinese Encyclopedia of Practical Traditional Chinese Medicine is an extensive series of twenty—one volumes, Based on the fundamental theories of Traditional Chinese Medicine(TCM) and with emphasis on the clinical practice of TCM, it is a semi—advanced English—Chinese academic works which is quite comprehensive, systematic, concise, practical and easy to read. It caters mainly to the following readers: senior students of colleges of TCM, young and middle—aged teachers of colleges of TCM, young and middle—aged physicians of hospitals of TCM, personnel of scientific research institutions of TCM, teachers giving correspondence courses in TCM to foreigners, TCM personnel going abroad in the capacity of lecturers or physicians, those trained in western medicine but wishing to study TCM, and foreigners coming to China to learn TCM or to take refresher courses in TCM.

Because Traditional Chinese Medicine and Pharmacology is unique to our Chinese nation, putting TCM into English has been the crux of the compilation and translation of this encyclopedia. Owing to the fact that no one can be proficient both in the theories of Traditional Chinese Medicine and Pharmacology and the clinical practice of every branch of TCM, as well as in English, to ensure that the English versions express accurately the inherent meanings of TCM, collective translation measures have been taken. That is, teachers of English familiar with TCM, professional medical translators, teachers or physicians of TCM and even teachers of palaeography with a strong command of English were all invited together to co-translate the Chinese manuscripts and, then, to co-deliberate and discuss the English versions. At last English-speaking foreigners studying TCM or teaching English in China were asked to polish the English Versions. In this way, the skills of the above trans lators and foreigners were merged to ensure the quality of the English versions. However, even using this method, the uncertainty that the English versions will be wholly accepted still remains. As for the Chinese manuscripts, they do reflect the essence, and give a general picture, of Traditional Chinese Medicine and Pharmacology. It is not asserted, though, that they are perfect. I whole heartedly look forward to any criticisms or opinions from readers in order to make improvements to future editions.

More than 200 people have taken part in the activities of compiling, translating and revising this encyclopedia. They come from twenty-eight institutions in all parts of China. Among these institutions, there are fifteen colleges of TCM: Shandong, Beijing, Shanghai, Tianjin, Nanjing, Zhejiang, Anhui, Henan, Hubei, Guangxi, Guiyang, Gansu, Chengdu, Shanxi and Changchun, and scientific research centers of TCM such as China Academy of TCM and Shandong Scientific Research Institute of TCM.

The Education Commission of Shandong Province has included the compilation and translation of this encyclopedia in its scientific research projects and allocated funds accordingly. The Health Department of Shandong Province has also given financial aid together with a number of pharmaceutical factories of TCM. The subsidization from Jinan Pharmaceutical Factory of

TCM provided the impetus for the work of compilation and translation to get under way.

The success of compiling and translating this encyclopedia is not only the fruit of the collective labor of all the compilers, translators and revisers but also the result of the support of the responsible leaders of the relevant leading institutions. As the encyclopedia is going to be published. I express my heartfelt thanks to all the compilers, translators and revisers for their sincere cooperation, and to the specialists, professors, leaders at all levels and pharmaceutical factories of TCM for their warm support.

It is my most profound wish that the publication of this encyclopedia will take its role in cultivating talented persons of TCM having a very good command of TCM English and in extending, rapidly, comprehensive knowledge of TCM to all corners of the globe.

Xu Xiangcai,
Shandong College of TCM,
March, 1990.

# Contents

# Notes

GYNECOLOGY is the twelfth volume of The English
—Chinese Encyclopedia of Practical Traditional Chinese Medicine.

This volume consists of six chapters: Introduction, Inflam-
mations in the Female Reproductive System, Menopathy,
Pathologic Pregnancy, Perverse Labor and Abnormal
Puerperium, and Miscellaneous Gynecopathy.

Mordern medical classifications of gynecological disorders
are adopted in this volume for the convenience of world—wide
readers, but its contents are based on the general theories and
therapies of Traditional Chinese Medicine, (TCM)

The Chinese manuscript was first examined by Miss Wang
Wenyu, of the Shandong Journal of TCM, then checked and approved by Prof. Ha Litian, the late authority in the field of
gynecology of TCM in China. The English version was
collectively discussed and deliberated by a group of scholars,
some of whom are English professors having been trained in
TCM, others are TCM professors having a good command of the
English language, and they have made every effort to make it ac-
curate.

editor

# 1. Introduction

## 1.1 A General Survey of Traditional Chinese Gynecology

Traditional Chinese Gynecology (TCG) is a branch of clinical medical science based on the general theories of traditional Chinese medicine (TCM), which enables one to make out the anatomical, physiological and pathological features of the female, to grasp its diagnostic principles and to study various diseases inflicted specifically by women.

The scope of TCG covers the regulation of menstruation, conception, pregnancy, labor, puerperium, metrorrhagia, metrostaxis, leukorrhea and miscellaneous gynecological diseases. For the sake of convenience, they are classified into five categories: menstruation, leukorrhea, pregnancy, parturition and miscellaneous diseases.

TCG is an important and inseparable component of Chinese medicine. It has a long history and is rich in experience. For thousands of years, it has played a significant role in the health and care of Chinese womanhood and contributed a great deal to the revival and prosperity of the whole nation.

As the extant documentation shows, TCG can be traced back as far as 3,000 years ago. The records about sterility can be seen in the inscriptions on bones or tortoise shells of the Shang Dynasty. (16 century−1066BC) Such commonly used medicinal herbs as Luru (Rubia cordifolia L), Tui (Herba Leonuri) Fouyi (Herba Plantaginis) were collected and utilized, as stated in *Shijing*(The book of Songs) composed in the early Zhou Dynasty.*Shanhaijing* (The Book of Mountains and Seas. a geographical work in ancient China) asserts that *You* (a species of cormorant) is beneficial for pregnancy while *Gurong* (a sort of ancient medicinal herb) will make one sterile. The harm of consanguineous marriage is pointed out in *Quli* (The Book of Rites. a Confucian classic): "Don't marry one who has the same surname." "The married couple who have one and the same family name will bear few healthy children."

Huangdi *Neijing* (the Yellow Emperor's Internal Classic, 221BC) describes the anatomy and physiology of the female and the diagnoses of gynecological diseases. It indicates that the first menstruation of a female may take place at the age of 14 and she becomes an adult at 21 and the menstruation is to cease around the age of 49. The generating mechanism of menstruation and the life cycle of the female sex from birth to old age are described in detail. The first prescription of Chinese gynecology *Siwuzeigu—luruwan* (a pill composed of four portions of Os Sepiella seu Sepiae and one portion of Radix Rubiae) was given in that classic. Gynecologists began to emerge in the late Warring States. The *Biographies of Bian Que and Cang Gone in Shiji*(Historical Records) narrates the deeds of the famous physician Bian Que who, on hearing of the dignified position of noblewomen in Handan, presented himself as a "doctor underneath the skirts". Such a physician was no other than a gynecologist or an obstetrician.

The earliest monograph of TCG among the existing medical

classics is *Jinkui Yaolue* (Synopsis of Prescriptions of the Golden Chamber) by Zhang Zhongjing in the Han Dynasty. His dissertations on the pulse conditions, syndromes and therapies of gravidic, puerperal and miscellaneous diseases of gynecology have so far exerted a prominent influence on later generations. The method of external treatment by means of vaginal douche and vaginal suppository was registered in that book. With the aid of pulse conditions of the patient, Hua Tuo, a magic surgeon of the same period, made a correct diagnosis of a couple of fetuses in the maternal womb, one of which was alive and he succeeded in getting rid of the dead fetus by way of acupuncture and drugs.

In the third century, a celebrated physician of the Jin Dynasty Wang Shuhe compiled *Mai Jing* (The Pulse Classic) Which relates how to take the pulse and differentiate symptoms and signs of women's diseases that are associated with pregnancy, puerperium, leukorrhea, menstruation and miscellaneous gynecopathy. He discovered " the abnormally rapid or slow pulse" during parturition and perceived the abnormal phenomena of menstruation: *Ju j ing* (seasonal menses) and *Binian* (annual menses)

Chu Deng of the Southern Qi Dynasty left behind a book entitled *Chushi Yishu* (Chu's Posthumous Papers). In the chapter of "Asking for offsprings", he exclaims that a man "should not marry until thirty" "Not until twenty can a woman get married and then she will have her baby healthy and long-lived." Besides, it is expounded that if a woman has excessive sexual intercourses with the male, she will surely be "poor in health and debilitated because of the deficiency of essence of life", "Excessive delivery and feeding of the infants will shorten her life owing to blood depletion." His views of late marriage, continence and birth control have played an important role in protecting the health of Chinese women and securing a flourishing prospect for our nation.

Xu Zhicai of the Northern Qi Dynasty wrote *Shiyue Yangtai Fang* (The Method of Nourishing the Fetus during Ten Months' Pregnancy), which describes the gradual growth and development of the fetus month by month, stresses the problems to be noted in the daily accommodations of the gravid woman and designates the forbidden areas of acupuncture and moxibustion. A list of recipes for preserving the fetus from abortion is presented in the annex.

In 610, a group of imperial physicians of the Sui Dynasty headed by Chao Yuanfang set forth *Zhubing Yanhou Lun* (A General Treatise on the Causes and Symptoms of Diseases which deals extensively with 283 kinds of gynecopathy in all. It is clearly indicated that pregnancy lasts for ten months and that a pregnant woman, when sick, must not keep mourishing the fetus or it will be harmful to herself. If it is the case, it is totally necessary to have artificial abortion in order to secure the safety of the mother.

Sun Simiao of the Tang Dynasty composed *Beij iQiangj in Yaofang* (Prescriptions Worth a Thousand Gold for Emergencies)in 652. Those prescriptions adaptable for women were put in the first and foremost place. It is defined that gynecology should be studied as a speciality. Sterility is considered to be concerned with both sexes. Generally speaking, sterility results "from consumptive diseases or internal injuries caused by overstrain" or "from general debility and emaciation of the married couple". It is desirable that the delivery room should be clean and quiet and that people are not allowed to go about and look on while the woman is in labour. Care must be taken of the key point that "sexual intercourse is not permitted until one hundred days after childbirth, otherwise the woman will became weak, frail and sickly all the life. One should be prudent about this." The hygiene of puerperium is also taken seriously.

*Tj ingxiao Chanbao* (Tested Treasures in Obstetrics) is the earliest extant work of obstetrics in China, compiled by Zan Xin of the Tang Dynasty in 852. It consists of three volumes and the supplement, where gravidic, puerperal and postpartum diseases are defined and treated.

In the Song Dynasty (11—13 centuries), the Bureau of Imperial Physicians was established to administer the medical affairs. The obstetrical department was then one of the nine departments with professors in that speciality, so it became the earliest division to take obstetrics as an independent branch in the medical system of the world. Tremendous progress in gynecology and obstetrics was made in the Song Dynasty and there were quite a number of gynecological writings, the most famous of which are Yang Zijian's *Shi Chan Lun* (Ten Problems in Obstetrics) and Chen Ziming's *Furen Liangfang Daguan* (The Complete Effective Prescriptions for Women).

TCM entered into a new era in the Jin and Yuan Dynasties from the thirteenth to fourteenth century. During that period, different academic schools thrived and contended in the field of medicine. Four major schools headed by Liu Wansu, Li Dongyuan, Zhu Danxi and Zhang Zihe had their individual views on gynecology. Liu put forward the theory that the physician should attach importance to the kidney channel of the female in her girlhood, to the liver channel in her prime and to the spleen channel in her old age. His experience influenced the later generations a great deal. Li advocated the method of reinforcing the spleen to send up the lucid *Yang* while invigorating *Qi* and enriching the blood. His method has been widely applied in Chinese gynecology. Based on the belief that *Yang Qi* which denotes functional activity tends to be excessive while *Yin Qi* which denotes substance is often insufficient, Zhu suggested "the woman big with child should eliminate the heat and nourish the blood" and "to ensure a successful gestation, Radix Scutellariae and Rhizoma Atractylodis Macrocephalae should be taken as miraculous medicine" Those herbs are still used in China today. Zhang maintained the doctrine that preserving health depends on dietetic therapy while curing illness depends on drug treatment. Therefore he liked to adopt the emetic and purgative therapies of dispelling retained water and removing phlegm when he dealt with diseases of menstruation.

A large quantity of gynecological writings were produced in the Ming Dynasty. Among them there were Wang Kentang's *Zhengzhi Zhun Sheng Nüke* (Standards for Diagnosis and Treatment of Women's Diseases), Xue Lizhai's *Nüke Zhaiyao* (Extracts of Obstetrics and Gynecology), Wan Quan's *Guangsi Jiyao* (Synopsis for Breeding More Kids) and Zhang Jinyue's *Furen Gui* (Principles of Gynecology). Wan suggested, "Before the sexual activity the male should clear away the heart—fire and check sexual desires so as to replenish vital essence, the other sex should be quiet and calm to nourish the blood." He classified the cases of infertility caused by the congenital physiological defects of the female as follows: *Luo* (spiral vagina), *Wen* (stricture of vagina),

*Gu* (imperforate hymen), *Jiao* (elongated clitoris) and *Mai* (amenorrhea or menoxenia). They are normally known as the five types of the female sterility. Zhang Jingyue's enunciation of *Tiangui* (the kidney—*Yin*) is in great detail. It is described as a sort of innate *Yin* fluid that is replenished by the gradual nourishment of the human body after its birth and it can exercise a direct influence on the growth, maturity, menarche and menopause. In the Ming Dynasty, the great pharmacist Li Shizhen compiled a monumental work —— *Bencao Gangmu* (Compendium of Materia Medica, 1587) in which he expounds that the female menstruation is almost as regular as the waxing and waning of the moon or the ebb and flow of the tide. He points out that menstruation has its own rule, that is to say, it takes place regularly, once in a month.

Gynecology in the Qing Dynasty is commonly known as the department of women's diseases. There were numerous writings on the subject. Among them the most influential are *Fu Qingzhu Nüke* (Fu Qingzhu's Obstetrics and Gynecology,) *Yizong Jinjian, Fuke Xinf a Yaojue*(The Golden mirror of medicine: Essentials of Treating Gynecopathy,) *Dasheng Pian* (Knowledge for labour) *Nüke Jiyao* (Summary for Women's Diseases )Jizhai Jushi (a lay Buddist) suggests in *Dasheng Pian* that when a pregnant woman is going to labour, she should "sleep for longer time, make efforts to bear delivery pain and try to delay the starting moment of labour as long as possible". These knacks have protected the parturient in body and spirit.

From the concluding years of the Qing Dynasty to the early years of the Republic of China, with the introduction of the Western medicine came the integration of the traditional Chinese and Western medicines. The representative works of that period are Tang Rongchuan's *Xue Zheng Lun* (A Treatise on Blood Troubles ), Zhang Xichun's *Yixue Zhong Zhong Chan Xi Lu* (Practical Records of Traditional Chinese Medicine with Reference to Western Medicine), Zhang Shanlei's *Shenshi Nüke Jiyao Jianzheng* (Shen's Summary of Women's Diseases Annotated).

Since the founding of The People's Republic of China in 1949, TCG has won tremendous achievements including the nonoperative treatment of ectopic pregnancy through the integration of Chinese and Western Medicines, the induction of labour by Chinese medicinal herbs, the rectification of the fetal position by acupuncture and moxibustion. In 1956 TCM colleges were set up, Since then *Zhongguo Yixue Baike Quanshu* (Encyclopedia of Traditional Chinese Medicine) and various textbooks of TCG have been compiled and published. Traditional Chinese gynecologists and obstetricians have been trained in large quantities. They have made significant contributions to the health and welfare of womanhood.

## 1.2 Anatomy and Physiology of the Female Reproductive System

### 1.2.1 The Internal and External Genital Organs

Different terms are used in traditional Chinese medicine to mean one and the same thing—uterus; they are *Baogong* (the cell where the fetus grows),*Nüzibao* (the bag for the fetus),

*Baozang* (viscera that contain the fetus), *Zizang* (viscera that breed the fetus), *Zichu* (the place where the fetus stays) but the uterus may simply be called *Zang* or *Bao* . Just as the uterus can periodically store and remove the menses and the fetus and no other *Zang—Fu* can be interior—exteriorly related with it, so it is denominated an extraordinary *Fu*—organ.

*Baomai* and *Baoluo* both of which denote uterine collaterals are appendant to the uterus. They have a close connection with *Zang—Fu* . Working along with the uterus, they perform the function of regulating the menses and breeding the fetus.

*Zimen* refers to the cervical orifice of the uterus.

*Chandao* refers to the vagina.

*Zichang* refers generally to the uterus and the vaginal wall. Zichang Bushou refers to hysteroptosis, rectocele or cystocele.

*Yinhu* refers to the vulva.

*Yinmen* or *Chanmen* refers to the vaginal orifice.

*Yinqi* refers to external genitals.

*Maqi* refers to the upper edge of pubes of the vulva.

*Jiaogu* refers to the sacrococcygeal joint, the region of pubic symphysis.

## 1.2.2 The *Chong, Ren Du* and *Dai* channels

The *Chong* channel originates from the interior of the uterus, ascends along the perineum to the head and descends to the feet. It runs forward to the abdomen and travels backward to the interior of the vertebrae where 12 regular channels gather and meet. The *Chong* channel functions to control and regulate the menses.

The *Ren* channel is in charge of the embryo in the uterus. It starts from the interior of the uterus, emerges at the perineum, then along the midline of the abdomen ascends to the lip and the lower part of the orbit. Semen (reproductive essence), blood and body fluids are all controlled by the *Ren*channel. Only when *Qi* goes smoothly through the channel can one's menstruation and fertility become regular and orderly.

The *Du* channel functions like a governor. It starts from the interior of the uterus, runs down through the perineum as *Ren* does and then along the vertebrae ascends to the head. The *Du* channel penetrates the vertebrae and is appendant to the kidney. In TCM the kidney is considered to be the origin of congenital constitution, the source of primordial *Qi*. So *Du* is concerned with primordial *Qi*, the primary motive force of the life activities. *Ren* and *Du* converge at the acupoint of *Yinj iao* . They govern the balance between *Yin* and *Yang* and the flow of *Qi* in the channels and regulate the methodical flow of menstruation.

The *Dai* channel originates from the hypochondrium, runs transversely around the body like a waistband. So it is also known as the belt channel. Its function is to control all those channels and collaterals and make them work properly along with *Qi* and blood.

The *Chong*,*Ren*,*Du* channels originate altogether from the interior of the uterus. They are bound by the *Dai* channel, joining with *Zang* and *Fu* by way of 12 regular channels. They work jointly, regulating the flow of menstruation and keeping up the normal physiological functions.

### 1.2.3 Menstruation and its Generating Mechanism

Menstruation refers to regular, periodic endometrorrhagia, which emerges once in a month like the wax and wane of the moon or the ebb and flow of the tide.it is a constant, unchanging phenomenon, so itmis also termed in Chinese medicine *Yuexun* (monthly tide), *Yuexin* (monthly information) and *Yueshui* (monthly liquid).

As early As 2000 years ago, some records about menstruation can be found in *Huangdi Neijing* (The Yellow Emperor's Internal Classic) ,"The kidney−*Qi* of a female is getting vigorous at the age of 7, her teeth renewed and her hair growing longer. Menophania initiates at 14 as the *Ren* channel is put through, and the *Taichong* channel is replenished. Menstruation attends regularly, so it is possible for the female to reproduce....At the age of 49, the *Ren* channel becomes void, the *Taichong* channel is attenuated, leading to menopause and amenorrhea. Since the genitals have withered, the female cannot reproduce any more". The process of growth, maturation and senility of the female genitality is fully described in that classic. For healthy girls,the menstrual onset occurs at the age of 14 or so, also known as menophania or menarche. It marks the advent of adolescence. In different regions, climates, nations and on different levels of nourishment, the age of menophania may change from 11 to 18. Except for the period of pregnancy and lactation, menstruation will not cease until the age of 49.

Under normal conditions the cycle of menstruation lasts for 28 days It should not precede nor delay longer than 7 days. The menstrual cycle persists for 3 to 7 days. Its volume is about 50—80 ml. It is dark red in color but at the start and in the end, it turns pink. The menstrual flow is ample on the second and third days. It is neither thin nor thick, having no blood clots nor special odor. *Bingyue* (bimonthly menses) refers to the menstruation that attends regularly once in two months. *Jujing* (delayed menses) or *Jijing* (seasonal menses) refers to that which attends once in 3 months *Binian* (annual menses). refers to that which attends only once in a year, *Anjing* (latent menses) refers to the symptom that a female has no menses all the life but is conceptive, *Jijing* (agitated menses) or *Goutai* (unclear pregnancy) or *Shengtai* (exuberant pregnancy) refers to the symptom that the female has a little blood shed per month after the conception with little harm to the fetus.

The generation of menstruation is a physiological phenomenon caused by the joint action of *Tiangui, Zang—Fu, Qi* and blood, channels and collaterals upon the uterus. *Tiangui*, possessed by both sexes, is a kind of *Yin* essence which influences the growth, maturity and reproduction of the human body. It rises from the innate kidney—*Qi* and having been nourished and supplied by the essential substances from water and food, it gradually becomes mature. *Tiangui* inherits from the parents, but it functions only when the kidney —*Qi* is plentiful and reaches the climax at a definite age. It enriches semen, blood and body fluids which are governed by the *Ren* channel and replenishes the *Chong* channel and vise versa. Having been enriched by the kidney—essence, the *Chong* channel brings together the blood in *Zang* and *Fu*, which gets gradually full and overflows the uterus regularly, so comes the menstrual flow of the female. The chief element of menstruation is blood, which is produced and transformed by *zang* and *f u* . According to the theory of TCM, the essence of life is stored in the kidney; blood stems from acquired essence. The heart governs the blood circulation;blood is stored in the liver and governed by the spleen. The lung is in charge of *Qi, Qi* commands blood. So the rise of menstruation is closely related with the kidney, liver, spleen and stomach. Blood is the basic element of menstruation while *Qi* is the motive force for blood circulation. Only when *Qi* and blood match with each other perfectly well can menstruation show itself in a sound manner. Channels and collaterals are joined with *Zang* and *Fu* in the interior and connected externally with the extremities of the body. They convey all sorts of information from outside to inside, from upper to lower. They make the various parts of the human body into an organic unit, circulating *Qi* and blood, nourishing the whole body. The *Chong, Ren, Du* and *Dai* channels are most closely related to the physiological and pathological features of the female, regulating the flow of *Qi* and blood in 12 regular channels. They play a tremendous role in the formation of menstruation.

The kidney is the base where menstruation is produced. *Qi* and blood are the essential substances of menstruation. The *Chong* and *Ren* channels are the spot where menstruation is transformed. The uterus is the place where menstruation flows. Only when the kidney–*Qi* is abundant, the information of *Tiangui* has come, the *Ren* channel is put through and the *Taichong* channel is replenished, can menstruation attend punctually.

## 1.3　Summary of Therapeutic Methods

Starting from the view that the human body is an organic whole, TCG holds that different diseases should be treated by different methods. Followingthe principles of four diagnostic methods and eight principal syndromes ofTCM,they try their best to make an overall analysis of symptoms and signs on the basis of physiological characteristics of the female, and discerns carefully the etiology and pathogenesis in conjunction with menstruation, leukorrhea, pregnancy, parturition and miscellaneous diseases. The following maxims should be obeyed: The primary cause of a disease must be searched out before medical treatment. Treat the outstanding syndromes when the illness is critical; treat the fundamental syndromes if the illness is steady. Treat deficiency syndromes by tonification;treat excess syndromes by purgation and reduction. Treat the cold syndromes by hot—natured drugs, treat the heat syndromes by cold—or cool—natured drugs. A general disease should be cured chiefly by internal treatment. For a local disease, external treatment may simultaneously be adopted.

### 1.3.1　Internal Treatment

#### 1. Tonification of the kidney

Tonification is the most important therapeutic method to reinforce the weak kidney. The importance of the kidney in the physiology of the female delermines the use of the kidney—tonifying method. When the kidney—$Qi$ is insufficient, the essence and blood will wear out, When the *Chong* and *Ren* channels will be disturbed and go out of order, various diseases including those concerned with menstruation, leukorrhea, pregnancy, parturition and miscellaneous diseases will be induced successively. By means of tonification, Yin and Yang of the kidney will work in equilibrium and in harmony, so as to keep on their normal physiological functions.

(1)Tonifying the kidney—Yang

When the kidney—Yang is deficient and the uterus can't get enough warmth, the private parts (pudenda) will lose warmth, and the female will lessen the interest in sexual activity, thus resulting in sterility due to the cold uterus, or in retarded growth of the fetus or in abortion within three to seven months.

Commonly used drugs:

Cortex Cinnamomi
Radix Aconiti Praeparata
Fructus Psoraleae
Herba Epimedii
Rhizoma Curculiginis
Semen Cuscutae
Radix Morindae Officinalis
Herba Cynomorii
Fructus Rubi

Typical recipes:

Shenqi Wan
Yougui Wan
Yougui Yin

(2):Replenishing the kidney—Yin

When the kidney—Yin is deficient, the Chong and Ren channels will lose enough nourishment, resulting in scanty menstruation, amenorrhea, vaginal dryness and roughness, metrorrhagia and metrostaxis, preceded or delayed menstrual cycle, sterility, retarded growth of the fetus.

Commonly used drugs: Radix Rehmanniae
Rhizoma Polygonati
Colla Corii Asini
Fructus Corni
Fructus Ligustri Lucidi
Radix Polygoni Multiflori
Colla Plastri Testudinis
Fructus Lycii
Cordyceps

Typical recipes:
*Liuwei Dihuang Wan*
*Zuogui Wan*

When using tonics to reinforce the kidney, no matter what the purpose is, to invigorate *Yang* or to nourish *Yin* or to reinforce both *Yin* and *Yang*, the prescription must be made up on the basis of differentiation of clinical symptoms and signs. The principle stated below should be followed: Don't forget to reinforce *Yang* while replenishing *Yin*; nor forget to enrich *Yin* while tonifying *Yang*. That is to say, several adjuvant drugs for warming *yang* should be added in the formula of nourishing *Yin* and vice versa. In so doing, the mutuality of *Yin* and *Yang* will be beneficial to the patient's recovery from the disease.

## 2. Regulation of the liver

This method is used to regulate the function of the liver and restore it to the normal state. Blood is stored in the liver which governs the normal flow of *Qi*. When the liver works properly, menstruation will attend regularly. The liver troubles in gynecology are manifested by the stagnation of the liver—$Qi$ and the deficiency of the liver—$Yin$. The basic remedy is to disperse the depressed liver—$Qi$ and nourish the liver.

(1)Soothing the liver

① Relieving the depressed liver and promoting the flow of stagnant $Qi$.

The blood of a female is constantly and repeatedly dissipated by menstruation, leukorrhea, pregnancy, parturition, thus resulting in deficiency of blood and excess of $Qi$, so gynecological diseases are chiefly induced by spiritual and emotional factors. If the female is depressed or angered, the liver—$Qi$ will run in the morbid state, characterized by the stagnation of the liver—$Qi$ and the obstruction of blood circulation in the channels and collaterals, leading to dysmenorrhea, amenorrhea, breast—pain before menses and agalactia after delivery. If the flow of liver—$Qi$ is excessive and out of control, the menstrual cycle will become irregular. Under such conditions, liver—soothing is the correct method of treatment.

Commonly used drugs :

Radix Bupleuri

Rhizoma Cyperi

Radix Curcumae

Fructus Meliae Toosendan

Radix Linderae

Pericarpium Citri Reticulatae Viride

Folium Citri Reticulatae

Herba Mentae

Typical recipes:

*Xiao Yao San*

*Chaihu Shugan San*

②Purging the liver of pathogenic fire

The stagnant liver—*Qi* will turn into pathogenic fire, characterized by the upward invasion of the hyperactive liver—*Qi* and the forced extravasion of blood, leading to the preceded menstrual cycle, menorrhagia, menostaxis, metrorrhagia and metrostaxis, hematemesis and headache during menstruation. Treatment must be based on soothing the liver by using several drugs for removing fire from the liver.

Commonly used drugs:

>Cortex Moutan Radicis
>
>Fructus Gardeniae
>
>Flos Chrysanthemi
>
>Spica Prunellae

Typical recipe:

>*Dan Zhi Xiaoyao San*

③Clearing away heat and promoting diuresis

The damp—heat of the liver channel surges downward, resulting in leukorrhagia, vulval pruritus and erosion. Recommended remedy is to eliminate damp—heat in the liver channel.

Commonly used drugs:

>Radix Gentianae
>
>Herba Artemisiae Scopariae
>
>Semen Plantaginis
>
>Cortex Phellodendri

Typical recipe: *Longdan Xiegan Tang*

(2)Nourishing the liver

①Enriching the blood and softening the liver

The deficiency of the liver—*Yin* will lead to delayed menstrual cycle, scanty menstruation, amenorrhea, metrorrhagia and metrostaxis, and other various diseases around menstruation and menopause.

Commonly used drugs:

Fructus Lycii
Radix Paeoniae Alba
Fructus Ligustri Lucidi
Herba Ecliptae
Fructus Mori
Fructus Schisandrae
Radix Angelicae Sinensis
Radix Rehmanniae

Typical recipes:

*Erzhi Wan*
*Yiguan Jian*
*Qi Ju Dihuang Wan*

② Calming the liver, suppressing the hyperactivities of the liver—*Yang* and subduing the endogenous wind to relieve convulsions

The deficiency of the liver—*Yin* and the hyperactivity of the liver—*Yang* will induce headache during menstruation, preeclampsia, eclampsia gravidarum due to the up—stirring of the liver—wind. The prescription will be made up on the basis of nourishing the liver—*Yin*, by using drugs for calming the liver, suppressing the hyperactivity of the liver—*Yang* and subduing the endogenous wind.

Commonly used drugs:

Ochra Haematitum

Radix Paeoniae Alba

Os Draconis

Concha Ostreae

Concha Margaritifera Usta

Plastrum Testudinis

Fructus Tribuli

Lumbricus

Ramulus Uncariae Cum Uncis

Cornu Antelopis

Calculus Bovis

Typical recipes:

*Sanj ia Fumai Tang*

*Lingyang Gouteng Tang*

*Lingyang Jiao Tang*

### 3.Strengthening of the spleen

The strengthening of the spleen is the most important method to reinforce the weak spleen. The spleen governs the blood and has the function of digesting, transporting and transforming nutrients. It is the source of growth and transformation of $Qi$ and blood, the pivot of metabolism of water and liguids. The insufficiency of the spleen—$Qi$ will bring about many gynecological diseases that must be cured by way of strengthening the spleen.

(1)Invigorating the spleen and replenishing $Qi$

The weakness of the spleen—$Qi$ will lead to the deficiency of both $Qi$ and blood in their growth and transformation, thus often resulting in delayed menstrual cycle, scanty menstruation, amenorrhea, agalactia, and morning sickness.

Commonly used drugs:

Radix Ginseng

Radix Codonopsis Pilosulae

Radix Astragali seu Hedysari

Rhizoma Dioscoreae

Fructus Ziziphi Jujubae

Radix Glycyrrhizae

Typal recipes:

*Si Junzi Tang*

*Shenling Baizhu San*

(2) Invigorating the spleen and removing dampness

The dysfunction of the spleen in transportation gives rise to the retention of water and dampness within the body, thus leading to leukorrhagia, edema of pregnancy, diarrhea and edema during menstruation, amenorrhea and sterility induced by the accumulation of phlegm from retained dampness.

Commonly used drugs:

Rhizoma Atractylodis

Poria

Polyporus Umbellatus

Rhizoma Pinelliae

Rhizoma Atractylodis Macroce Phalae

Semen Plantaginis

Pericarpium Arecae

Semen Coicis

Semen Phaseoli

Herba Agastachis

Cortex Magnoliae Officinalis

Typical recipes:

*Wandai Tang*

*Quansheng Baizhu San*

*Qigong Wan*

(3)Invigorating the spleen and elevating the sinking *Qi*

The weak spleen and the sinking *Qi* in middle—Jiao are powerless to govern the blood and to control *Qi*, giving rise to metrorrhagia and metrostaxis, menorrhagia, fetal abortion, habitual abortion, lochiorrhea, prolapse of the uterus. Recommended treatment is to strengthen the spleen and elevate *Qi* in middle—*Jiao*.

Commonly used drugs:

Radix Codonopsis Pilosulae

Radix Astragali seu Hedysari

Rhizoma Atractylodis Macrocephalae

Radix Bupleuri

Rhizoma Cimicifugae

Typical recipes:

*Buzhong Yiqi Tang*

*Juyuan jian*

*Guben Zhibeng Tang*

(4)Invigorating the spleen and normalizing the stomach

The spleen and the stomach are interior—exteriorly related. The incoordination between them will fail to make the stomach—*Qi* descend, and instead it will invade upward, resulting in belching and vomiting. Recommended treatment is to strengthen the spleen and regulate the stomach so as to lower the adversely flowing *Qi*. For those whose liver—*Qi* is stagnant or hyperactive in attacking the stomach, drugs for checking the hyperfunction of the liver should be given.

Commonly used drugs:Pericarpium Citri Reticulatae

Rhizoma Pinelliae

Fructus Amomi

Folium Perillae

Rhizoma Coptidis

Ochra Haematitum

Caulis Bambusae in Taeniam

Fructus Euodiae

Rhizoma Zingiberis Recens .

Typical recipes:

*Xiangsha Liuj unzi Tang*

*Suye Huanglian Tang*

## 4. Harmoniousness of *Qi* and blood

*Qi* and blood are the basic materials and motive forces to keep up the activities of the human life. If *Qi* and blood are in harmony, the physiological functions of the human body are normal; if they are in derangement, the *Chong* and *Ren* channels will be impaired, resulting in various diseases concerned with menstruation, leukorrhea, pregnancy and parturition. Regulating *Qi* and treating blood disorders are one of the important problems in TCG.

The first thing to do in the course of regulating *Qi* and blood is to differentiate the symptoms and signs according to the concrete state and nature of the illness. Only then can suitable methods be chosen. There are different types of *Qi* illnesses including deficiency, stagnation, sinking and upward invasion. The illness of *Qi*–deficient type should be treated by tonification, the illness of *Qi*–stagnant type treated by alleviation. The illness of sinking type will be healed by elevating *Qi*; the illness of adversely rising type by lowering *Qi* . Discussions about the deficiency, collapse and reversed flow of $Qi$ are omitted here, as the topic has been dealt with in the preceding section.

(1)Regulating the flow of $Qi$ and removing stagnation

Owing to the stagnation of $Qi$, the blood flow within the *Chong* and *Ren* channels are hindered, resulting in amenorrhea, dysmenorrhea, irregular menstruation, lump in the abdomen, sterility, embarrassment of the fetus. Recommended treatment is to regulate the flow of $Qi$, to remove stagnation and to resolve the lump by promoting the circulation of $Qi$.

Commonly used drugs:

> Rhizoma Cyperi
> Fructus Aurantii
> Cortex Magnoliae Officinalis
> Radix Aucklandiae
> Radix Linderae
> Pericarpium Citri Reticulatae Viride
> Fructus Meliae Toosendan
> Semen Citri Reticulatae
> Semen Litchi
> Fructus Citri Sarcodactylis

Typical recipe:

> *Jiawei Wuyao San*

(2)Tonifying and enriching the blood

If the *Chong* and *Ren* channels are impaired due to the deficiency of blood, there will appear scanty menstruation, delayed menstrual cycle, amenorrhea, embarrassment of the fetus, postpartum general aching.

Commonly used drugs:

> Radix Angelicae Sinensis

Radix Rehmanniae Praeparata

Radix Paeoniae Alba

Radix Polygoni Multiflori

Colla Corii Asini

Arillus Longan

Caulis Spatholobi

Fructus Lycii

Fructus Mori

Fructus Ziziphi Jujubae

Typical recipes:

*Siwu Tang*

*Danggui Buxue Tang*

*Renshen Zixue Tang*

(3)Removing pathogenic heat from the blood

When the pathogenic heat is accumulated in the blood system and harasses the *Chong* and *Ren* channels and compels the blood to escape from vessels and channels due to the affection of heat—evil, frequently leading to menorrhagia, preceded menstrual cycle, menostaxis, metrorrhagia and metrostaxis, vaginal bleeding during pregnancy, lochiorrhea after delivery. Recommended treatment is to remove heat from the blood so as to arrest bleeding.

Commonly used drugs:

Radix Rehmanniae

Radix Scrophulariae

Cortex Moutan Radicis

Radix Arnebiae seu Lithospermi

Radix Cynanchi Atrati

Fructus Gardeniae

Radix Sanguisorbae

Cacumen Biotae

Radix Paeoniae Alba

Radix Ophiopogonis

Typical recipes:

*Qingj ing Tang*

*Liangdi Tang*

(4)Warming the channels to promote blood flow

The cold—evil has the nature of shrinkage, convulsion and stagnation. When the pathogenic cold is accumulated in the uterus, the blood circulation is obstructed, giving rise to scanty menstruation,delayed menstrual cycle, amenorrhea, dysmen—orrhea, embe..rassment of the fetus, and lochiostasis.

Commonly used drugs:Cortex Cinnamomi

Radix Aconiti Praeparata

Ramulus Cinnamomi

Folium Artemisiae Argyi

Fructus Foenicuii

Fructus Euodiae

Rhizoma Zingiberis Praeparata

. Radix Linderae

Typical recipes:

*Wenj ing Tang*

*Af u Nuangong Wan*

(5)Promoting blood circulation by removing blood stasis

Blood stasis may be caused by the stagnation of *Qi*, the ac—cumulation of pathogenic cold or the scorching of body fluids by blood—heat. When the *Chong* and *Ren* channels are obstructed by blood stasis,there appear dysmenorrhea,amenorrhea,

metrorrhagia and metrostaxis, lump in the abdomen, postpartum
pyrexia, lochiorrhea after delivery.

Commonly used drugs:Radix Angelicae Sinensis

Rhizoma Ligustici Chuanxiong

Herba Leonuri

Pollen Tyhae

Faeces Trogopterorum

Flos Carthami

Semen Persicae

Radix Salviae Miltiorrhizae

Herbs Lycopi

Radix Schyranthis Bidentatae

Radix Notoginseng

Resina Olibani

Myrrha

Semen Vaccariae

Typical recipes:

*Taohong Siwu Tang*

*Shafu Zhuyu Tang*

*Shenghua Tang*

## 5.Removal of the heat and toxic materials

When the human body is invaded by pathogenic heat–evil
which gathers and produces toxic materials, such diseases as
leukorrhagia, vulval pruritus and erosion, postpartum pyrexia
and convulsion may occur.

Commonly used drugs:Flos Lonicerae

Herba Taraxaci

Herba Violae

Herba Patriniae

Herba Houttuyniae

Caulis Sargentodoxae

Rhizoma Smilacis Glabrae

Radix Sophorae Flavescentis

Flos Chrysanthemi Indici

Cortex Phellodendri

Radix Isatidis

Folium Isatidis

Rhizoma Dryopteris

Typical recipes:

*Wuwei Xiaodu Yin*

*Yinqiao Hongj iang Jiedu Tang*

If the heat−evil consumes *Yin*, drugs for replenishing the vital essence such as Radix Rehmanniae, Radix Scrophulariae, Radix Glehniae, Radix Ophiopogonis, Rhizoma Phragmitis should usually be added to the prescription of clearing away the heat and toxic materials. If the toxic heat accumulates and forms blood stasis, then such drugs as *Radix Paeoniae Rubra, Cortex Moutan Radicis, Carapax Trionycis, Sargassum,* Thallus Laminariae, Herba Artemisiae Anomalae, Concha Ostreae, Resina Olibani, Myrrha should be used to promote blood circulation, to remove blood stasis and to soften and resolve the hard mass in the abdomen. This therapy will produce better curative effects.

## 1.3.2 External Treatment

In the book *Jinkui Yaolue* (Synopsis of Prescriptions of the Golden Chamber) compiled in the year of 219, Zhang Zhongjing cured the miscellaneous diseases of gynecology by the method of external treatment. *She Chuang Zi San* (The powder of Cnidium fruit) was used as suppository to heal leukorrhagia of cold—damp type, *Langy a Tang* was used for vaginal douche to treat the pathogenic damp—heat inside the lower—*Jiao* and vulval erosion. Alum was placed into the vagina to cure blood clots in the uterus and frequent drippings of leukorrhea from the vagina. *Gaof aJian Dao Tang* was applied in the case of flatus vaginalis. Since then, external treatment of gynecopathy has achieved great progress in later generations. Chief methods are as follows:

### 1. Fumigating and bathing

Therapeutic method:Clear away heat and toxic materials, promote blood circulation by removing blood stasis; soften and resolve the hard lump in the abdomen, disperse pathogenic wind; destroy parasites and relieve itching.

Administration: Put a dose of Chinese medicinal herbs into a basin, add 2000—2500 ml. of water and submerge the herbs for half an hour. After that, have the dose heated, boiling for 15—20 min. and then remove the dregs. At the start, fumigate the local affected part by hot steam;when the water temperature is fit, have a sitz—bath for 15—20min, once a day.

Indications: Vulval pruritus, vulvitis, cystis and abscess of Barthdin's glands, vulval furunculosis, chronic malnutrition of the vulva, trichomonal vaginitis, colpomycosis, senile vaginitis.

### 2. External application

Therapeutic method:Promote blood circulation by removing blood stasis;soften and resolve hard mass in the abdomen; clear away the heat and toxic materials.

Administration: Crush the medicinal herbs into small pieces and put them into a bag. After decocting on a stove, place the bag on the topical region as a hot compress, or make the medicinal herbs into an adhesive plaster and compress it on the affected region or certain acupoints.

Indications: dysmenorrhea,pelvic inflammation mass, hydrosalpinx, abnormal menstruation.

### 3.Pressing into the vagina

Therapeutic method:Clear away the heat and toxic materials; remove the necrotic tissue and promote granulation; destroy parasites and relieve itching.

Administration: Before going to bed, wash the vulva and vagina clean, press the stype or tablet or medicinal powder into the depth of the vagina. Place a cushion under the buttock to prevent the vaginal fluid out to foul the bed. It is to be done in the late evening. If drugs are erosive, the operation must be done by the physician. First protect well the surrounding normal tissues by cotton balls. Then choose a lined cotton ball, dip it in the prepared medicinal powder, press it on the affected region and the ball will be taken out on a scheduled date.

Indications: vaginitis, cervicitis, cervical carcinoma.

### 4.Loosening the bowels by topical application of drugs

Therapeutic method:Clear away the heat and toxic materials; promote blood circulation by removing blood stasis and dampness; loosen the bowels and moisten *Fu*—organs.

Administration: Press the stype into the anus or inject the decoction into the rectum. Before the application, it is best to defecate or adopt the clearing enema so that drugs can be better absorbed. The temperature of the decoction is 37°C. The dosage is 100—200ml, once per day. The longer the docoction stays inside the rectum, the better the effect will be.

Indications: postpartum infective pyrexia, pelvic inflammation, flatus vaginalis.

**Caution:**

Drugs are not applicable until 3 to 7 days after the end of menstruation. It is forbidden to use drugs during menstruation or shortly after delivery.

The methods of enema and topical application on the lower abdomen should not be applied to pregnant women.

Sexual activities and sitz baths are not permitted with medicine within the vagina.

All tools and drugs must be disinfected and sterilized perfectly.

# 2. Inflammations in the Female Reproductive System

## 2.1 Vulvitis and Bartholinitis

### 2.1.1 Vulvitis

The inflammation of the progenital skin and mucosa is known as vulvitis. It can be classified into the acute and chronic types. It results from the increased secretion of the vagina, the stimulation of menstrual blood and the menstruous pad, the action and immersion of the diabetic's glycuresis and of the fecal or urinary fistula patient's feces and urine, the mixed infection brought forth by the above factors. Clinically, it manifests itself by vulval pruritus, painful and burning sensation, local swelling and ulceration. In TCM, this syndrome falls into the category of vulval pruritus and vulval ulcer (also known as *Yinshi* which means vulval erosion and *ni* which refers to the ulcer on the female external genitals.)

TCG holds that the liver channel of foot—*Jueyin* revolves round the external genitals and that the pudendum is governed by the liver channel. Hence, progenital diseases are induced by the damp—heat of the liver channel or by the fire and dampness produced by the depressed liver—Qi and the weak spleen. The pathogenic damp—heat flows downward by channels and accumulates in the pudendum.

**Clinical manifestations:** Inflammation, itching and pain on the progenital skin, a burning sensation which becomes drastic when the sick is urinating or having physical or sexual activities. The case may also be marked by vexation and irritation, spastic pain in the lower abdomen or distention in the hypochondria. The patient has a dry throat and bitter taste in the mouth, feeling fevers or chills at times; a reddened tongue with a yellowish, greasy coating; a rapid, slippery pulse. Gynecological examination finds out local congestion and swelling of the vulva, distinct scratch marks and at times ulceration . In severe cases, the swelling of inguinal lymph–nodes and tenderness can be perceived. The chronic vulvitus has an effect on thickening the skin and mucosa, making them rough and lichenized.

Therapeutic method: Clear away the heat and promote diuresis; detoxicate and relieve itching.

Recipe: *Longdan Xiegan Tang* (38)

Ingredients: Radix Gentianae    6 g

Fructus Gardenia    9 g

Radix Scutellariae    12 g

Semen Plantaginis    12 g(in a parcel)

Caulis Akebiae    6 g

Rhizoma Alismatis    9 g

Radix Rehmanniae    15 g

Radix Angelicae Sinensis    12 g

Radix Bupleuri    9 g

Radix Glycyrrhizae    6 g.

Administration: Decoct the above drugs in an adequate amount of Water to get 200–300ml of decoction. Divide it into two equal portions. Take one half in the morning and the other half in the evening.

Modification: In case of fever or leukocytosis
in the laboratory findings, add the following drugs to the recipe:

        Flos Lonicerae   30 g

        Rhizoma Smilacis Glabrae   15 g

        Cortex Moutan Radicis   15 g

.In case of difficulty and pain in micturition, scanty and
deep–colored urine, add

        Talcum   15 g

        Herba Lophatheri   12 g.

In case of constipation, add

        Radix et Rhizoma Rhei   6g (to be added later)

        Aloe   9 g.

External treatment: Clear away the heat and eliminate
dampness; detoxicate and relieve itching.

Recipe: Progenital detergent No.1

Ingredients:Flos Chrysanthemi Indici   30 g

        Radix Sophorae Flavescentis   30 g

        Fructus Cnidii   30 g

        Flos Lonicerae   30 g

        Cortex Phellodendri   15 g

        Rhizoma Smilacis Glabrae   15 g

        Pericarpium Zanthoxyli   12 g

        Cortex Moutan Radicis   12 g

        Borneolum  3 g  (to be infused in hot
decoction).

Administration:Put the above drugs except Borneolum in
2000–2500 ml of water, submerged for half an hour and then
have them heated, boiling for 15–20min, then pour the hot
decoction into the bath–tub, remove the dregs, infuse borneol in

the tub. First fumigate the vulva by its vapour and when the temperature of water becomes appropriate, have a sitz bath for 15—20min, once per day.

Modification: In case of scratches or ulcers on the skin or mucosa, deduct Pericarpium Zanthoxyli but add

Radix Arnebiae seu Lithospermi   15 g

Rhizoma Bletillae   12 g.

In case of severe itching and lichenoid skin and mucosa, add

Radix Paeoniae Rubra   15 g

Radix Angelicae Sinensis   15 g

Herba Schizonepetae   9 g

Radix Ledebouriellae   9 g.

## 2.1.2  Bartholinitis

Bartholinitis occurs mostly in the child—bearing age, rarely in the infant period or after menopause. It is generally caused by the mixed infection of staphylococci, streptococci, colibacillus and enterococci. Clinically, it is mainly characterized by swelling and aching of the greater lip of pudendum on one side. This syndrome falls into the category of vulval swelling.

The swelling of the vulva is induced by the pathogenic damp—heat which flows downward through the liver channel and is retained in the vulva. Its entanglement with blood and *Qi* results in the distention of striae of skin, muscles and viscera with little excretion of damp—heat.

**Clinical manifestations:** Aching and swelling on one side of the vulva, physical activities restricted. In severe cases, the sick has fever and a bitter taste; a yellowish, greasy fur; a wiry and rapid pulse. Gynecological examination finds out red—swelling, high temperature and noticeable tenderness on the skin under the greater lip of pudendum on one side. The diameter of the lump is about 5—6 cm, having an undulatory sensation.

Therapeutic method: Clear away the heat and toxic materials;subside the swelling and evacuate the pus.

Recipe: *Chai Cen Zhi Ju Tang*

Ingredients:Radix Bupleuri   9 g

Radix Scutellariae   12 g

Rhizoma Smilacis Glabrae   15 g

Semen Coicis   30 g

Fructus Forsythiae   15 g

Radix Angelicae Sinensis   15 g

Radix Angelicae Dahuricae   12 g

Radix Platycodi   9 g

Caulis Akebiae   6 g

Radix Glycyrrhizae   6 g.

Administration:The above drugs are decocted in an adequate amount of water. Take one half of the decoction in the morning and the other half in the evening.

External treatment: Clear away the heat and toxic materials; promote blood circulation by removing blood stasis and subside the swelling.

Recipe: Progenital detergent No.2

Ingredients:Flos Chrysanthemi Indici   30 g

Herba Taraxaci   30 g

Fructus Forsythiae   15 g

Radix Angelicae Sinensis   15 g

Cortex Moutan Radicis   15 g

Radix Paeoniae Rubra   15 g

Lignum Sappan    15 g

Radix Angelicae Dahuricae    12 g

Cortex Phellodendri    12 g

Squama Manitis    9 g

Spina Gleditsiae    9 g

Borneolum (to be infused in hot decoction)
3 g.

Decoct the above medicinal herbs in water. Fumigate the affected part by its vapour and then have a sitz bath, once per day. The method used is just the same as the preceding.

**Simple Recipe and Proved Prescription:**

Ingredients:Pericarpium Zanthoxyli    15 g

Folium Artemisiae Argyi    15 g

Flos Chrysanthemi Indici    30 g.

Decoct the above drugs in water. Fumigate and wash the affected part once or twice per day. Use the same method as the preceding. Its function is to relieve itching.

Indigo Naturalis    30 g

Gecko    30 g

Cortex Phellodendri    15 g.

Grind them into powder. After mixing with vegetable oil uniformly, apply it to the affected region. It is used for the treatment of the progenital ulcer.

Folium Artemisiae Argyi    30 g

Radix Ledebouriellae    15 g

Radix Euphorbiae Pekinensis    12 g.

Decoct the drugs in water for fumigation and washing. In addition,use

Pericarpium Citri Reticulatae    30 g

Fructus Aurantii Immaturus    30 g.

Having ground, baked and filled in a bag, it can be applied to the affected region for detumescence and alleviation of pain.

**Caution:**Don't eat pungent,stimulating food.Wash the vulva frequently. Keep it clean and dry. Often change the underwear. The Menstruous pad and the sanitary tissues should be disinfected before use. Foster a good habit of personal hygiene.

Take an active attitude toward the treatment of vaginitis, cervicitis, diabetes, urinary and fecal fistulae. Prevent the stimulation of excessive secretion.

## 2.2  Vaginitis

When the female has entered into adolescence the acid—base scale (pH) of the vagina amounts to $4.2 \sim 5.0$, so the vagina has the capability to purify itself. If the defense function is impaired, the pathogenic bacteria will invade, resulting in vaginitis. Clinically it is characterized by the burning sensation and pain of the vagina, pruritus vulvae and profused leukorrhea. In TCM, it falls into the category of"leukorrhagia"and "vulval pruritus."

The term" leukorrhea" can be defined in two ways. In the broad sense, it refers to gynecological diseases concerned with menstruation, leukorrhea, pregnancy and parturition; in the narrow sense, it refers only to the small quantity of vaginal secretion which is whitish or colourless, sticky and odorless. It is a normal physiological phenomenon, an expression of abundance and exuberance of the kidney—$Qi$ , of the excellent functioning of the spleen as well as the $Ren$ and $Dai$ channels..It marks the adolescence of the female.

But if the leukorrhea is incessant, large in quantity, abnormal in color, odor and quality, accompanied by general or local symptoms, it can be regarded as "morbid leukorrhea".This disease is chiefly induced by damp—evil, As the spleen fails to function in transportation, the phlegm—dampness is accumulated in the body and the damp—heat flows downward in the liver channel,the weak kidney cannot control nocturnal emission, as the uterine collaterals become weak and void after the menstrual or puerperal period, or as the vulva and vagina are unclean or injured in surgical operation, so damp—evil takes advantage of this opportunity to invade. Having been stored up, it transforms into pathogenic heat and impairs the *Ren* and *Dai* channels, resulting in their failure in control. Such is the etiology of morbid leukorrhea. In ancient medical documentation, vaginal discharges were grouped into greenish, yellowish, reddish (or bloody), white, black and multicolored ones. But clinically, white and yellowish vaginal discharges are commonly seen. If reddish or multicolored discharge is discovered, careful examination must be made to prevent and eliminate canceration.

## Type and treatment

### 1)Spleen—insufficiency

**Clinical manifestations:** The vaginal discharge is white or yellowish, thick and viscid, odorless and incessant. The patient has a sallow complexion, weary and tired, anorectic and with loose stools. Her limbs are cool, the insteps swollen. The tongue is pale with a whitish, greasy fur. The pulse is moderate and feeble. But little abnormality can be found in gynecological examination.

Therapeutic method: Strengthen the spleen and replenish

*Qi* , elevate the *Yang* and remove dampness.

    Recipe: *Wandai Tang* (81)

    Ingredients:Rhizoma Atractylodis Macrocephalae  15 g

                Rhizoma Dioscoreae  12 g

                Radix Ginseng (to be decocted first)  9 g

                Radix Paeoniae Alba  12 g

                Rhizoma Atractylodis  9 g

                Pericarpium Citri Reticulatae  12 g

                Radix Glycyrrhizae  6 g

                Semen Plantaginis (in a parcel)  12 g

                Radix Bupleuri  9 g

                Spica Schizonepetae  6 g.

Decoct the above drugs in an adequate amount of water to get 200–300ml of decoction. Divide it into two equal portions. Take one in the morning and the other in the evening.

    Modifications: In case of yellowish morbid leukorrhea, add to the recipe:

                Semen Coicis  30 g

                Cortex Phellodendri  9 g

    In case of lumbodynia, add

                Semen Euryales  30 g

                Semen Cuscutae  15 g

                Cortex Eucommiae  15 g.

    In case of a long–standing morbid leukorrhea with incessant drippings of discharge from the vagina, add

                Os Sepiella seu Sepiae  30 g

                Fructus Rosae Laevigatae  15 g

                Semen Ginkgo  9 g.

    Proprietary: *Bai Dai Wan.*Take one bolus with water, thrice per day.

**2. Damp—heat**

(1)The downward flow of damp—heat

**Clinical manifestations:** The vaginal discharge is yellow or whitish ,yellow profuse and sticky, having bad odor. The patient has an oppressed sensation in the chest, a greasy taste in the mouth and pain in the lower abdomen. In other cases, the white, viscid discharge may look like soya—bean residue or coagulating cheese. This disease is also characterized by pruritus vulvae, oliguria, difficulty and pain in micturition. The coating of the tongue is yellowish, thick or greasy. The pulse is soft and rapid, or wiry and slippery. Gynecological examinations find white membranoid substance on the labia minora and the vaginal mucosa and when it is rubbed off, there appear local reddening and swelling or even ulcers and in the secretion white *candida albicans* can be detected. Such case should be diagnosed as colpomycosis.

Therapeutic method: Eliminate pathogenic dampness and heat.

Recipe: *Zhi Dai Fang* (104)

Ingredients: Polyporus Umbellatus   12 g

Poria   18 g

Semen Plantaginis  (in a parcel)   12 g

Rhizoma Alismatis   9 g

Herba Artemisiae Scopariae   12 g

Radix Paeoniae Rubra   15 g

Cortex Moutan Radicis   12 g

Cortex Phellodendri   9 g

Fructus Gardeniae   9 g

Radix Achyranthis Bidentatae　12 g.

The decoction of a dose is 200—300ml. Take one half in the morning and the other half in the evening.

Modifications: In case of scanty, deep—colored urine or having difficulty and pain in micturition, add

Talcum　15 g

Herba Lophatheri　9 g.

In case of having an oppressed sensation in the chest and a greasy taste in the mouth with a greasy, yellowish coating on the tongue, add

Semen Coicis　30 g

Rhizoma Dioscoreae Hypoglaucae　12 g

Rhizoma Atractylodis　9 g.

External Treatment: Clear away heat and promote diuresis; destroy parasites and relieve itching.

Recipe: Progenital detergent No.1.

Ingredients:　Fructus Kochiae　30 g

Cortex Hibisci　30 g

Radix Sophorae Flavescentis　30 g

Rhizoma Smilacis Glabrae　30 g

Fructus Cnidii　15 g

Pericarpium Zanthoxyli　12 g

Flos Chrysanthemi Indici　30 g

Folium Artemisiae Argyi　9 g

Borneolum (to be infused in hot decoction)
3 g.

Decoct the drugs in water for fumigation and washing in a sitz bath, one dose per day. The method is the same as that of treating vulvitis.

(2)Dampness and heat in the liver and the gall bladder

**Clinical manifestations:** Hypersecretion of morbid leukorrhea,yellow or greenish yellow in color, sticky or foamy, stinking in odor. The patient feels itching and pain in the pudendum as well as a burning sensation. She is mentally depressed, having a bitter taste and a dry throat. The case is also marked by dysphoria and insomnia, constipation, dark urine and hypochondriac pain.The tongue is reddened with a yellowish, thin fur. The pulse is slippery, thready and rapid. These symdromes get more serious just around the menstrual cycle or during the gestational and puerperal periods. Gynecological examination finds out reddening and swelling of the vaginal and cervical mucosa which is often scattered with hemorrhagic spots or fragiform processes, and a large quantity of frothy or puriform secretion existing in the posterior fornix. The laboratory examination of leukorrhea finds trichomonas. This case should be diagnosed as trichomonal vaginitis.

Therapeutic method: Purge heat from the liver, destroy parasites and relieve itching.

Recipe:*Longdan Xiegan Tang*(38) (see 2.1.1). Add to the recipe

Ingredients:   Radix Stemonae   15 g

Rhizoma Smilacis Glabrae   15 g.

External treatment: Clear away the heat and toxic materials; destroy parasites and relieve itching.

Recipe: Progenital detergent No.2.

Radix Pulsatillae   30 g

Radix Sophorae Flavescentis   30 g

Radix Stemonae   30 g

                    Pericarpium Granati    15 g
                    Fructus Cnidii    15 g
                    Cortex Phellodendri    12 g
                    Alumen    15 g
                    Folium Artemisiae Argyi    9 g
                    Borneolum ( to be infused in hot decoction)    3 g
                    Flos    Chrysanthemi Indici    30 g.

Decoct the drugs in water for fumigation and washing in a sitz bath, one dose per day. The method taken is the same as that of treating vulvitis.

Proprietary:*Longdan Xiegan Wan*.Take 9g of medicine with boiled water, twice a day.

(3)The toxic heat

**Clinical manifestations:** Hypersecretion of morbid leukorrhea, with either reddish white or multicolored vaginal discharge. It is sticky and greasy, or pyoid in appearance, stinking or unpleasantly foul in odor. The patient feels pain in the lower abdomen and dizzy in the head, having paroxysmal fevers and a dry throat. The case is also characterized by dyschesia and oliguria. The stools are dry and offensive in odor, the urine is dark—colored and scanty. The patient has a reddened tongue with dry, yellowish fur; a rapid pulse. Gynecological examination discovers cervical edema, congestion and tubercular, cauliflowerlike or cavernous canceration. Then the above cases should be diagnosed respectively as acute inflammation or cervical carcinoma.

Therapeutic method: Clear away the heat and toxic materials

Recipe: *Wuwei Xiaodu Yin*(86), Augmented

Ingredients:Herba Taraxaci    15 g
                    Flos Lonicerae    15 g

Flos Chrysanthemi Indici   30 g

Herba Violae   30 g

Radix Semiaquilegiae   15 g

Herba Hedyotis Diffusae   30 g

Semen Coicis   15 g

Rhizoma Paridis   15 g

Radix Ailanthi Altissimae   30 g

Rhizoma Smilacis Glabrae   15 g

Rhizoma Cyperi   12 g

Herba Lobeliae Radicantis   30 g.

Decoct the above drugs in an adequate amount of water to get 200—300ml of decoction. Divide it into two equal portions. Take one half in the morning and the other half in the evening.

Modifications: In case of constipation which lasts for a few days, add to the recipe :

Radix et Rhizoma Rhei (to be infused in hot decoction)   6 g

Natrii Sulphas (to be taken with boiled water)   3 g.

In case of a dry mouth and a dry fur of the tongue in addition to difficulty and pain in micturition and oliguria, add

Radix Rehmanniae   15 g

Herba Lophatheri   12 g

Rhizoma Coptidis   6 g

Radix Glycyrrhizae   9 g.

In case of pyoid vaginal discharge and drastic pain in the abdomen, add

Herba Houttuyniae   30 g

Rhizoma Corydalis   12 g

Herba Plantaginis   15 g.

### 3.Kidney—deficiency

(1)Insufficiency of the kidney—*Yang*

**Clinical manifestations:** Cold, watery and profuse leukorrhea with incessant drippings all day long. The patient feels cold in the lower abdomen and so much pain in the waist as if it were cracked. The urine is colorless, more frequent and greatly increased in volume, especially at night. The stools are loose and scarce.The patient has a pale tongue with white, thin fur; a deep, slow pulse. But no abnormality is found in gynecological examination.

Therapeutic method: Warm the kidney, strengthen the vital essence and arrest leukorrhagia.

Recipe: *Nei Bu Wan* (43)

Ingredients:Cornu Cervi Pantotrichum    9 g

Semen Cuscutae    24 g

Semen Astragali Complanati    15 g

Radix Astragali seu Hedysari    15 g

Cortex Cinnamomi    6 g

Oötheca Mantidis    30 g

Herba Cistanchis    15 g

Radix Aconiti Praeparata    6 g

Fructus Tribuli    15 g

Radix Asteris    9 g.

The 200—300ml of decoction is divided into two portions. Take them respectively in the morning and evening.

Modifications: In case of frequent micturition at night and loose stools, add to the recipe:

Fructus Alpiniae Oxyphyllae    30 g

Fructus Psoraleae    15 g

Rhizoma Atractylodis Macrocephalae   18 g.

In case of oppressed chest, loss of appetite and hypodynamia, add

Poria   15 g
Pericarpium Citri Reticulatae   12 g
Cortex Magnoliae Officinalis   9 g
Fructus Amomi   6 g.

(2)Insufficiency of the kidney—*Yin*

**Clinical manifestations:** A dry, burning sensation in the vulva where there is itching or pain, with little discharge either yellow or palish red. The leukorrhea is viscid and odorless. The patient feels dizzy in the head, dry in the mouth and sore in the waist, characterized in addition by tinnitus, paroxysmal fever with perspiration and dysphoria with a fiery sensation in the chest, palms and soles. The stools are dry, the urine deep—colored.The patient has a red tongue with little fur. a slippery, thready and rapid pulse. Gynecological examination detects atrophy of the vulva with much vaginal secretion which is sanguinous or purulent and looks like yellowish water. The vaginal rugae have disappeared and the mucosa is congested with petechial hemorrhage and ulceration.

Therapeutic method:   Tonify the kidney and nourish *Yin* , reduce fever and arrest leukorrhagia.

Recipe: *Zhi  Bai Dihuang Tang*(103)

Ingredients:Radix Rehmaniae Praeparata   18 g
Cortex Moutan Radicis   12 g
Poria   15 g
Rhizoma Alismatis   9 g
Fructus Corni   12 g
Rhizoma Dioscoreae   15 g

Rhizoma Anemarrhenae   6 g

Cortex Phellodendri   9 g.

The 200—300ml of decoction is divided into two portions,to be taken respectively in the morning and evening.

Modifications: In case of abundant and incessant vaginal discharge, add to the recipe:

Semen Euryales   30 g

Fructus Rosae Laevigatae   15 g

Stamen Nelumbinis   12 g.

In case of dizziness, dysphoria and insomnia, add

Flos Chrysanthemi   9 g

Radix Ophiopognis   12 g

Fructus Schisandrae   12 g

Os Draconis   30 g.

In case of sanguinous leukorrhea, add

Herba Ecliptae   18 g

Radix Sanguisorbae   15 g.

External treatment: Clear away pathogenic heat from the blood and toxic materials from the body; tonify the kidney and arrest morbid discharge.

Recipe: Progenital detergent No.3.

Ingredients:  Flos Chrysanthemi Indici   30 g

Flos Lonicerae   30 g

Herba Epimedii   30 g

Radix Arnebiae seu Lithospermi   15 g

Cortex Phellodendri   15 g

Radix Angelicae Sinensis   15 g

Fructus Cnidii   30 g

Radix Paeoniae Rubra   15 g

Cortex Moutan Radicis  12 g

Fructus Mume  15 g

Folium Artemisiae Argyi  9 g

Borneolum (to be added later)  3 g.

Decoct the drugs in water for fumigation and washing in a sitz bath, one dose per day. The method used is the same as that of treating vulvitus.

**Proprietary, Simple Recipe and Proved Prescriptions:**

In case of colpomycosis, take a tube of *Bing Peng San* and mix it with glycerin in a uniform way. Using a cotton stick, spread the oilment newly made upon the vagina and the vulva, once or twice a day.

Or the following drugs can be decocted in water for fumigation and washing in a sitz bath, once a day:

Fructus Kochiae  45 g

Flos Chrysanthemi Indici  30 g.

In case of trichomonal vaginitis, decoct the following drugs in water for fumigation and washing, once a day:

Radix Stemonae  30 g

Radix Pulsatillae  30 g

Radix Sophorae Flavescentis  30 g.

*Ta Yang Tang* (79) is used to cure pruritus genitalium. Decoct the following drugs in water for fumigation and washing, once a day:

Fructus Carpesii  30 g

Radix Sophorae Flavescentis  30 g

Radix Clematidis  15 g

Tip of Radix Angelicae Sinensis  30 g

Herba Agrimoniae  9 g

Fructus Cnidii    15 g

Pig's Bile 2 galls.

In case of senile vaginitis, decoct the following drugs for fumigation and washing, once a day.

Herba Epimedii    30 g

Radix Arnebiae seu Lithospermi    15 g

Cortex Phellodendri    15 g

Flos Chrysanthemi indici    30 g.

**Caution:**

The menstruous pad and the underwear should frequently be washed and dried up in the sun. Keep them clean and dry.

Use your private bathtub and towels instead of public ones to prevent infection.

Aseptic manipulation must be carried out rigorously in gynecological examination to avoid cross infection.

# 2.3   Cervicitis

Cervicilis is a common disease for women at the child—bearing age. It can be acute or chronic. The acute cervicitis occurs simultaneously with puerperal infection, septic abortion or acute vaginitis. Clinically, it is characterized by profuse leukorrhea, cervical hypertrophy, congestion, erosion and Naboth's cysts. It falls into the category of leukorrheal disease in the TCM. As to its type and treatment, please refer to 2.1.1 (Vulvitis). The local treatment of cervicitis is fully discussed here in this section.

**Clinical manifestations:** Profuse, purulent leukorrhea, soreness in the loin and sacrococcyx and strained pain in the lower abdomen. It gets more drastic during menstruation and defecation or after sexual activity. At times, it is characterized by dysuria and oliguria with a deep color. Or the patient has a history of sterility. Gynecological examination detects cervical edema and congestion in the acute cases. As for chronic inflammation, there appear cervical erosion of different degrees in simple, follicular or papillary form, cervical hypertrophy and eversion, cervical polyp—us and Naboth's cysts with purulent leukorrhea in the cervical canal.

Therapeutic method: Clear away the heat and toxic materials; to activate blood flow; remove the necrotic tissues and promote granulation.

Recipe: Powder No.1 for cervicitis.

Functions: Clear away the heat and toxic materials, eliminate dampness and arrest leukorrhagia.

Ingredients:  Cortex Phellodendri   30 g
                Radix Coptidis   30 g
                Radix Scutellariae   30 g
                Radix eu Rhizoma Rhei   15 g
                Borneolum   3 g.

Administration: Grind the first 4 kinds of baked drugs into powder, mix the complex fully with fine—granulated Borneolum and fill them into a powder—blower in preparation for use. Then expose the uterine neck with a vaginal speculum, clean out the secretion with dry cotton balls, sprinkle the medicinal powder evenly over the uterine neck by the blower or compress the powdery cotton balls on the surface of the affected region and take them out in 24 hours. The application is to be done once a day. The course of treatment lasts 7 days.

This prescription is adapted to simple—typed erosion which

is superficial and obviously congested. It can also be applied to the case of distinct congestion when necrotic tissues have been removed by Powder No.2.

Powder No.2 for cervicitis.

Functions: Activate the blood flow and eliminate blood stasis; remove the necrotic tissues and promote granulation.

Ingredients: Alumen   30 g

Sal Ammoniacum   6 g

Resina Olibani   9 g

Myrrha   9 g

Catechu   15 g

Sulfur   15 g

Borax   1.5 g

Borneolum   3 g.

Grind the above drugs in preparation for use. Expose the uterine neck, clean out the vaginal secretion, protect the fornix and vagina well with cotton balls, compress the powdery cotton balls on the affected region and take them out in 24 hours. Caution: Don't sprinkle the medicinal powder on the surrounding skin and mucosa. This application is to be done once in a day. Two or three times are needed.

Powder No.2 is well adapted to the case of granular or papillary erosion of the uterine neck.

Powder No.3 for cervicitis.

Functions: Astrict the erosion and promote granulation.

Ingredients:   Gecko   30 g

Rhizoma Bletillae   12 g

Galla Chinensis   9 g

Cortex Phellodendri Glabrae   30 g

Os Sepiellae Seu Sepiae   30 g

Corium Elephatis    15 g

Borneolum    3 g.

Grind the above drugs into powder in preparation for use. The method used is the same as that of Powder No.1 for cervicitis.

The preceding three sorts of medicinal powders can be used alternately according to the concrete conditions of cervical erosion. Powder No.1 is fit for conspicuous inflammation, Powder No.2 for tubercular and papillary erosion. Powder No.3 is applicable when congestion and edema of the uterine neck have been subdued. After the removal of the necrotic tissues, both Powders No.1 and 3 can be used.

**Proprietary, Simple Recipe and Proved Prescription:**

*Kushen Shuan* has the function of clearing away heat, promoting diuresis, dispelling wind, destroying parasites and relieving itching. Place a stype directly into the depth of the vagina every evening.

*Baidai Wan*.Take one bocus with boiled water, twice a day.

**Caution:**

In case of childbirth or artificial labor, abortion or other related operations, the working regulations and aseptic manipulations must be followed strictly to prevent the injury and infection of the uterine neck.

Pay attention to personal hygiene. Wash the underwear frequently. Keep the vulva clean and dry to avoid infection.

## 2.4  Pelvic Inflammation

When the female's internal genital organs and the surrounding connective tissues and pelvic peritoneum are infected, the case is known as pelvic inflammation. One or several sections can be invaded at the same time. According to the process of the disease, it can clinically be classified into three:acute, chronic and tuberculous. It is caused mainly by the failure of strict disinfection in childbirth, abortion and other related manipulations or by the neglect of personal hygiene during the menstrual cycle or after delivery. Clinically, the patient is characterized by fever and pain in the lower abdomen, soreness in the loin and sacrococcyx, profuse leukorrhea and menstrual disorder and sterility. In TCM, the pelvic inflammation is defined as "the invasion of the blood chamber by heat", "leukorrheal disease", "menstrual disorder", "mass in the lower abdomen" and "sterility".

As the uterine collaterals are weak and void during the menstrual cycle and after delivery, the evil toxins seize this opportunity to enter. Toxic damp—heat accumulates in the lower—*Jiao*, stays in the uterus and attacks *Qi* and blood, thus resulting in this illness. The struggle between the vital energy and the pathogenic evil, the disharmony between *Ying* and *Wei* and the blockage of channels by pathogenic factors and toxic substances lead to the aversion to cold and fever, the accumulation of blood stasis and toxins in the interior, and the formation of abdominal mass.

## Type and Treatment

### 1. Damp-heat

**Clinical manifestations:** Hyperpyrexia, chills, pain and tenderness in the lower abdomen. Yellowish or pyoid leukorrhea, viscid, profuse and stinking. The patient has difficulties in micturition and defecation due to oliguria and the tenesmus of anus; a dry mouth with a bitter taste; a reddened tongue with yellowish, thin or greasy coating; a slippery, rapid pulse or a wiry, thready and rapid pulse. Gynecological examination finds a normal vulva but a congested vagina with much purulent secretion. The fornix feels great pain when touched; the uterine neck is marked by hyperemia and edema and also by tenderness when raised. The uterus is normal in size or slightly larger, having tenderness when pressed. Its movements are limited. In some cases, the mass or patchy thickening of the mucosa may be found in the uterus. Or encysted mass may be touched upon in the posterior fornix. As the laboratory examination of blood shows that the number of white cells is $10 \sim 20 \times 10^9 / L$.

**Therapeutic method:** Clear away the heat and toxic materials, promote diuresis with the assistance of activating blood circulation and removing blood stasis.

Recipe: *Ji Pen Tang*.

Ingredients:Radix Bupleuri    12 g

        Radix Scutellariae    15 g

        Flos Lonicerae    30 g

        Herba Patriniae    30 g

        Fructus Forsythiae    24 g

        Cortex Moutan Radicis    15 g

Cortex Phellodendri   9 g

Radix Salviae Miltiorrhizae   15 g

Rhizoma Corydalis   12 g

Resina Olibani Praeparata   9 g

Resina Commiphorae Myrrha Praeparata   9 g

Radix Paeoniae Rubra   15 g

Fructus Meliae Toosendan   9 g.

Decoct the above drugs in an adequate amount of water to get 200–300ml of decoction. Take one dose in the morning and a second dose in the evening. After the abatement of fever, one dose is enough for the whole day.

Modifications: In case of constipation, add to the recipe,

Radix eu Rhizoma Rhei (to be added later)   6 g

Natrium Sulfuricum Exsiccatum (infused in hot decoction)   3 g.

In case of urodynia and urgency  of  micturition, add

Herba Lophatheri   12 g

Radix Glycyrrhizae   9 g

Talcum   12 g.

In case of profuse, purulent leukorrhea, add

Semen Benincasae   30 g

Herba Houttuyniae   24 g

Semen Coicis   15 g.

In case of mass in the abdomen, add

Fructus Grataegi   15 g

Endothelium Corneum Gigeriae Galli   9 g

Rhizoma Sparganii   12 g

Rhizoma Zedoariae   12 g.

In case of vexation, thirsty, a crimson tongue and skin eruption, add

> Cornu Rhinoceri Asiatici (infused in hot decoction)  3 g
>
> Radix Rehmanniae  18 g
>
> Fructus Gardeniae  12 g
>
> Rhizoma Imperatae  30 g
>
> Radix Coptidis  6 g.

Deduct Radix Bupleuri

Resina Olibani Praeparata

Resina Commiphorae Myrrha Praeparata

Fructus Meliae Toosendan.

## 2. *Qi* —stagnancy and Blood—stasis

**Clinical manifestations:** Soreness in the loin, tenesmic or distending pain and tenderness in the lower abdomen. The case gets more drastic after fatigue or sexual intercourse and around the menstrual cycle. It is also characterized by profuse menstruation and blood clots. When they are out, the pain abates. The patient feels a sort of distending pain in the chest and breasts. Leukorrhea is abundant, white or yellowish. A wiry, uneven pulse. A dark tongue dotted with ecchymoses; a white, thin fur. Gynecological examination finds the uterus retroverted and its movement restrained, due to fixation adhesion or tenderness. In some cases, pachynsis adnexa, funiculus, lump or cystic mass may be perceived. B—type ultrasonic examination is very helpful in diagnosing this illness.

Therapeutic method: Promote blood circulation and remove blood stasis; regulate the flow of *Qi* and alleviate the pain.

Recipe: *Man Pen Tang*  No.1.

Ingredients:  Pollen Tyhae  12 g

Faeces Trogopterori   12 g

Radix Angelicae Sinensis   15 g

Semen Persicae   12 g

Flos Carthami · 12 g

Resina Olibani   9 g

Myrrha   9 g

Radix Paeoniae Rubra   15 g

Radix Salviae Miltiorrhizae   30 g

Rhizoma Cyperi   12 g

Caulis Lonicerae   30 g

Rhizoma Smilacis Glabrae   15 g.

The decoction of a dose is 200—300ml. Take one half in the morning and the other half in the evening.

Modification: In case of severe pain in the chest and breasts, add

Folium Citri Reticulatae   12 g

Fructus Meliae Toosendan   12 g.

In case of profuse and yellowish leukorrhea, add

Semen Plantaginis (in a parcel)   12 g

Rhizoma Alismatis   9 g.

In case of distress in the loin, add

Radix Achyranthis Bidentatae   15 g

Radix Dipsaci   15 g.

### 3.Blood—stasis due to accumulation of cold

**Clinical manifestations:**   Cold and painful sensation in the lower abdomen, which gets drastic when compressed and which can be relieved by warmth. The  menstruation is scanty, delayed and dark in color, mixed with blood clots. The pulse is deep, either wiry or tense. The fur of the tongue is whitish and thin.

Gynecological examination has the same findings as those of *Qi* —stagnant and blood—stasis.

Therapeutic method: Warm the channels and expel pathogenic cold; promote blood circulation and remove blood stasis.

Recipe: *Man Pen Tang* No.2.

Ingredients: Fructus Foenicuii   9 g

Ramulus Cinnamomi   9 g

Poria   15 g

Radix Angelicae Sinensis   15 g

Rhizoma Ligustici Chuanxiong   9 g

Cortex Moutan Radicis   9 g

Radix Linderae   12 g

Semen Persicae   12 g

Caulis Spatholobi   15 g.

The decoction made is about 200—300ml. Take one half in the morning and the rest in the evening.

Modifications: In case of severe cold in the abdomen, add

Rhizoma Zingiberis Praeparata   6 g

Fructus Euodiae   9 g.

In case of severe pain in the abdomen scanty and delayed menstruation with blood clots, add to the recipe

Radix Achyranthis Bidentatae   15 g

Cortex Cinnamomi   9 g

Caulis Spatholobi   30 g.

4. *Yin*—deficiency and blood—heat

**Clinical manifestations:** Decreasing menstruation or menostasis,with tenesmic pain in the lower abdomen which gets more drastic after menstruation. The case is also characterized by tidal fever in the afternoon, hypodynamia, anorexia, night sweat and feverish sensation in the palms and soles. The tongue is reddish, either with yellow thin fur or no fur at all. The pulse is thready and rapid . Most patients have a history of primary sterility or tuberculosis. Gynecological examination detects the poor development of the womb, which is restricted in its movement or characterized by fixation and adhesion. In the appendicular region, uneven and irregular lumps can be detected, which are stiff and tubercular on the surface. The laboratory examination of blood shows that the blood sedimentation rate is normal or quickened. Typical tubercles can be observed in the pathological sections by uterine curettage. The iodized oil roentgenograph betrays calcific spots in the pelvic cavity, the stricture or deformity of the uterine cavity with its edge saw—toothed, and a rigid, stenosed or toruboid oviduct.

Therapeutic method: Replenish the vital essence and clear away the heat; activate blood flow and remove blood stasis.

Recipe: *Man Pen Tang* No.3.

Ingredients: Radix Rehmanniae    15 g

Carapax Trionycis    30 g

Plastrum Testudinis    30 g

Flos Chrysanthemi Indici    30 g

Radix Stemonae    15 g

Radix Sanguisorbae    15 g

Spica Prunellae    12 g

Caulis Spatholobi    15 g

Cortex Lycii Radicis    12 g

Herba Artemisiae Chinghao    9 g

Cortex Moutan Radicis    9 g

Radix Scrophulariae   15 g.

Decoct the above drugs in an adequate amount of water to get 200—300 ml of decoction. Take equal shares in the morning and evening.

Modifications: In case of hydrosalpinx, add to the recipe:

Semen Phaseoli   30 g

Radix Stephaniae Tetrandrae   12 g

Semen Plantaginis   12g (in a parcel)

Rhizoma Alismatis   9 g

Cortex Cinnamomi   6 g.

In case of encysted mass in the abdomen, add

Concha Ostreae   30 g

Bulbus Fritillariae Thunbergii   12 g

Fractus Forsythiae   24 g

Endothelium Corneum Gigeriae Galli   9 g

Fructus Grataegi   15 g.

In case of obstruction of the oviduct in the tubal patent test by liquid instillation, the following drugs may be used.

Radix Salviae Miltiorrhizae   30 g

Fructus Forsythiae   24 g

Cortex Moutan Radicis   15 g

Radix Angelicae Sinensis   15 g

Rhizoma Ligustici Chuanxiong   9 g

Lignum Sappan   15 g

Semen Plantaginis (in a parcel)   12 g

Semen Vaccariae   12 g

Squama Manitis   12 g

Cortex Cinnamomi   9 g

Radix Achyranthis Bidentatae   15 g

                    Caulis Spatholobi   30 g
                    Fructus Meliae Toosendan   12 g.
The decoction made is 200—300 ml. Take equal shares in the morning and evening. since the dag when menstruation has paused. It is requested to take the same drugs for a period of two or three months. That is to say, one has to take 18—24 doses in one month.

**Other Therapies:**

①Retention—enema of traditional Chinese drugs.

Ingredients:Radix Salviae Miltiorrhizae   30 g

                    Herba Patriniae   30 g

                    Fructus Forsythiae   30 g

                    Herba Violae   30 g

                    Radix Paeoniae Rubra   15 g

                    Resina Olibani Praeparata   15 g

                    Resina Commiphorae myrrha Praeparata   15 g

                    Fructus Meliae Toosendan   15 g.

Administration:Boil the above drugs into a 100—200ml decoction and cool it to 37°C. The operation is performed before the patient's sleep. She is asked to take the left lateral position. First insert the anal canal into the anus, then inject the drug extract slowly by a 100ml syringe through the canal into the rectum. The course of treatment lasts 10 days, one injection for each day. In order to promote the absorption of the medicinal liquid, it is recommended to use cleaning enema or to take a little mild purgative for the evacuation of stools. The longer the retention of the drugs, the better the result will be.

②Topical application of traditional Chinese drugs.The drugs used include

Natrii Sulfas 250 g

Garlic Bulb 6—7 Massae

Radix et Rhizoma Rhei   250 g

Vinegar   200 g.

Administration: Crush the peeled garlics with Natrii Sulfas. Cover a piece of gauze on the inflammatory mass, spread the crushed drugs evenly on the gauze to scorch the mass for 5—10 minutes. As the skin of the inflammatory mass is marked by the first—degree scald(reddened, having a burning sensation), remove the drugs. Mix Radix et Rhizoma Rhei with vinegar into a paste. Apply it on the mass for more than half an hour. The method is well adapted to the inflammatory mass and abscess.

③Injection of the extract of Radix Salviae Miltiorrhizae

Inject the 2ml of extract of Radix Salviae Miltiorrhizae intramuscularly , twice a day. The course of treatment lasts 10 days. An alternative method is to add 10ml of extract of red sage root into 500ml of 10% glucose solution. Inject the mixed liquid in intravenous drips. A course of treatment consists of 10 days. For common cases, two or three courses are needed.

*Jinji ChongJi.*Take one parcel at a time, twice a day. A course of treatment lasts 10 days. For common cases, two or three courses are needed. Or take *Jinji PianJi* three times a day, 6 pills at a time.

*Kongfu Xiaoyen Shuan.*Before going to bed， take the left lateral position and then press the stype into the anus. The operation is to be repeated for 10 days as a course of treatment.

**Caution:**

Take good care of personal hygiene during the menstrual and puerperal periods. Have no sitz baths nor sexual activity. The menstrual pad and sanitary tissue should keep clean and dry without pollution.

The aseptic manipulation in the uterine cavity must be followed strictly.

## Annex:Chronic Malnutrition of the Vulva

The chronic malnutrition of the vulva refers to a group of diseases which are marked by the degeneration of tissues and the modification of pigments due to the dystrophy of the vulval skin and mucosa. In the traditional Chinese medicine, this case is treated under the category of "vulval pruritus". As the external genitals are surrounded by the liver channel and the kidney governs the two private parts, so the deficiency of liver—*Yin* and kidney—*Yin* will lead to the insufficiency of vital essence and blood. As a result, vulval pruritus is induced by the dryness and endogenic wind due to the deficiency of Yin and blood.

### Type and Treatment

1. *Yin* —deficiency

**Clinical manifestations:** A dry, burning sensation in the private parts, acutely itching. The leukorrhea is scarce, yellowish or sanguinous. The case is also characterized by dizziness, tinnitus, soreness in the waist, dysphoria with a feverish sensation in the chest, palms and soles,and paroxysmal fever with perspiration. The patient has a red tongue with little coating; a small, feeble and rapid pulse. Gynecological examination finds the vulval skin and mucosa whitish and thin, chapped and lacking elasticity. The clitoris or the pudendal lip is withered and the vaginal orifice stenosed.

Therapeutic method: Tonify the kidney and subdue the pathogenic fire; nourish the blood and disperse the endogenic wind.

Recipe: *Zhi Bai Dihuang Tang* (103), augmented.

Ingredients:  Rhizoma Anemarrhenae   6 g

Cortex Phellodendri   9 g

Radix Rehmanniae   15 g

Rhizoma Dioscoreae   12 g

Cortex Moutan Radicis   9 g

Fructus Corni   12 g

Rhizoma Alismatis   9 g

Poria   15 g

Radix Polygoni Multiflori   30 g

Cortex Dictamni Radicis   15 g

Radix Angelicae Sinensis   15 g.

The decoction made is 200—300 ml. Take one half of it in the morning and the other half in the evening.

External treatment: Tonify the kidney and nourish the blood; remove toxic substances and relieve itching.

Recipe: Progenital detergent No.4.

Ingredients:  Herba Epimedii   15 g

Radix Angelicae Sinensis   15 g

Radix Arnebiae seu Lithospermi   15 g

Cortex Phellodendi   12 g

Cortex Moutan Radicis   12 g

Herba Hedyotis Diffusae   30 g

Paridis Rhizoma   30 g

Caulis Spatholobi   15 g

Folium Artemisiae Argyi　15 g

Borneolum (to be infused in the hot decoction)　3 g.

Decoct the above drugs in water for fumigation and washing in a sitz bath, one dose per day. The method used is the same as that of treating vulvitus.

### 2.Endogenic wind due to blood—deficiency

**Clinical manifestations:** The patient is characterized by vulval pruritus, listlessness, insomnia, anorexia and magersucht. The tongue is pale with white, thin fur. The pulse is weak and thready. If the illness lasts a long time, the vulval skin and mucosa will be thickened and become rough. Gynecological examination shows that the skins of the greater lip of pudendum, the labial ditch, the clitoris and post—labial commissure are thickened. They look pink or dark red in color, scattered with distinct white spots.

Therapeutic method: Nourish the blood and promote blood circulation; expel the endogenic wind and relieve itching.

Recipe: *Danggui Yinzi*(17).

Ingredients:Radix Angelicae Sinensis　15 g

Rhizoma Ligustici Chuanxiong　9 g

Radix Paeoniae Alba　15 g

Radix Rehmanniae　15 g

Radix Ledebouriellae　9 g

Herba Schizonepetae　9 g

Radix Astragali seu Hedysari　30 g

Radix Glycyrrhizae　6 g

Semen Astragali　30 g

Radix Polygoni Multiflori Praeparata　30 g.

Decoct the above drugs in an adequate amount of water to get 200—300ml of decoction. Take equal shares in the morning and evening.

External treatment: Promote blood circulation, dispel the wind and arrest itching.

Recipe: Progenital detergent No.5.

Ingredients: Herba Schizonepetae    9 g
Radix Ledebouriallae    9 g
Herba Speranskiae Tuberculatae    15 g
Radix Salviae Miltiorrhizae    30 g
Caulis Spatholobi    30 g
Lignum Sappan    15 g
Radix Paeoniae Rubra    15 g
Cortex Moutan Radicis    12 g
Pericarpium Zanthoxyli    12 g
Folium Artemisiae Argyi    12 g
Borneolum (to be infused in hot decoction)    3 g
Radix Angelicae Sinensis    15 g.

Decoct the above drugs in water for fumigation and washing in a sitz bath, one dose per day. The method used is the same as before.

Simple Recipe and Proved Prescription:

Ingredients: Herba Epimedii    30 g
Herba Pyrolae    30 g.

Decoct them in water for washing, once a day.

*Zhouhongjun Ruangao.* Apply it on the affected region and then radiate by the phototherapy unit for 30–40min once a day. A course of treatment consists of 30 days. Its effects are to relieve itching and to recover its original color and softness.

# 3. Menopathy

## 3.1 Dysfunctional Endometrorrhagia

This term denotes the abnormal bleeding of endometrium caused by cryptorrhea when one's menstruation is abnormal and gynecological examination detects no symptom of pregnancy, no tumor, no inflammation, no trauma and no general bleeding. Clinically, the disease can be classified into two types: ovulatory and anovulatory. The former occurs mostly to females of child−bearing age, the latter to those at the age of puberty or climacter. In TCM, this disease belongs to the category of "metrorrhagia and metrostaxis", which refers to massive uterine bleeding or incessant drippings of blood from the uterus beyond the menstrual cycle. Metrorrhagia is acute, drastic and profuse in bleeding; metrostaxis is chronic, mild and scanty. One of the two cases can change into the other, as both of them are induced by blood−heat, blood stasis and the weak kidney and spleen, resulting in the impairment of the *Chong* and *Ren* channels that can no longer govern menstruation and blood.

### Type and Treatment

The therapeutic principle of metrorrhagia and metrostaxis is: Treat the outstanding syndromes when the illness is critical; treat the fundamental syndromes when the illness is steady. Three methods must be handled in a flexible way. They are: "stopping up the gap" which refers to hemostasis, "clearing up the source" which means searching for the primary cause and treating the fundamental, "restoring the function" which refers to strengthening the liver and kidney and nursing one's health after the disease. Emphasis may be put on any one of the three aspects, but one aspect should never be isolated from others.

### 1. Blood—heat

(1)Heat of excess

**Clinical manifestations:** Massive uterine bleeding or incessant drippings of blood from the uterus. The blood is viscid and crimson in color. The patient is thirsty and feverish, restless and sleepless, also characterized by constipation and deep—colored urine; a scarlet tongue with yellowish or greasy fur; a full and rapid pulse. The menstruation is usually preceded or profuse.

Therapeutic method: Remove the pathogenic heat from the blood, arrest bleeding and regulate menstruation.

Recipe: *Qingre Guj ing Tang*(53)

Ingredients: Radix Scutellariae       12 g

              Fructus Gardeniae       12 g

              Radix Rehlmanniae       30 g

              Cortex Lycii Radicis       12 g

              Radix Sanguisorbae       30 g

              Colla Corii Asini   (to be dissolved in the decoction)       12 g

              Nodus Nelumbinis Rhizomatis       9 g

              Petiolus Trachycarpi Carbonisatiotis       12 g

              Plastrom Testudinis       30 g

              Concha Ostreae       30 g

Radix Glycyrhizae    6 g.

Decoct the above drugs in water to get 200—300ml of decoction. Take equal shares in the morning and evening. In case of profuse bleeding. take two doses a day. Take them separately in the morning and evening.

Modification: In case of high fever and thirst, marked by a flushed face and congested eyes, add to the recipe:

Gypsum Fibrosum    30 g

Rhizoma Anemarrhenae    6 g

Rhizoma Imperata    30 g.

In case of constipation which persists for several days, add

Radix et Rhizoma Rhei    6 g(to be added later)

Natrii Sulfas (to be infused in hot

decoction)    3 g.

In case of a burdened chest and a bitter taste in the mouth, vexation and irritation, add

Radix Bupleuris    9 g

Radix Paeoniae Alba    15 g.

In case of abdominal distention, viscid menses with a stinking smell and a yellowish, greasy fur, add

Herba Houttuyniae    15 g

Semen Coicis    15 g

Cortex Phellodendri    9 g.

(2)Fever due to deficiency

**Clinical manifestations:** Irregular menses, scarce, viscid and scarlet in color. The case manifests itself by vexation and hectic fever, a burning sensation in the palms and soles, a deep—colored urine and dry stools. A reddened tongue with yellowish, thin fur. A rapid, thready pulse.

Therapeutic method: Nourish the vital essence and clear away the heat; arrest bleeding and regulate menstruation.

Recipe: *Bao Yin Jian*(5), augmented.

Ingredient: Radix Rehmanniae     30 g

       Rhizoma Rehmanniae Praeparata    15 g

       Radix Paeoniae Alba    18 g

       Rhizoma Dioscoreae    15 g

       Radix Dip'saci    15 g

       Radix Scutellariae    12 g

       Cortex Phellodendri    9 g

       Radix Glycyrrhizae    6 g

       Cortex Lycii Radicis    12 g

       Radix Scrophulariae    15 g

       Cortex Moutan Radicis    9 g

Decoct the above drugs in water to get 200—300ml of decoction. Take one half of it in the morning and the other half in the evening. In case of profuse bleeding, take two doses a day. Drink them separately in the morning and evening.

Modification: In case of vexation and insomnia, add

       Os Draconis    30 g

       Concha Ostreae    30 g

       Fructus Schisandrae    12 g.

In case of profuse bleeding, add

       Radix Sanguisorbae    30 g

       Herba Agrimoniae    15 g

       Os Sepiellae seu Sepiae    30 g.

In case of dyspnea and lassitude, dizziness and palpitation due to prolonged bleeding from the uterus, add

       Radix Astragali seu Hedysari    30 g

Radix Pseudostellariae　　12 g.

## 2. Blood-stasis

**Clinical manifestations:** Abnormal, intermittent bleeding from the uterus or abrupt, massive uterine bleeding after a few month's amenorrhea. The menses are dark purplish, mingled with blood clots. The patient feels abdominal pain and tenderness which will be relaxed when blood clots are discharged. The tongue is a dark purplish and spotted with ecchymoses. The pulse is deep and uneven.

Therapeutic method: Promote blood circulation by removing blood stasis; arrest bleeding and regulate menstruation.

Recipe: *Siwu Tang*(69) plus *Shixiao San*(70), augmented.

Ingredients: Radix Rehmanniae Praeparata　　15 g

　　　　　　　Radix Angelicae Sinensis　　15 g

　　　　　　　Rhizoma Ligustici Chuanxiong　　12 g

　　　　　　　Radix Paeoniae Rubra　　15 g

　　　　　　　Pollen Typhae　　12 g

　　　　　　　Faeces Trogopterorum　　12 g

　　　　　　　Herba Leonuri　　30 g

　　　　　　　Radix Rubiae　　12 g

　　　　　　　Flos Carthami　　12 g

　　　　　　　Rhizoma Corydalis　　9 g.

Decoct the above drugs in water to get 200-300ml of decoction. Divide it into two equal portions. Take one portion in the morning and the second portion in the evening. In case of profuse uterine bleeding. take two doses for a day.

Modification: In case of distending pain in the chest, breasts and lower abdomen, add to the recipe:

　　　　　　　Fructus Meliae Toosendan　　9 g

Rhizoma Cyperi    12 g.

In case of drastic abdominal pain and numerous blood clots, add

Radix Achyranthis Bidentatae    15 g

Herba Siphonostegia    15 g.

In case of a dry mouth with bitter taste, a flushed face and excessive uterine bleeding, add

Spica Prunellae    12 g

Radix Salviae Miltiorrhizae    15 g

Radix Sanguisorbae    30 g

In case of abdominal pain caused by cold and dark, viscid menses, add

Folum Artemisiae Argyi    12 g

Radix Linderae    12 g.

Proprietary: *Bao Kun Dan*. Take 30 pills once a day. Avoid raw, cold, pungent and stimulating food in the course of treatment.

*San Qi Pian*. The daily dose is 5—10 pills: don't exceed 30 pills in number. In case of incessant uterine bleeding. a second dose may be taken 6 hours later.

*Yimucao Gao*. Take one spoon(about 10ml) of the extract at a time, thrice a day.

*Yunnan Baiyao*. Take 0.2—0.3 g every 4 hours. The maximum amount of a dose is 0.5g.

### 3. Spleen—deficiency

**Clinical manifestations:** Abrupt and profuse uterine bleeding or incessant drippings of blood from the uterus. It is thin and light—colored. The patient looks languid and weary with a pale and puffy face. looking languid and weary. The case is also characterized by palpitation, loss of appetite , cool limbs and loose stools. A pale, corpulent tongue with whitish, thin fur. A feeble and moderate pulse.

Therapeutic method: Invigorate $Qi$, to arrest bleeding and regulate menstruation.

Recipe: *Guben Zhibeng Tang*(24), modified

Ingredients: Radix Ginseng(to be decocted first)    15 g

Radix Astragali seu Hedysari    30 g

Rhizoma Atractylodis Macroce Phalae    18 g

Radix Rehmanniae Praeparata    15 g

Rhizoma Zingiberis Praeparata    9 g

Plumula Nelumbinis    30 g

Os Draconis    30 g

Cocha Ostreae    30 g

Rhizoma Cimicifugae    6g.

The decoction made is 200—300ml. Take equal shares in the morning and evening. In case of massive bleeding, take two doses for a day, one dose at a time.

Modification: In case of abdominal distention, loss of appetite and loose stools, deduct Radix Rehmanniae Praeparata, but add:

Radix Bupleuri    9 g

Radix Paeoniae Alba    15 g

Semen Amomi    6 g.

In case of prolonged and incessant uterine bleeding, add

Os Sepiellae seu Sepiae    30 g

Fructus Mume    12g.

In case of palpitation and short breaths, add

Fructus Schisandrae    12 g

Radix Ophiopogonis    12 g.

**Proprietary and Simple Recipe:** *Guipi Wan*.Take one bolus, thrice a day.

*Buzhong Yiqi Wan* . Take one bolus, three times a day.

*Renseng Guipi Wan.* Take one bolus, thrice a day.

Ginseng, 30 g. Soak the medicinal herb in water for some time and then decoct it. Eat the herbt together with the soup.

**4. Kidney—deficiency**

(1)Deficiency of kidney—*Yin*

**Clinical manifestations:** The menses are disorderly and irregular, incessant or profuse, scarlet and viscid. The patient is characterized by dizziness and tinnitus: sore loins and weak knees; dysphoria with a feverish sensation in the chest, palms and soles; a reddened tongue with little or no coating; a rapid, thready pulse.

Therapeutic method: Nourish the kidney and replenish vital essence; arrest bleeding and regulate menstruation.

Recipe: *Zuo Gui Wan*(105) plus *Erzhi Wan*(22), modified.

Ingredients:Radix Rehmanniae        15 g

Radix Rehmanniae Praeparata      15 g

Rhizoma Dioscoreae      15 g

Fructus Lycii        18 g

Fructus Corni        12 g

Semen Cuscutae        24 g

Colla Plastri Testudinis(to be melted )      15 g

Fructus Ligustri Lucidi      15 g

Herba Ecliptae        30 g

Colla Cornus Cervi        12 g

Radix Scrophulariae        12 g

Cortex Moutan Radicis    12 g

Radix Sanguisorbae    15 g.

Decoct the above drugs in water to get 200—300ml of decoction. Divide the decoction into two equal portions. Take one in the morning and the other in the evening. In case of massive bleeding, take two doses for a day, one dose at a time.

Modification: In case of a dry throat, dizziness and tinnitus, add to the recipe

Oncha Ostreae    30 g

Spica Pranelae    12 g.

In case of aching hypochondria and distending breasts, vexation and irritability, add

Fructus Meliae Toosendan    12 g

Radix Paeoniae Alba    15 g

Radix Bupleuri    9 g.

In case of yellowish fur, dark—colored urine and constipation, add

Cortex Phellodendri    6 g

Radix Adenophorae Strictae    15 g.

Proprietary: *Liuwei Dihuang Wan*. Take one bolus at a time, twice a day. The dosage of pellets is 9 g at a time, twice a day.

(2)Insufficiency of kidney—*Yang*

**Clinical manifestations:** Irregular menses, massive uterine bleeding or incessant drippings of blood from the uterus, which is thin and light—colored. The patient is characterized by a dim, gloomy complexion; lassitude in loins and knees; polyuria and nocturia; a pale tongue with whitish, thin coating; a small ,deep pulse.

Therapeutic method: Warm the kidney and reinforce the *Chong* and *Ren* channels; arrest bleeding and regulate menstruation.

Recipe: *Yougui Wan* (96), modified.

Ingredients:

Radix Aconiti Praeparata    6 g

Cortex Cinnamomi    6 g

Radix Rehmanniae Praeparata    15 g

Rhizoma Dioscoreae    15 g

Fructus Corni    12 g

Fructus Lycii    15 g

Semen Cuscutae    24 g

Colla Cornus Cervi    12 g

Cortex Eucommiae    30 g

Halloysitum Rubrum    30 g

Fructus Rubi    30g.

Decoct the above drugs in water to get 200—300ml of decoction. Take one half of it in the morning and the other in the evening. In case of massive uterine bleeding, take two doses a day, one at a time.

Modification: In case of profuse bleeding, deduct Cortex Cinnamomi, but add

Radix Astragali seu Hedysari    30 g

Os Sepiella seu Sepiae    30g.

In case of abdominal pain caused by cold, and dark—colored, copious uterine bleeding with blood clots, add

Resina Olibani    9 g

Myrrha    9 g

Fructus Foenicuii    6 g.

In case of edema and anorexia with cool limbs, add

> Poria    15 g
>
> Rhizoma Zingiberis Praeparata    6 g
>
> Semen Amomi    6 g.

Proprietary: *Jingui Shenqi Wan*. Infuse one bolus in hot, dilute salt water. Take the prepared decoction of a bolus at a draught, twice a day.

*Ai Fu Nuangong Wan*. Take one bolus at a time, twice a day.

**Application of the Artificial Menstrual Cycle with traditional Chinese Drugs**

When the dysfunctional uterine bleeding is arrested, the regulation of menstrual cycle must be taken into consideration. Abundant clinical practice and experiments have proved that according to the clinical symptoms and signs, kidney—tonifying should be regarded as the chief therapy, supported by regulating the liver function, invigorating the spleen and promoting blood circulation. This kind of comprehensive treatment is beneficial to the follicular development, regular ovulation. normalized luteoidism and endometrial denudation.

(1)Postmenstruum (6th—10th day of the menstrual cycle)

Therapeutic method: Reinforce the *Chong* and *Ren* channels by tonifying the kidney and nourishing the blood.

Recipe: *Cu Luanpao Tang*.

> Radix Rehmanniae Praeparata    15 g
>
> Rhizoma Dioscoreae    15 g
>
> Radix Dipsaci    30 g
>
> Semen Cuscutae    24 g
>
> Radix Polygoni Multiflori    30 g
>
> Fructus Lycii    15 g

> Radix Astragali seu Hedysari    30 g
>
> Radix Angelicae Sinensis    15 g
>
> Rhizoma Cyperi    12 g.

The decoction of a dose is 200—300ml. Take equal shares in the morning and evening. 5 or 6 doses are needed.

Modification: In case of delayed and scanty menstruation combined with insufficiency of the kidney—*Yang*, add to the recipe:

> Herba Epimedii    15 g
>
> Rhizoma Curculiginis    12 g
>
> Placenta Hominis    12 g
>
> Cortex Cinnamomi    6 g.

In case of preceded and profuse menstruation combined with deficiency of the kidney—*Yin* exchange Radix Rehmanniae Praeparata for Radix Rehmanniae and add

> Fructus Ligustri Lucidi    15 g
>
> Herba Ecliptae    15 g
>
> Plastrum Testudinis    30 g
>
> Carapx Trionycis    30 g.

In case of exhaustion and lack of appetite combined with deficiency of *Qi*. deduct Radix Rehmanniae Praeparata but add

> Radix Codonopsis Pilosulae    30 g
>
> Rhizoma Atractylodis Macrocephalae    18 g
>
> Semen Amomi    9 g.

(2)Preovulatory and ovulatory phases (11th—16th day of the menstrual cycle)

Therapeutic method: Tonify the kidney and nourish the blood, assisted by removing blood stasis to promote blood circulation.

Recipe: *Cu Pailuan Tang*.

Ingredients: Rhizoma Dioscoreae   15 g
              Radix Dipsaci   30 g
              Semen Cuscutae   24 g
              Fructus Lycii   15 g
              Herba Cistanchis   30 g
              Herba Epimedii   15 g
              Radix Salviae Miltiorrhizae   15 g
              Radix Paeoniae Rubra   12 g
              Flos Carthami   12 g
              Herba Siphonostegia   12 g
              Rhizoma Ligustici Chuanxiong   9 g
              Rhizoma Cyperi   12 g.

The decoction of a dose is 200—300ml. Take one half in the morning and the other half in the evening. 6 doses are needed.

(3)Postovulatory phase (17th—25th day of the menstrual cycle)

Therapeutic method: Tonify the liver and kidney, invigorate the spleen and reinforce the *Chong* and *Ren* channels.

Recipe: *Zhu Huangti Tang*.

Ingredients: Radix Astragali seu Hedysari   30 g
              Rhizoma Dioscoreae   15 g
              Radix Paeoniae Alba   15 g
              Radix Dipsaci   30 g
              Herba Ecliptae   15 g
              Fructus Ligustri Lucidi   15 g
              Os Draconis   30 g
              Concha Ostreae   30 g
              Radix Polygoni Multiflori   15 g

Semen Cuscutae     24 g

Fructus Rubi     30 g

Radix Salviae Miltiorrhizae     12 g.

The decoction of a dose is 200—300ml. Take one half in the morning and the other half in the evening. 6—8 doses are needed.

(4)Premenstruum (25th—28th day of the menstrual cycle)

Therapeutic method: Promote blood flow and induce menstruation.

Recipe: *Tong Jing Tang*.

Ingredients: Radix Angeliae Sinensis     15 g

Rhizoma Ligustici Chuanxiong     12 g

Radix Paeoniae Rubra     15 g

Flos Carthami     12 g

Radix Salviae Miltiorrhizae     30 g

Herba Lycopi     15 g

Radix Achyranthis Bidentatae     15 g

Caulis Spatholobi     30 g

Pollen Typhae     12 g

Fructus Leonuri     12 g

Rhizoma Cyperi     12 g

Cortex Cinnamomi     6 g.

The decoction of a dose is 200—300ml. Take equal shares in the morning and evening. 3—5 doses are needed.

# 3.2 Dysmenorrhea

If in the menstrual period or around it there appears abdominal pain or other distresses which exert an influence on the daily life and work, this syndrome is termed dysmenorrhea. Clinically, there are two sorts of dysmenorrhea, primary and secondary. The former refers to the case that the genitals have no organic disease, it is also known as functional dysmenorrhea. The latter is caused by distinct organic disease, and in most cases, it is induced by endometriosis, acute or chronic inflammation of pelvic organs, stenosis and blockage of the cervix.

TCM holds that pain is caused by the blockage of channels. The emotional depression, imprudence in daily life or invasion of six climatic factors (including wind, cold, summer—heat, dampness, dryness and fire) may lead to the blood stasis in the *Chong* and *Ren* channels or accumulation of cold—evil in the channels and vessels, resulting in the impediment of the flow of *Qi* and blood as well as the stagnation of menses. Thus dysmenorrhea occurs. Besides, it may be brought about by deficiency of *Qi* and blood due to the excessive consumption of the liver—*Yin* and kidney— *Yin* as they fail to nourish the uterine collaterals.

## Type and Treatment

Clinically, it is necessary to distinguish between syndromes of cold and heat, deficiency and excess according to the time, position, nature and degree of the pain and by making reference to the cycle, nature, amount, color of the menses, and other symptoms such as the tongue and pulse conditions. Generally speaking, if the pain occurs in the premenstrual or menstrual period and it is severe with tenderness, the disease lies in sthenia. If the pain occurs in the postmenstrual period and it is dull latent, and able to be relieved by pressing or stroks, the disease lies in asthenia. If the pain is colic due to coldness and it can be abated by warmth, the disease lies in cold; if the pain is scorching and it gets aggravated by warmth, the disease lies in heat. If distention is more serious than pain, the disease lies in the stagnation of $Qi$; if pain is more drastic than distention and it is a kind of stabbing or throbbing pain which can be relieved by discharge of blood clots, the disease lies in blood stasis. If the position of pain is at the two sides of the lower abdomen, the disease lies in the liver; if the loin is entangled in pain, the disease lies in the kidney.

### 1. $Qi$—Stagnation and blood stasis

**Clinical manifestations:** Abdominal pain, distention and tenderness in the lower abdomen, just one or two days before menstruation or during the menstrual cycle; purplish dark, scarce menses mixed with blood clots, the excretion of which can alleviate the pain. The patient feels a kind of distending pain in the chest and breasts. The tongue is purplish dark and specked with ecchymoses on its margin. The pulse is taut and uneven.

Therapeutic method: Soothe the liver and regulate the flow of $Qi$; alleviate the pain by removing blood stasis.

Recipe: *Gexia Zhuyu Tang* (25), augmented.

Ingredients:  
  Radix Angelicae Sinensis        15 g  
  Rhizoma Ligustici Chuanxiong      12 g  
  Radix Paeoniae Rubra       15 g  
  Semen Persicae       12 g  
  Flos Carthami       12 g  
  Fructus Aurantii       9 g  
  Rhizoma Corydalis       12 g  
  Faeces Trogopterorum       12 g  
  Cortex Moutan Radicis       9 g

Radix Linderae          12 g

Rhizoma Cyperi          12 g

Radix Glycyrrhizae       6 g

Herba Siphonostegia       15 g

Radix Achyranthis Bidentatae    15 g

Radix Salviae Miltiorrhizae     30 g.

Decoct the above drugs in water to 200—300 ml of decoction. Take one half of it in the morning and the other half in the evening, starting from 7—10 days previous to menstruation till the menstrual onset.

Modification: In case of nausea and vomiting, add to the recipe:

Fructus Euodiae          12 g

Caulis Bambusae in Taeniam     9 g

Rhizoma Coptidis        6 g.

In case of yellowish fur, rapid pulse and a bitter taste in the mouth, add

Fructus Gardeniae        9 g

Spica Prunellae        12 g.

In case of chest distress and loss of appetite, add

Fructus Crataegi        15 g

Endothelium Corneum Gigeriae Galli       6 g

Rhizoma Atractylodis Macrocephalae    12 g.

Proprietary: *Yuanhu Zhitong Pian*. Take 4 pills at a time, thrice a day.

*Yimucao Gao*. Take 10 ml at a time after mixing it with water, thrice a day.

**2. Accumulation of cold and dampness**

**Clinical manifestations:**  Cold—pain in the lower abdomen just before menstruation or during the menstrual period, which becomes aggravated by pressing and relieved by warmth. The case is also marked by dark—colored, scanty menses mixed with blood clots, by loose stools and by aversion to cold. The patient has a whitish, greasy fur and a deep and tense pulse.

Therapeutic method: Warm the channels, expel cold and dampness, remove blood stasis and alleviate the pain.

Recipe: *ShaofuZhuyu Tang* (60) plus Rhizoma Atractylodis, Poria.

Ingredients: Fructus Foeniculi        6 g
            Rhizoma Zingiberis        6 g
            Rhizoma Corydalis         9 g
            Myrrha        12 g
            Radix Angelicae Sinensis        15 g
            Rhizoma Ligustici Chuanxiong        9 g
            Cortex Cinnamomi        6 g
            Radix Paeoniae Rubra        12 g
            Pollen Typhae        12 g
            Faeces Trogopterorum        12 g
            Rhizoma Atractylodis        9 g
            Poria        12 g
            Radix Linderae        12 g
            Fructus Euodiae        12 g.

The decoction of the above drugs is 200—300ml. Take equal shares in the morning and evening, starting from 7—10 days previous to menstruation till the menstrual onset.

Modification: In case of severe pain and cold limbs accompanied by profuse perspiration of cold sweat, add
            Radix Aconiti Praeparata        9 g

Folium Artemisiae Argyi    12 g.

In case of lumbago and scarce dischaige, add

Radix Achyranthis Bidentatae    15 g

Cortex Eucommiae    15 g

Caulis Spatholobi    30 g.

Proprietary: *Ai Fu Nuangong Wan*. Take one bolus at a time with warm water, twice a day.

### 3. Deficiency of *Qi* and blood

**Clinical manifestations:** The case is characterized by dull and patent pain with a straining sensation in the lower abdomen and vagina just one or two days after menstrual onset or during the menstrual period, which can be lessened by pressing and stroking. The menses are scarce, dilute and dim in shade. The patient looks weary and languid with dim complexion, poor appetite and loose stools. She is also marked by a pale tongue and a deep, feeble pulse.

Therapeutic method: Replenish *Qi* and blood and alleviate the pain.

Recipe:*Sheng Yu Tang* (72), modified.

Ingredients: Radix Ginseng (to be decocted first)    15 g

Radix Astragali seu Hedysari    30 g

Radix Angelicae Sinensis    15 g

Rhizoma Ligustici Chuanxiong    9 g

Radix Rehmanniae Praeparata    15 g

Radix Paeoniae Alba    18 g

Rhizoma Cyperi    9 g

Rhizoma Corydalis    9 g

Radix Glycyrrhizae Praeparata    9 g

Caulis Spatholobi    15 g

Flos Carthami    12 g.

The decoction of the above drugs is 200–300ml. Take one half in the morning and the other half in the evening.

Modification: In case of dizziness, palpitation and insomnia, add

Semen Biotae    15 g

Semen Ziziphi Spinosae    30 g.

In case of anorexia and loose stools, add

Rhizoma Atractylodis Macrocephalae    18 g

Fructus Crataegi    15 g

Poria    15g.

In case of scanty and light–colored menses, add again

Caulis Spatholobi    30 g

Radix Polygoni Multiflori    30 g

Colla Corii Asini    12 g.

(to be infused in hot decoction)

Proprietary: *Bazhen Yimu Wan.*Take one bolus at a time, twice a day.

*Jixueteng Pian.* Take 5 pills at a time, thrice a day.

**4. Impairment of the liver and kidney**

**Clinical manifestations:**   Dull and persistent pain in the lower abdomen one or two days after the menstrual onset, accompanied by lumbodynia. The menses are scanty, dilute and dim in shade. The case is also characterized by dizziness, tinnitus and hectic fever; a feeble and thready pulse; a thin, whitish or yellowish fur.

Therapeutic method: Tonify the liver and kidney, and relieve the pain.

Recipe:*Tiao Gan Tang*(73), augmented.

Ingredients:   Radix Angelicae Sinensis   12 g

Radix Paeoniae Alba   15 g

Fructus Corni   12 g

Radix Morindae Officinalis   15 g

Colla Corii Asini (to be infused)   12 g

Rhizoma Dioscoreae   12 g

Radix Glycyrrhizae   6 g

Fructus Lycii   30 g

Radix Rehmanniae Praeparata   15 g

Cortex Moutan Radicis   9 g

Rhizoma Cyperi   12 g.

The decoction of a dose is 200—300ml. Take equal shares in the morning and evening.

Modification: In case of distending pain in the lower abdomen and hypochondria, add to the recipe.

Fructus Meliae Toosendan   12 g

Rhizoma Corydalis   9 g

Semen Citri Reticulatae   9 g.

In case of flushed cheeks, dry mouth and hectic fever, add

Herba Artemisiae Chinghao   9 g

Carapax Trionycis   30 g

Cortex Lycii Radicis   12 g.

but deduct Radix Morindae Officinalis from the recipe.

In case of lumbosacral pain and abundant polyuria at night, add

Fructus Alpiniae Oxyphyllae   15 g

Oötheca Mantidis   30 g.

**Caution**

During the menstrual period, keep from showers and swimming. Don't eat too much of cold food. Pay attention to personal hygiene. Keep the vulva clean by daily washing. Sexual activity is forbidden.

## 3.3 Amenorrhea

Amenorrhea refers to the case of no menstrual onset of a female who should have had menses as she has reached the adult age, excluding those physiological conditions before adolescence, in the period of pregnancy and lactation, and after menopause. Clinically, two types of pathogenic amenorrhea should be distinguished: primary and secondary. The former refers to no menses over the age of 18; the latter to the stoppage of regular menstruation for more than 3 months. TCM holds this disease may be caused by various factors——disorder, environmental changes, general chronic wasting diseases, cryptorrhea, uterine hypoplasia and serious injury of endometrium.

According to clinical symptoms and signs, two sorts of amenorrhea should be distinguished. One lies in asthenia due to blood depletion, and the other in sthenia due to blood stagnation. For most cases, the illness of deficiency type results from the excessive consumption of the liver and kidney, scarcity of $Qi$ and blood, $Yi$-deficiency and blood dryness, so that there is no blood to go down. On the other hand, the illness of excess type is induced mostly by the stagnant $Qi$ and blood stasis, the blockage of phlegm—dampness and the obstruction of channel $Qi$, so that menses are kept from descending.

### Type and Treatment

#### 1. Deficiency of the liver and kidney

Clinical manifestations: The female has no menses over the age of 18, or the menses are delayed or scanty or gradually suppressed. The case manifests itself by dizziness and tinnifus, soreness of the loins and weakness of the legs. The patient has a dim complexion or flushed cheeks; a palish red tongue with little coating; a deep, feeble pulse. Gynecological examination detects uterine hypoplasia or infantile uterus. The cytological examination of the vagina finds that estrogenic hormones are slightly affected or slightly depressed.

Therapeutic method: Tonify the liver and kidney, nourish the blood and restore regular menstruation.

Recipe:*Gui Shen Wan* (26), augmented.

| | |
|---|---|
| Radix Rehmanniae Praeparata | 15 g |
| Rhizoma Dioscoreae | 15 g |
| Fructus Corni | 12 g |
| Poria | 15 g |
| Radix Angelicae Sinensis | 15 g |
| Fructus Lycii | 30 g |
| Cortex Eucommiae | 30 g |
| Semen Cuscutae | 24 g |
| Radix Dipsaci | 30 g |
| Herba Epimedii | 15 g. |

Decoct the above drugs in water to get 200—300ml of decoction. Take equal portions in the morning and evening.

Modification: In case of aversion to cold with cool limbs, clear and copious urine and loose stools, add

| | |
|---|---|
| Radix Morindae Officinalis | 12 g |
| Radix Aconiti Praeparata | 9 g. |

In case of abdominal distention, poor appetite and loose stools, deduct

> Radix Rehmanniae Praeparata

but add

> Semen Dolichoris    30 g
>
> Fructus Crataegi    15 g
>
> Semen Amomi    9 g.

In case of a dry mouth and throat, a rapid and thready pulse, exchange Radix Rehmanniae Praeparata for Radix Rehmanniae and add

> Herba Ecliptae    15 g
>
> Fructus Ligustri Lucidi    15 g
>
> Radix Ophiopogonis    12 g.

Proprietary:*Liuwei Dihuang Wan*. Take one bolus at a time, thrice a day.*Wuj i Bai Feng Wan*. Take one bolus at a time, twice a day.

**2.** *Yin* **−deficiency and blood dryness**

**Clinical manifestations:** The menstruation is delayed, scarce or gradually drawn to a close. The patient is marked by flushed cheeks, dry mouth and throat, a feverish sensation in the palms and soles as well as night sweat or spitting blood at coughing; a reddened tongue with little or no coating; a wiry, rapid and thready pulse. For most cases, the patient has a history of tuberculosis. Gynecological examination may find nothing abnormal but it is also probable to perceive some encysted mass in the pelvic cavity, which is hard in quality, adherent to the surrounding tissues and has no distinct tenderness. The arrested growth of the uterus can always be found.

Therapeutic method: Restore normal menstruation by nourishing blood and removing heat.

Recipe: *Jia Jian Yi Yin Jian*(102), modified.

Ingredients:
| | |
|---|---|
| Radix Rehmanniae | 15 g |
| Radix Paeoniae Alba | 15 g |
| Radix Ophiopogonis | 12 g |
| Rhizoma Anemarrhenae | 9 g |
| Cortex Lycii Radicis | 12 g |
| Radix Glycyrrhizae Praeparata | 6 g |
| Radix Stemonae | 15 g |
| Radix Sanguisorbae | 15 g |
| Radix Scrophulariae | 12 g |
| Carapax Trionycis | 30 g |
| Plastrum Testudinis | 30 g. |

The decoction of the above drugs is 200—300ml. Take one half of it in the morning and the other half in the evening.

Modification: In case of unproductive cough and hymoptysis, add to the recipe

| | |
|---|---|
| Radix Adenophorae Strictae | 30 g |
| Bulbus Fritillariae Cirrhosae | 12 g |
| Bulbus Lilii | 30 g |
| Rhizoma Bletillae | 12 g |
| Fructus Schisandrae | 12g. |

In case of palpitation and insomnia, add

| | |
|---|---|
| Caulis Polygoni Multiflori | 15 g |
| Semen Biotae | 15 g. |

In case of encysted mass, add

| | |
|---|---|
| Endothelium Corneum Gigeriae Galli | 9 g |
| Fructus Forsythiae | 30 g |
| Spica Prunellae | 15 g |

Concha Ostreae      30 g.

### 3. Scarcity of *Qi* and blood

**Clinical manifestations:** The menstruation is delayed, scarce, dilute and light colored and finally drawn to a close. The patient is characterized by dizziness and palitation, short breaths and poor appetite. She looks weary and languid, with a dim complexion, sparse hair and a meagre body; a pale tongue with thin, whitish coating; a feeble, moderate pulse. Uterine hypoplasia or atrophy is perceivable in the gynecological examination.

Therapeutic method: Restore regular menstruation by invigorating *Qi* and nourishing blood.

Recipe: *Renshen Yangrong Tang* (58), augmented.

Ingredients:Radix Ginseng (to be decocted first)      15 g

Radix Astragali seu Hedysari      30 g

Rhizoma Atractylodis Macrocephalae      30 g

Poria      15 g

Radix Polygalae      9 g

Pericarpium Citri Reticulatae      12 g

Fructus Schisandrae      12 g

Radix Angelicae Sinensis      15 g

Radix Paeoniae Alba      15 g

Radix Rehmanniae Praeparata      15 g

Cortex Cinnamomi      9 g

Radix Glycyrrhizae Praeparata      6 g

Radix Polygoni Multiflori      30 g

Semen Biotae      15 g

Caulis Spatholobi      30 g

Arillus Longan      12 g.

The decoction of a dose is 200—300ml. Take equal shares in

the morning and evening.

Modification: In case of insomnia or excessive dreaming, add

Semen Ziziphi Spinosae    30 g.

In case of dry mouth with a reddened tongue or oral ulceration, add

Radix Scutellariae    9 g

Rhizoma Coptidis    9 g.

In case of amenorrhea caused by serious postpartum hemorrhage, accompanied by aversion to cold, hyposexuality and atrophy of genital organs, add

Herba Epimedii    30 g

Placenta Hominis    15 g

Cornu Cervi Degelatinatum    12 g

Semen Cuscutae    30 g.

Proprietary: *Danggui Wan*. Take one bolus at a time, thrice a day.

*Shouwu Pian*. Take 3—5pills at a time, thrice a day.

**4.*Qi*–Stagnantion and blood stasis**

**Clinical manifestations:**    The menses have ceased for several months. The patient is characterized by mental depression, restlessness and irritability, accompanied by distention over the chest, abdominal pain and tenderness; a purplish dark tongue specked with ecchymoses; a deep and uneven pulse.

Therapeutic method:Regulate the flow of *Qi* and promote blood circulation; remove blood stasis and restore normal menstruation.

Recipe: *Xuef u Zhuyu Tang* (90),augmented.

Ingredients: Semen Persicae    12 g

Flos Carthami    12 g

Radix Angelicae Sinensis     15 g

Radix Rehmanniae     15 g

Rhizoma Ligustici Chuanxiong     9 g

Radix Paeoniae Rubra     15 g

Radix Achyrantis Bidentatae     15 g

Radix Platycodi     12 g

Radix Bupleuri     9 g

Fructus Aurantii     9 g

Radix Glycyrrhizae     6 g

Radix Salviae Miltiorrhizae     30 g

Lignum Sappan     15 g

Herba Lycopi     18 g.

The decoction of the above drugs is 200—300ml. Take equal shares in the morning and evening.

Modification: In case of oppressive distention in the chest and lower abdomen, add

Pericarpium Citri Reticulatae Viride     12 g

Fructus Meliae Toosendan     12 g.

In case of severe abdominal pain and tenderness, add

Herba Leonuri     30 g

Rhizoma Sparganii     12 g

Herba Siphonostegia     15 g.

In case of cold—pain with cool limbs, a whitish fur and a deep, tense pulse, add

Cortex Cinnamomi     6 g

Fructus Foeniculi     9 g.

and deduct

Radix Salviae Miltiorrhizae

Radix Rehmanniae.

In case of burning pain in the lower abdomen, profuse yellowish leukorrhea, a yellowish fur and a rapid pulse, add

    Herba Patriniae    30 g

    Cortex Moutan Radicis    12 g

    Cortex Phellodendri    9 g.

Proprietary: *Bao Kun Dan*. Take 30pills at a time daily.

*Danshen Gao*. Take one spoon of medicine which is melted in hot water, thrice a day.

### 5. Blockage of phlegm—dampness

**Clinical manifestations:**  Stoppage of menstruation, profuse leukorrhea, nausea and vomiting with productive sputa. The patient looks plump, weary and listless with a turgid face and swollen feet and a full, oppressive sensation in the chest and hypochondria. She has also a greasy fur and a slippery pulse. Gynecological examination detects the hypoplasia of the uterus or the enlargement of the ovary which is tenacious in quality. The uterus is normal in size but the lab tests show the endocrine function is often abnormal.

Therapeutic method: Eliminate phlegm—dampness, regulate the flow of *Qi*, invigorate the blood and restore normal menstruation

Recipe: *Qi Gong Wan*(47), augmented.

Ingredients: Poria    18 g

    Rhizoma Pinelliae    12 g

    Pericarpium Citri Reticulatae    12 g

    Rhizoma Atractylodis    15 g

    Rhizoma Cyperi    12 g

    Massa Fermentata Medicinalis    12 g

    Rhizoma Ligustici Chuanxiong    9 g

Herba Epimedii     30 g
Caulis Spatholobi     30 g
Radix Dipsaci     30 g
Radix Achyranthis Bidentatae     15 g
Semen Persicae     12 g
Semen Plantaginis     12 g (in a parcel)
Cortex Cinnamomi     6 g
Semen Vaccariae     12 g.

Decoct the drugs in water to get 200—300 ml of dcoction. Take one half of it in the morning and the other half in the evening.

Modification: In case of scanty leukorrhea and uterine hypoplasia, add

Semen Cuscutae     24 g
Herba Cistanchis     30 g.

In case of ovarian enlargement on both sides, add

Radix Salviae Mitiorrhizae     15 g
Concha Ostreae     30 g
Lignum Sappan     15 g
Rhizoma Sparganii     12 g.

In case of profuse, yellowish leukorrhea and a yellowish, greasy fur, add

Rhizoma Alismatis     9 g
Cortex Phellodendi     6 g.

# 3.4   Premenstrual Tension Syndrome

Premenstrual Tension Syndrome refers to a series of symptoms appearing periodically before the menstrual onset, such as mental tension, emotional lability, distractibility, either restlessness and irritability or depression and anxiety, insomnia, dizziness and headache, distending pain over the chest and breasts, general dropsy and diarrhea. Generally speaking, the syndrome turns up 7—14 days before menstruation and becomes aggravated 2—3 days before it and retreats after the menstrual onset. Various factors may give rise to this syndrome. They are: retention of water and sodium due to the decrease of progestogen and the relative increase of estrogenic hormones in the body; excessive profusion of prolactin in the blood caused by mental tension; different sensitivity of the organism to the rise of aldosterone prior to menstruation.

The syndrome of premenstrual tension is normally discussed in ancient medical classics under the topic of "Various syndromes concerning menstruation" . It results from stagnation of the liver—$Qi$, from $Yang$—deficiency of both spleen and kidney, and from blood deficiency and hyperactivity of the liver.

## Type and Treatment

### 1. Stagnation of the liver—$Qi$
**Clinical manifestations:**  Distending pain over the nipples and breasts which, in serious cases, feel extremely hurt when touched slightly on the dress;an oppressive sensation in the chest and hypochondria and fullness in the lower abdomen.The patient is also characterized by either mental depression or restlessness and irritability. The tongue is light—colored with a thin and whitish fur. The pulse is taut. Gynecological examination finds the breasts hard and distending with tubercula and tenderness.

Therapeutic method: Soothe the liver and promote the flow of *Qi*, invigorate the blood and regulate the menstruation.

Recipe:*Chaihu Shugan San*(9), augmented.

Ingredients:Radix Bupleuri          9 g

Radix Paeoniae Alba          15 g

Rhizoma Ligustici Chuanxiong          9 g

Rhizoma Cyperi          12 g

Pericarpium Citri Reticulatae          12 g

Fructus Aurantii          9 g

Radix Glycyrrhizae Praeparata          6 g

Folium Citri Reticulatae          12 g

Fructus Meliae Toosendan          12 g

Radix Curcumae          9 g

Radix Salviae Miltiorrhizae          15 g.

The decoction of the above drugs is 200—300ml. Take equal shares in the morning and evening. Start administration before the occurrence of symptoms and stop it at the menstrual onset. The same prescription can be used again for the next cycle.

Modification: In case of obstruction of the menses with abdominal pain, add

Radix Achyrantis Bidentatae          15 g

Semen Persicae          12 g

Lignum Sappan          15 g.

In case of dry mouth with a bitter taste, a thin and yellowish fur, headache and fever, dark—colored urine and constipation, deduct

Rhizoma Ligustici Chuanxion g

but add

Cortex Moutan Radicis          9 g

Fructus Gardeniae          9 g
Concha Haliotidis          15 g.

In case of hard and distending breasts with encysted mass, add

Semen Vaccariae          12 g
Semen Citri Reticulatae          12 g
Semen Litchi          12 g
Fructus Liquidambaris          12 g.

In case of mental depression and sleeplessness with deep sighs, add

Flos Albiziae          15 g.

Proprietary:*Xiao Yao Wan*. Take 6−9g at a time, twice a day, Start it 7−10 days prior to the menstrual onset.

*Qi Zhi Xiangfu Wan*. Take one bolus at a time, thrice a day. Start administration 7−10 days before the menstrual onset.

2.*Yang*−**deficiency of both the spleen and kidney**

**Clinical manifestations:**   The patient has a turgid face, weary and listless, with swollen eyelids and limbs in the premenstrual or menstrual stage, accompanied by abdominal distention, diarrhea, anorexia and distress in the loins and knees. The menses are abundant and light−colored. The patient has a whitish, greasy fur and a deep, moderate pulse.

Therapeutic method:Warm the kidney and invigorate the spleen.

Recipe: Jiangu Tang(32) , augmented.

Ingredients: Radix Codonopsis Pilosulae          30 g
Rhizoma Atractylodis Macrocephalae          15 g
Poria          15 g

Semen Coicis 15 g

Radix Morindae Officinalis 15 g

Cortex Cinnamomi 6 g

Fructus Psoraleae 15 g

Semen Dolichoris 30 g

Rhizoma Disoscoreae 12 g

Plumula Nelumbinis 12 g

Radix Platycodi 9 g

Semen Amomi 9 g

Semen Plantaginis 12 g (in a parcel)

Radix Glycyrrhizae 6 g.

The decoction of a dose is 200–300 ml. Take equal portions in the morning and evening, by starting administration on the day when the symptom occurs and by stopping it at the menstrual onset. The same prescription can be used again for the next cycle.

Modification: In case of aversion to cold with cool limbs, add

Ramulus Cinnamomi 9 g.

In case of serious swelling of lower limbs, add

Radix Stephaniae Tetrandrae 15 g

Semen Phaseoli 30 g.

In case of diarrhea right after abdominal pain, accompanied by distention of hydochondria, add

Radix Paeoniae Alba 15 g

Radix Ledebouriellae 9 g.

*Tongxie Yaofang* can be used as an alternative.

Rhizoma Atractylodis Macrocephalae 18 g

Radix Paeoniae Alba 15 g

Pericarpium Citri Reticulatae 12 g

Radix Ledebouriellae     9 g.

In case of protracted diarrhea or diarrhea at dawn, add

Fructus Schisandrae     12 g

Semen Myristicae     15 g.

### 3. Hyperactivity of the liver—*Qi* due to blood deficiency

**Clinical manifestations:**   The case is characterized by dizziness, headache, pantalgia, restlessness and insomnia around or during the period; cycle. a pale tongue with a thin fur; a taut, rapid and thready pulse.

Therapeutic method: Nourish the blood and the liver.

Recipe:*Qi Ju Dihuang Tang*(49), augmented.

Ingredients: Radix Rehmanniae Praeparata     15 g

Fructus Corni     15 g

Rhizoma Disoscoreae     12 g

Rhizoma Alismatis     9 g

Cortex Moutan Radicis     9 g

Poria     12 g

Fructus Lycii     15 g

Flos Chrysanthemi     9 g

Radix Paeoniae Alba     15 g

Os Draconis     30 g

Concha Ostreae     30 g

Concha Haliotidis     15 g

Herba Menthae     6 g.

The decoction of the above drugs is 200—300ml. Take equal portions in the morning and evening, by start administration on the day when the symptom occurs and stopping it at the menstrual onset. The same prescription can be used again for the next cycle.

Modification: In case of a dry throat with a bitter taste, a redden tongue with a yellowish coating, add

    Spica Prunelae        12 g
    Fructus Gardeniae      9 g.

In case of bodily pain and numbness in the menstrual period, add

    Caulis Spatholobi          30 g
    Radix Astragali seu Hedysari      30 g
    Radix Angelicae Sinensis      15 g.

In case of restlessness, palpitation and insomnia, add

    Arillus Longan        12 g
    Radix Polygoni Multiflori      15 g
    Semen Ziziphi Spinosae      30 g.

Proprietary: *Qi Ju Dihuang Wan*. Take one bolus at a time, thrice a day, for dizziness during the menstrual period.

*Jixueteng Qingao Pian*. Take 5pills at a time, thrice a day, for general aching during menstruation.

*Xiao Yao Wan*. Take one parcel at a time, twice a day, for distending pain over the breasts in the premenstrual period.

## 3.5  Menopausal Syndrome

The female climacteric is a transitional period in which the function of the ovary deteriorates gradually to a total loss. The stoppage of menstruation in the climacteric is termed menopause, which generally occurs at the age of 45–55. To some females, around this physiological process of manopause there appear menstrual disorder, vexation, palpitation, insomnia, general dropsy and diarrhea, distress in the loins and knees, and dysphoria with a feverish sensation in palms and soles. These and other symptoms of a person may vary from others in number, diversity and intensity. In TCM, menopausal syndrome is referred to as "various syndromes around the menopausal period". They are considered to be induced by gradual consumption of kidney—*Qi*, emptiness of the *Ren* and *Chong* channels, exhaustion of Tienqui, breakdown of *Yin—Yang* equilibrium in the body and disorders of *Zang—Fu, Qi* and blood. Its treatment is chiefly based on tonifying the kidney, supported by soothing the liver and strengthening the spleen.

## Type and Treatment

### 1. *Yin*—deficiency of the kidney.

**Clinical manifestations:** Dizziness and tinnitus, eye distress and dim eyesight, paroxysmal fever with perspiration on the face and dysphoria with a feverish sensation in palms and soles along with soreness in the loins and knees. The menses are preceded or irregular, copious or scarce, scarlet in color. The urine is small in quantity and deep in color, associated with constipation. The tongue is reddened with little coating. The pulse is rapid and thready.

Therapeutic method: Replenish the kidney, supported by checking the exuberance of *Yang*.

Recipe:*Zhuogui Ying* (106), augmented.

Ingredients: Radix Rehmanniae Praeparata     15 g
            Rhizoma Disoscoreae      15 g
            Fructus Lycii      18 g
            Fructus Corni      12 g
            Poria      12 g

Radix Glycyrrhizae    6 g

Os Draconis    30 g

Concha Ostreae    30 g

Radix Paeoniae Alba    15 g.

Decoct the above drugs in water to get 200—300ml of decoction. Take one half of it in the morning and the other half in the evening.

Modification: In case of profuse and scarlet menstruation, add

Herba Ecliptae    18 g

Fructus Ligustri Lucidi    15 g

Radix Sanguisorbae    30 g.

In case of incessant drippings of blood and purplish dark menses with blood clots, add

Herba Leonuri    30 g

Radix Rubiae    12 g.

In case of a dry mouth with bitter taste, distending and congested eyes, along with headache, exchange Radix Rehmanniae Praeparata for Radix Rehmanniae, and add

Flos Chrysanthemi    9 g

Concha Margaritifera Usta    30 g

Spica Prunellae    12 g.

In case of abrupt, unrestrained sensations, deduct Radix Glycyrrhizae but add

Fructus Tritici Levis    30 g

Radix Glycyrrhizae Praeparata    12 g

Fructus Ziziphi Jujubae    7 dates

Cortex Albiziae    15 g.

In case of paroxysmal fever associated with copious perspiration, add

> Radix Astragali seu Hedysari    30 g
> Fructus Tritici Levis    15 g.

## 2. *Yang*–deficiency of the kidney

**Clinical manifestations:** The patient looks weary and dejected with a gloomy complexion and cool limbs. The case is also characterized by aversion to cold, poor appetite, abdominal distention, general edema, loose stools, nocturia and urinary incontinence. The menses are massive or mixed with metrorrhagia and metrostaxis. The uterine blood is dim in shade. The leukorrhea is clear and dilute. The tongue is, thick and tender with thin, whitish fur and with teeth–prints on its margin. The pulse is deep, feeble and thready.

Therapeutic method: Warm the kidney–*Yang*, with the aid of strengthening the spleen.

Recipe: *Yougui Wan* (96) (see 3.1 Dysfunctional Endometrorrhagia) The decoction of a dose is 200–300ml. Take equal shares in the morning and evening.

Modification: In case of nocturia and urinary incontinence, add

> Fructus Alpiniae Oxyphyllae    30 g
> Os Sepiella seu Sepiae    15 g
> Fructus Rubi    15 g.

In case of a turgid face and swollen limbs, add

> Semen Plantaginis    12 g (in a parcel)
> Rhizoma Alismatis    9 g.

In case of sexual hypoesthesia, add

> Herba Epimedii    30 g
> Rhizoma Curculiginis    15 g.

In case of protracted diarrhea, add

> Rhizoma Zingiberis Praeparata     6 g
> Semen Myristicae     15 g
> Plumula Nelumbinis     12 g
> Halloysitum Rubrum     15 g.

**Proprietary, Simple Recipe and Proved prescription:**

(1)*Geng Nian Kang*. Take 4 pill at a time, twice a day.

(2)*Yi Shen Ning*. Take 2 pills at a time, twice a day.

(3)Fructus Tritici Levis     30 g

> Fructus Ziziphi Jujubae     7 dates
> Radix Glycyrrhizae     12 g.

The decoction of a dose is 200ml. Take equal shares in the morning and evening. It is used for emotional depression or capricious moods.

# 3.6 Other Menstrual Diseases

## 3.6.1 Preceded Menstrual Cycle

If the menstrual period occurs 7 days or even 10 days earlier than the normal date, this syndrome is known as" preceded menstrual cycle" and in most cases it is caused by *Qi*–deficiency and blood–heat. Owing to improper diet, overfatigue or extreme anxiety, the spleen–*Qi* is impaired, leading to the hypofunction of *Qi* of middle–*Jiao* in controlling the blood and protecting the *Chong* and *Ren* channels. The other cause is that the excess of *Yang* in the exterior of the body, the extravangence in eating pungent and stimulating food or the consumption of *Yin*–blood lead to water–deficiency and fire–exuberance, so that pathogenic heat attacks the *Chong* and *Ren* channels and forces the blood to go astray.

## Type and Treatment

### 1. *Qi*–deficiency

**Clinical manifestations:** The menses are preceded, profuse, light in color and low in consistency. The patient looks tired, sleepy and languid, she is characterized also by poor appetite, loose stools and hollow tenesmus of the lower abdomen; a pale tongue; a feeble, thready pulse.

Therapeutic method: Invigorate *Qi* and control the blood; reinforce the *Chong* and *Ren* channels.

Recipe: *Buzhong Yiqi Tang* (7), modified.

Ingredients: Radix Ginseng(to be decocted first)     15 g
Radix Astragali seu Hedysari     30 g
Rhizoma Atractylodis Macrocephalae     15 g
Radix Glycyrrhizae Praeparata     9 g
Os Draconis     30 g
Concha Ostreae     30 g
Crinis Carbonisatus     12 g
Pericarpium Citri Reticulatae     12 g
Radix Bupleuri     6 g
Rhizoma Cimicifugae     6 g.

The decoction of a dose is 200–300ml. Take equal portions in the morning and evening.

Modification: In case of palpitation, insomnia and dreaminess, deduct

                    Radix Bupleuri
                    Rhizoma Cimicifugae

but add

                    Arillus Longan        12 g
                    Semen Ziziphi Spinosae        30 g
                    Radix Polygalae        9 g.

In case of polyuria and loose stools with pain in the loins and coldness in the abdomen, deduct

                    Radix Bupleuri
                    Rhizoma Cimicifugae

but add

                    Fructus Alpiniae Oxyphyllae        15 g
                    Fructus Psoraleae        15 g
                    Rhizoma Zingiberis Praeparata        6 g.

Proprietary: *Renshen Guipi Wan* . Take one bolus at a time, thrice a day.

### 2. Blood—heat

(1) Heat of excess

**Clinical manifestations:** The menses are preceded, copious and viscid, scarlet or purplish red in color. The patient has a flushed face and a dry mouth and likes to have cold drinks. The case is also characterized by vexation, constipation and scanty, dark—colored urines; a reddened tongue with thin, yellowish coating; a rapid, forceful and slippery pulse.

Therapeutic method: Remove pathogenic heat from the blood and regulate the menstrual cycle.

Recipe:*Qing Jing Tang*(51), modified.

Ingredients: Cortex Moutan Radicis        12 g
                    Cortex Lyii Radicis        12 g

Radix Paeoniae Alba        15 g

Radix Rehmanniae           15 g

Herba Artemisiae Chinghao        9 g

Cortex Phellodendri        9 g

Herba Cephalanoploris           15 g

Radix Scutellariae         9 g

Radix Sanguisorbae         30 g.

The decoction of a dose is 200—300 ml. Take one half in the morning and the other half in the evening.

Modification: In case of high fever and thirst with a flushed face, dry stools and deep—colored urines, add

Gypsum Fibrosum        15 g

Radix eu Rhizoma Rhei (to be added

later)     6 g.

(2) Stagnation of the liver—*Qi* and blood—heat

**Clinical manifestations:** The menstruation is preceded, viscid, copious or scarce, purplish red in color, mixed with blood clots. The case is characterized by dysphoria; irritability; distending pain over the breasts and the lower abdomen; an oppressive sensation in the chest; a dry throat with bitter taste in the mouth; a reddened tongue with thin, yellowish fur; a taut, rapid pulse.

Therapeutic method: Clear away pathogenic heat from the liver, relieve the depression of the liver—*Qi* and regulate the menstrual cycle.

Recipe: *Dan Zhi Xiaoyao San*(21), modified.

Ingredients: Cortex Moutan Radicis        12 g

Fructus Gardeniae        9 g

Radix Paeoniae Alba        15 g

Radix Angelicae Sinensis    12 g

Rhizoma Atractylodis Macrocephalae    12 g

Radix Bupleuri    9 g

Poria    12 g

Radix Glycyrrhizae Praeparata    6 g

Herba Menthae    9 g

Radix Rehmanniae    15 g

Fructus Meliae Toosendan    12 g

Rhizoma Cyperi    12 g.

Decoct the above drugs in water to get 200—300ml of decoction. Take one half of it in the morning and the other half in the evening.

Modification: In case of distending pain and hard mass in the breasts, add

Semen Vaccariae    12 g

Fasciculus Vascularia Luffae    9 g

Semen Litchi    12 g

Semen Citri Reticulatae    9 g.

In case of obstruction of the menses due to numerous blood clots, add

Radix Salviae Miltiorrhizae    15 g

Herba Lycopi    18 g

Rhizoma Ligustici Chuanxiong    9 g.

In case of thirst, dizziness and insomnia, add

Flos Chrysanthemi    9 g

Concha Haliotidis    15 g

Concha Ostreae    30 g.

(3) *Yin*—deficiency and blood—heat

**Clinical manifestations:** The menstruation is preceded,

viscid, scanty and red. The case manifests itself by thirst, dysphoria and insomnia, accompanied by a feverish sensation in palms and soles. The patient has a flushed face, a reddened tongne with little or no coating and a rapid, thready pulse.

Therapeutic method: Replenish the vital essence, clear away pathogenic heat and regulate the menstrual cycle.

Recipe: *Liang Di Tang*(37), augmented

Ingredients: Radix Rehmanniae        15 g
　　　　　　Cortex Lycii Radicis        12 g
　　　　　·　Radix Scrophulariae        15 g
　　　　　　Radix Ophiopogonis        12 g
　　　　　　Colla Corii Asini (to be infused) 12 g
　　　　　　Radix Paeoniae Alba        15 g
　　　　　　Radix Adenophorae Strictae        15 g
　　　　　　Cortex Moutae Radicis        9 g
　　　　　　Herba Ecliptae        15 g
　　　　　　Fructus Ligustri Lucidi        15 g
　　　　　　Radix Scutellariae        9 g.

The decoction of the above drugs is 200—300ml. Take equal portions in the morning and evening.

Modification: In case of scanty menstruation, hectic fever and insomnia, add
　　　　　　Radix Salviae Miltiorrhizae        15 g
　　　　　　Herba Artemisiae Chinghao        9 g
　　　　　　Plastrum Testudinis        30g
　　　　　　Semen Biotae        15 g.

## 3.6.2  Delayed Menstrual Cycle

If the menstrual cycle is delayed 7 days or even 40–50 days later than the normal date, this syndrome is known as "delayed menstrual cycle" which should be distinguished between asthenia and sthenia. The former type results from the consumption of Ying-blood or the decline of Yang-Qi, so that the source of blood is not powerful enough to refill the sea of blood regularly. The latter type is caused by stagnation of Qi and blood or by blood stasis due to accumulation of cold, so that the Chong and Ren channels are obstructed and the menses are delayed.

## Type and Treatment

### 1. Blood-cold

**Clinical manifestations:**  The menstruation is delayed, scarce in quantity, dark in color and mixed with blood clots. This type manifests itself by aversion to cold, cold pain in the lower abdomen which can be abated by warmth, cool limbs, a whitish fur and a deep, tense pulse.

Therapeutic method: Warm the channels and expel pathogenic cold;
promote blood circulation and remove blood stagnation.

Recipe: Wenjing Tang(82), augmented.

Ingredients: Radix Ginseng (to be decocted first)      15 g
   Radix Angelicae Sinensis      12 g
   Rhizoma Ligustici Chuanxiong      9 g
   Radix Paeoniae Alba      15 g
   Cortex Cinnamomi      6 g
   Radix Achyranthis Bidentatae      15 g
   Cortex Moutan Radicis      12 g

Rhizoma Zedoariae    12 g

Radix Glycyrrhizae    6 g

Caulis Spatholobi    30 g

Radix Linderae    12 g.

Decoct the above drugs in water to get 200—300ml of decoction. Take one half of it in the morning and the other half in the evening.

Modification: In case of abdominal pain and tenderness with numerous blood clots, add

Pollen Typhae    12 g

Herba Leonuri    30 g

Lignum Sappan    15 g

Rhizoma Cyperi    12 g.

In case of massive menses, deduct

Radix Achyranthis Bidentatae

Rhizoma Zedoariae

but add

Folium Artemisiae Argyi    12 g

Rhizoma Zingiberis    6 g.

Proprietary: *Wuj i Baif eng Wan* . Take one bolus at a time, twice a day

*Nü Jin Dan*. Take one bolus at a time, twice a day.

## 2. Deficiency—cold

**Clinical manifestations:** The menstruation is delayed, scarce, pink—colored and watery without blood clots. The case is marked by soreness and weakness of the loins and by a dull pain in the lower abdomen which can be lessened by strokes and warmth. The patient has a pale tongue with whitish fur and a deep and slow pulse.

Therapeutic method: Strengthen *Yang—Qi* and dispel the cold; nourish the blood and regulate the menstrual cycle.

Recipe: *Ai Fu Nuangong Wan*(1)

Ingredients:Folium Artemisiae Argyi    9 g

              Rhizoma Cyperi    12 g

              Radix Angelicae Sinensis    12 g

              Radix Dipsaci    15 g

              Fructus Euodiae    12 g

              Rhizoma Ligustici Chuanxiong    9 g

              Radix Paeoniae Alba    15 g

              Radix Astragali seu Hedysari    15 g

              Radix Rehmanniae Praeparata    12 g

              Cortex Cinnamomi    6 g.

The decoction of a dose is 200—300ml. Take one half in the morning and the other half in the evening.

Modification: In case of copious, clear urines and loose stools, add

              Fructus Psoraleae    15 g

              Rhizoma Atractylodis Macrocephalae    15 g.

In case of long—standing sterility caused by the cold of the uterus, add

              Fluoritum    30 g.

### 3. Blood—deficiency

**Clinical manifestations:** The menstruation is delayed, scarce, light in color and carries no clots. The case is marked by dull pain and hollow tenesmus of the lower abdomen, dizziness, palpitation and insomnia. The patient has a dim complexion, a pale tongue with thin, whitish coating and a small, feeble pulse.

Therapeutic method: Invigorate *Qi* and nourish the blood

Recipe: *Zi Xue Tang*(110), augmented.

Ingredients:Radix Ginseng (to be decocted first)　15 g

Rhizoma Disoscoreae　12 g

Radix Astragali seu Hedysari　30 g

Poria　12 g

Rhizoma Ligustici Chuanxiong　9 g

Radix Angelicae Sinensis　15 g

Radix Paeoniae Alba　18 g

Radix Rehmanniae Praeparata　30 g

Radix Polygoni Multiflori　30 g

Caulis Spatholobi　30 g

Semen Ziziphi Spinosae　15 g

Colla Corii Asini (to be infused in hot
decoction)　12 g.

Decoct the drugs to get 200—300ml of decoction. Take one half of it in the morning and the other half in the evening.

Modification: In case of thirst, dysphoria and a feverish sensation in the palms and soles, deduct

Radix Rehmanniae Praeparata

Radix Ginseng

but add

Radix Rehmanniae　15 g

Radix Pseudostellariae　15 g

Herba Ecliptae　15 g

Fructus Ligustri Lucidi　12 g.

In case of palpitation and insomnia, add

Semen Biotae　15 g

Fructus Schisandrae　12g.

In case of poor appetite and loose stools, deduct

Radix Rehmanniae Praeparata

but add

Rhizoma Atractyladis Macrocephalae      15 g

Semen Dolichoris    30 g

Plumula Nelumbinis      12 g.

Proprietary: *Shouwu Pian*. Take 5 pills at a time, thrice a day.

*Bazhen Yimu Wan.* Take one bolus at a time, thrice a day.

**4. Stagnation of *Qi***

**Clinical manifestations:** The menstruation is delayed, sparse, dark red with blood clots. The patient is characterized by mental depression and distending pain in the lower abdomen as well as in the breasts and chest. The tongue is in normal condition. The pulse is taut or uneven.

Therapeutic method: Improve the flow of *Qi* and readjust the menstrual cycle.

Recipe: *Jiawei Wuyao Tang*(87), modified.

Ingredients:  Radix Linderae      12 g

Semen Amomi      9 g

Rhizoma Corydalis      12 g

Rhizoma Cyperi      12 g

Radix Glycyrrhizae      6 g

Semen Arecae      9 g

Radix Aucklandiae      9 g

Radix Achyranthis Bidentatae      15 g

Cortex Cinnamomi      6g.

The decoction of a dose is 200–300 ml. Take equal shares in the morning and evening.

Modification: In case of severe abdominal pain and copious blood clots, add

Radix Angelicae Sinensis     15 g

Rhizoma Ligustici Chuanxiong     9 g

Caulis Spatholobi     15 g.

In case of oppressive detention in the chest and mental depression, add

Radix Bupleuri     9 g

Radix Curcumae     9g.

Proprietary: *Qizhi Xiangf u Wan*. Take one bolus at a time, thrice a day.

*Yuanhu Zhitong Pian*. Take 5 pills at a time, thrice a day.

### 3.6.3 Irregular Menstrual Cycle

If the menstrual cycle is over 7 days earlier or later than the scheduled date, this syndrome is known as "irregular menstrual cycle"or "menstrual disorder". This illness is closely related to the liver and kidney. The function of the liver is to govern the normal flow of $Qi$ and to control the blood sea. The kidney stores reproductive essence and food essence and acts as the source of menstruation. The dysfunction of the liver due to the stagnation of $Qi$ and the hypofunction of the kidney in storing essence will lead to derangement of $Qi$ and blood and to the irregularity of the blood sea in storing blood, thus resulting in menstrual disorders.

### Type and Treatment

**1. Stagnation of the liver–$Qi$**

**Clinical manifestations:** The menstrual cycle is preceded or delayed, profuse or scanty in quantity, purplish red in color and mixed with blood clots. The patient often gives out deep sighs or eructations, and complains of anorexia, oppressive sensation in the chest and distending pain in the breasts and the lower abdomen. The tongue has a thin, whitish or yellowish fur. and the pulse is taut.

Therapeutic method: Relieve the depression of the liver, promote the flow of *Qi* and readjust the menstrual cycle.

Recipe:*Xiaoyao San* (94), modified.

Ingredients:Radix Bupleuri          9 g

      Rhizoma Atractylodis Macrocephalae          15 g

      Poria          12 g

      Radix Angelicae Sinensis          12 g

      Radix Paeoniae Alba          15 g

      Herba Menthae          9 g

      Radix Achyranthis Bidentatae          15 g

      Lignum Sappan          15 g

      Rhizoma Cyperi          12 g

      Radix Curcumae          9 g.

Decoct the above drugs in water to get 200—300ml of decoction. Take one half of it in the morning and the other half in the evening.

Modification: In case of an oppressed chest and anorexia, add to the recipe

      Cortex Magnoliae Officinalis          9 g

      Semen Amomi          6 g

      Pericarpium Citri Reticulatae          12 g.

In case of massive menses, deduct

      Radix Achyranthis Bidentatae

      Lignum Sappan.

Proprietary: *Bao Kun Wan*. Take 30 pills once a day.

## 2. Deficiency of the kidney

**Clinical manifestations:** The menstruation is irregular, scarce, dilute and dark—colored. The patient is characterized by dizziness, tinnitus and distress in the loins. The tongue looks pale with little coating. The pulse is deep and thready.

Therapeutic method: Tonify the kidney and regulate the menstruation.

Recipe: *Gu Yin Jian*(27), augmented.

Ingredients: Radix Ginseng (to be decocted first)     15 g

Radix Rehmanniae Praeparata     15 g

Rhizoma Dioscoreae     12 g

Fructus Corni     15 g

Semen Cuscutae     24 g

Radix Polygalae     9 g

Fructus Schisandrae     12 g

Radix Glycyrrhizae Praeparata     6 g

Herba Cistanchis     15 g

Radix Dipsaci     30 g

Herba Epimedii     15 g.

The decoction of the drugs is 200—300ml. Take equal portions in the morning and evening.

Modification: In case of scanty, scarlet menses, a deep, rapid and thready pulse, a reddened tongue with little fur, add

Cortex Moutan Radicis     15 g

Herba Ecliptae     15 g

and substitute Radix Rehmanniae Praeparata by

Radix Rehmanniae     15 g.

In case of clear, copious urines and loose stools with cold—pain in the loins and knees, deduct

Herba Cistanchis

Radix Rehmanniae Praeparata

but add

Cortex Cinnamomi       6 g

Radix Morindae Officinalis       12 g

Fructus Psoraleae       15 g.

Proprietary: *Gui Fu Dihuang Wan.* Take one bolus at a time with dilute saline water, twice a day.

## 3.6.4 Menorrhagia

If the menstrual cycle is essentially regular but the discharge is noticeably increased in quantity, this syndrome is termed "menorrhagia".In most cases, it is caused by the deficiency of *Qi* in governing the blood flow or by the harassment of blood—sea by blood—heat, thus leading to the debility of the *Chong* and *Ren* channels and to the escape of the blood from the channels with the menses. The illness may also be caused by the obstruction of blood stasis in the interior.

### Type and Treatment

#### 1. *Qi*—deficiency

**Clinical manifestations:** Hypermenorrhea with thin, pale red discharges. The patient is characterized by a pale complexion, short breaths, feeble limbs, reserved moods, palpitation and restlessness, and hollow tenesmus in the lower abdomen. She has a pale tongue and a feeble, thready pulse.

Therapeutic method: Invigorate *Qi*,reinforce the *Chong* and *Ren* channels and regulate the menstruation.

Recipe: *Ju Yuan Jian*(35), augmented.

Ingredients: Radix Ginseng (to be decocted first)      15 g

Radix Astragali seu Hedysari      30 g

Rhizoma Atractylodis Macrocephalae      18 g

Rhizoma Cimicifugae      6 g

Radix Glycyrrhizae Praeparata      9 g

Os Draconis      30 g

Concha Ostreae      30 g

Fructus Schisandrae      15 g

Radix Paeoniae Alba      15 g.

Decoct the above drugs in water to get 200–300ml of decoction. Divide them into two equal portions. Take one in the morning and the other in the evening.

Modification: In case of massive discharge, add

Os Sepiela seu Sepiae      30 g

Folium Artemisiae Argyi      9 g

Rhizoma Zingiberis Praeparata      6 g.

In case of palpitation and insomnia, add

Semen Biotae      15 g

Semen Ziziphi Spinosae      30g.

Proprietary: *Buzhong Yiqi Wan*. Take one bolus at a time, thrice a day.

## 2. Blood—heat

**Clinical manifestations:** The menstruation is copious, viscid, crimson or scarlet, and frequently carries blood clots. The case manifests itself by thirst, dysphoria, dark—colored urine and constipation; a reddened tongue with yellowish coating; a rapid, slippery pulse.

Therapeutic method: Remove heat—evil from the blood and

subdue uterine bleeding.

Recipe: *Bao Yin Jian*(5), modified.

Ingredients: 
Radix Rehmanniae     18 g
Radix Scutellariae     12 g
Cortex Phellodendri     9 g
Radix Paeoniae Alba     15 g
Rhizoma Disoscoreae     12 g
Radix Dipsaci     15 g
Radix Sanguisorbae     30 g
Concha Ostreae     30 g
Rhizoma Imperatae     30 g
Herba Cephalanoploris     30 g.

Decoct the above drugs in water to get 200—300ml of decoction. Take one half of it in the morning and the other half in the evening.

Modification: In case of dysphoria, constipation and dark—colored urine, add

Herba Lephatheri     12 g
Fructus Gardeniae     9 g
Radixet Rhizoma Rhei (to be added later)     6 g.

In case of dry throat and hectic fever with perspiration in the afternoon and evening, add

Radix Adenophorae     15 g
Cortex Lyii Radicis     9 g
Radix Ophiopogonis     12 g.

In case of debility and lassitude with short breaths and reserved moods, add

Radix Astragali seu Hedysari     30 g
Rhizoma Atractylodis Macrocephalae     15g.

### 3. Blood stasis

**Clinical manifestations:** The menses are copious, purplish dark in color, mixed with blood clots and accompanied by abdominal pain and tenderness compression.The tongue looks purplish, specked with ecchymoses. The pulse is thready and uneven.

Therapeutic method: Activate the blood flow, remove blood stasis and subdue uterine bleeding.

Recipe: *Shixiao San*(70), augmented.

Ingredients:Faeces Trogopterorum    12 g
                Pollen Typhae    12 g
                Herba Leonuri    30 g
                Radix Rubiae    12 g
                Radix Salviae Miltiorrhizae    15 g
                Cortex Moutan Radicis    9 g
                Semen Persicae    12 g
                Radix Astragali seu Hedysari    15 g.

The decoction of a dose is 200–300ml. Take equal portions in the morning and evening.

Modification: In case of cold–pain in the lower abdomen, deduct

                Radix Salviae Miltiorrhizae

but add

                Folium Artemisiae Argyi    9 g
                Radix Linderae    12 g.

In case of distending pain in the chest and lower abdomen, add

                Pericarpium Citri Reticulatae Viride    12 g
                Fructus Maliae Toosendan    12 g.

Proprietary: *Sanqi Pian*.Take 5—10 pills at a time daily. The dosage should not exceed 30 pills. If the bleeding is profuse, another dose can be taken with an interval of six hours.

## 3.6.5  Hypomenorrhea

If the menstrual cycle is essentially normal but the discharge is noticeably reduced even to few drops or the cycle lasts less than 2 days and the discharge is scanty, this syndrome is termed " hypomenorrhea" , which should be distinguished between asthenia and sthenia. The former type is caused by the meagre supply of essence and blood which results in the vacancy of the blood—sea. The latter type is in most cases caused by the retention of blood stasis in the interior or the stagnation of phlegm—dampness, resulting in the blockage of blood in the channels.

### Type and Treatment

#### 1. Blood—deficiency

**Clinical manifestations:** The menstruation is greatly reduced in quantity, even to few drops. It is light—colored with no clots. The patient has a sallow complexion with pallid lips and a colorless tongue, lustreless nails and haggard skin, accompanied by dizziness, palpitation and hollow tenesmus of the lower abdomen. The tongue is pink with a thin, whitish fur and the pulse is thready.

**Therapeutic method:** Nourish the blood and regulate the menstruation.

**Recipe:** *Renshen Yangrong Tang*(58), augmented.

Ingredients: Radix Paeoniae Alba        18 g

　　　　　　Radix Angelicae Sinensis        15 g

　　　　　　Pericarpium Citri Reticulatae        12 g

　　　　　　Radix Astragali seu Hedysari        30 g

　　　　　　Cortex Cinnamomi        6 g

　　　　　　Radix Ginseng (to be decocted first)        15 g

　　　　　　Rhizoma Atractylodis Macrocephalae        15 g

　　　　　　Radix Glycyrrhizae Praeparata        9 g

　　　　　　Radix Rehmanniae Praeparata        15 g

　　　　　　Fructus Schisandrae        12 g

　　　　　　Poria        15 g

　　　　　　Radix Polygalae        9 g

　　　　　　Radix Polygoni Multiflori        30 g

　　　　　　Radix Salviae Miltiorrhizae        30 g

　　　　　　Caulis Spatholobi        30 g

　　　　　　Rhizoma Zingiberis Recens        6 g

　　　　　　Fructus Ziziphi Jujubae        7 dates.

Decoct the above drugs in water to get 200—300ml of decoction. Take one half of it in the morning and the other half in the evening.

　　　　　Modification: In case of palpitation and insomnia, add

　　　　　　Semen Biotae        15 g

　　　　　　Radix Ophiopogonis        12 g.

　　　　　Proprietary: *Renshen Jianpi Wan*. Take one bolus at a time, thrice a day.

### 2. Deficiency of the kidney

**Clinical manifestations:** The menophania is retarded. Afterwards, the menses are often delayed, scanty, dilute and light—colored. The patient has sore loins, weak knees and painful heels, accompanied by dizziness and tinnitus or by nocturia and a cold sensation in the lower abdomen. The tongue is pale. The pulse is deep, either slow or feeble.

Therapeutic method: Tonify the kidney, nourish the blood and enrich the menstruation.

Recipe: *Gui Shen Wan* (26), augmented.

Ingredients:  Radix Rehmanniae Praeparata       15 g

Rhizoma Disoscoreae       15 g

Cornus Officinalis       12 g

Poria       15 g

Radix Angelicae Sinensis       15 g

Semen Cuscutae       24 g

Cortex Eucommiae       30 g

Fructus Lycii       30 g

Herba Epimedii       30 g

Cortex Cinnamomi       9 g.

The decoction of the above drugs 200—300ml. Take equal shares in the morning and evening.

Modification: In case of reddened menses, a dry throat, a reddened longue with little fur and a hot sensation in palms and soles, deduct

Radix Rehmanniae Praeparata

Cortex Eucommiae

Cortex Cinnamomi

Herba Epimedii

but add

Radix Rehmanniae       15 g

Radix Scrophulariae       15 g

Fructus Ligustri Lucidi       12 g

Herba Ecliptae    15 g.

In case of profuse urine and cold abdomen, add

Radix Morindae Officinalis    15 g

Fructus Alpiniae Oxyphyllae    30 g.

Proprietary: *Liuwei Dihuang Wan*. Take one bolus at a time, twice a day. It is suitable for the deficiency of kidney—*Yin*.

*Gui Fu Dihuang Wan*. Take one bolus at a time, twice a day. It is fit for the deficiency of kidney—*Yang*.

### 3. Blood stasis

**Clinical manifestations:** The menses are sparse, purplish dark in color and mixed with blood clots. The distending pain in the lower abdomen refuses to be pressed but it can be abated by the removal of clots. The tongue is purplish dark and spotted with acchymoses. The pulse is uneven.

Therapeutic method: Activate the blood flow, remove blood stasis and regulate the menstruation.

Recipe:*Tao Hong Siwu Tang*(75), modified.

Ingredients:Semen Persicae    12 g

Flos Carthami    12 g

Radix Angelicae Sinensis    15 g

Rhizoma Ligustici Chuanxiong    9 g

Radix Paeoniae Alba    15 g

Herba Bycopi    15 g

Herba Leonuri    30 g

Radix Achyranthis Bidentatae    15 g

Rhizoma Sparganii    12 g.

The decoction of a dose is 200—300 ml. Take one half in the morning and the other half in the evening.

Modification: In case of oppressed chest and distending abdomen, add

> Rhizoma Cypori    12 g
> Radix Linderae    12 g
> Fructus Aurantii    9g.

In case of cold—pain in the abdomen, add

> Ramulus Cinnamomi    9 g
> Folium Artemisiae Argyi    12 g
> Fructus Euodiae    12 g.

## 4. Phlegm—dampness

**Clinical manifestations:** The menses are pink, viscid and scanty. The patient looks heavy and corpulent and is also characterized by an depressed sensation in the chest; nausea; vomiting; copious leukorrhea; a pale tongue with whitish, greasy fur; a slippery pulse.

Therapeutic method: Remove the phlegm, excrete dampness and promote blood circulation in the channels.

Recipe: *Cang Fu Daotan Wan*(10), augmented.

Ingredients: Poria    18 g

> Rhizoma Pinelliae    12 g
> Pericarpium Citri Reticulatae    12 g
> Rhizoma Atractylodis    12 g
> Rhizoma Cyperi    12 g
> Arisaema cum Bile    12 g
> Fructus Aurantii    12 g
> Massa Fermentata Medicinalis    12 g
> Radix Glycyrrhizae    6 g
> Rhizoma Zingiberis Recens    6 g
> Caulis Spatholobi    15 g
> Radix Achyranthis Bidentatae    12 g

> Rhizoma Ligustici Chuanxiong    9 g
>
> Semen Plantaginis (to be parcelled in
>
>    gauze)    12 g
>
> Cortex Cinnamomi    6 g.

The decoction of a dose is 200—300ml. Take equal shares in the morning and evening.

> Modification: In case of lumbago, add
>
>    Radix Dipsaci    30 g
>
>    Semen Cuscutae    24 g.
>
> In case of a turgid face and swollen limbs, add
>
>    Rhizoma Atractylodis Macrocephalae    15g
>
>    Radix Stephaniae Tetrandrae    12 g
>
>    Semen Phaseoli    30 g.

### 3.6.6   Stomatomenia

If hematemesis or epistaxis occurs regularly 2 or 3 days before the menstrual onset or during the menstrual period and it disappears by itself a few days after the menses, this syndrome is known as "stomatomenia" or "hematemesis or epistaxis during menstruation. " In most cases, it is caused by the adversely moving $Qi$ in the $Chong$ channel due to blood heat. In the premenstrual or menstrual stage, $Qi$ and blood are abundant in the $Chong$ channel which is subordinate to the $Yangming$ channel and whose large collaterals end in the nasopharnx, namely posterior naris. The nose is the orifice of the lungs. If pathogenic fire is generated from the stagnation of the liver—$Qi$ when one is depressed in feeling, if asthenic fire flames up due to consistent deficiency of $Yin$ , the heat and liver—$Qi$ carried by the $Chong$—$Qi$ will travel upward and scorch the collaterals and impair the blood, resulting in hematemesis or epistaxis.

## Type and Treatment

### 1. Fire generated from stagnation of the liver—$Qi$

Clinical manifestations: The case manifests itself by bleeding from the mouth and the nose in the premenstrual or menstrual period. The blood is profuse and scarlet with blood clots. The patient has a dry throat with a bitter taste in the mouth, distention of the breasts, hypochondriac pain, and scanty, preceded menses, accompanied by dizziness, dysphoria and irritability. The tongue is reddened with yellowish coating. The pulse is taut and rapid.

Therapeutic method: Soothe the depressed liver $-Qi$ clear away the heat and make the blood descend properly.

Recipe:*Qinggan Yinj ing Tang*(48), modified.

Ingredients:Radix Paeoniae Alba          15 g

Radix Rehmanniae          15 g

Cortex Moutan Radicis          12 g

Fructus Gardeniae          12 g

Radix Scutellariae          9 g

Fructus Meliae Toosendan          9 g

Radix Rubiae          12 g

Radix Achyranthis Bidentatae          15 g

Rhizoma Imperatae          30 g

Radix Glycyrrhizae          6 g

Herba Cephalanoploris          30 g

Nodus Nelumbinis Rhizomatis          12 g

Herba Agrimoniae        15 g.

Decoct the above drugs in water to get 200—300ml of decoction. Divide it into two equal portions. Take one in the morning and the other in the evening. When the patient is in normal conditions, take one dose every other day.

Modification: In case of sparse menses with abdominal pain,add

> Herba Leonuri        30 g
> Flos Carthami        12 g
> Radix Salviae Miltiorrhizae 15g.

### 2. *Yin*-deficiency of the lung and kidney

**Clinical manifestations:** Hematemesis and epistaxis in the premenstrual or menstrual period with scanty, dark red discharges; dizziness, tinnitus, thirst and hectic fever, emaciation and scanty, preceded menses. The patient has flushed cheeks, a feverish sensation in the palms and soles, and little or no sputa in coughing. The tongue is reddened or crimson without fur. The pulse is rapid and thready.

Therapeutic method: Nourish the kidney and moisten the lung; clear away the heat, subdue the adverse *Qi* and arrest the bleeding.

Recipe:*Shunj ing Tang* (62), augmented.

Ingredients:Radix Angelicae Sinensis      12 g
> Radix Rehmanniae      15 g
> Radix Adenophorae Strictae      18 g
> Radix Paeoniae Alba      15 g
> Poria      12 g
> Herba Schizonepetae      9 g
> Cortex Moutan Radicis      12 g

> Radix Achyranthis Bidentatae    15 g
> Radix Arnebiae seu Lithospermi    15 g
> Radix Cymanchi Atrati    12 g
> Herba Ecliptae    30 g
> Cortex Lycii Radicis    12 g
> Radix Scutellariae    9 g.

The decoction of a dose is 200—300ml. Take equal portions in the morning and evening for 7 days prior to the menstrual period. When the patient is in normal conditions, take one dose every other day.

Modification: In case of hectic fever and dry cough without sputa, add

> Radix Ophiopogonis    12 g
> Folium Mori    12 g
> Bulbus Lilii    15g.

In case of thirst and profuse bleeding, add

> Rhizoma Imperatae    30 g
> Cacumen Biotae    12 g.

### 3.6.7   Stomatoglossitis

If ulceration of the mouth and tongue occurs regularly and repeatedly each month as menstruation is approaching or is going on, this syndrome is termed "stomatoglossitis". The mouth is the threshold of the stomach; the tongue is the sprout or extension of the heart. In most cases, this illness is caused by the steaming of stomach—heat and by the flaring—up of heart—fire.

**Type and Treatment**

## 1. Hyperactivity of fire due to *Yin*-deficiency

**Clinical manifestations:** The case is marked by pain with aphthous stomatitis, thirst, dysphoria and sleeplessness, a feverish sensation in the chest, palms and soles, scanty and yellowish urine; a reddened tongue with little fur; a rapid, thready pulse.

Therapeutic method: Nourish *Yin* and subdue pathogenic fire.

Recipe:*Zhi Bai Dihuang Tang*(103), augmented.

| | |
|---|---|
| Radix Rehmanniae | 15 g |
| Cortex Moutan Radicis | 12 g |
| Poria | 12 g |
| Rhizoma Alismatis | 9 g |
| Fructus Corni | 12 g |
| Rhizoma Dioscoreae | 12 g |
| Rhizoma Anemarrhenae | 6 g |
| Cortex Phellodendri | 9 g |
| Radix Trichosanthis | 12 g |
| Radix Ophiopogonis | 12 g |
| Herba Lophatheri | 9 g |
| Radix Glycyrrhizae | 6 g. |

Decoct the above drugs in water to get 200—300ml of decoction. Take one half of it in the morning and the other half in the evening.

## 2. Steaming of Stomach-heat

**Clinical manifestations:** Erosion in the mouth and tongue during the menstrual cycle, halitosis, thirst, dark-colored urine and constipation. A thick, yellowish fur. A rapid and slippery pulse.

Therapeutic method: Clear away the heat from the stomach

and purge the pathogenic fire.

Recipe: *Liangge San*(39)

Ingredients:Radix et Rhizoma Rhei(to be added later)    6 g

Natrii Sulfas    6 g

Radix Glycyrrhizae    9 g

Fructus Gardeniae    12 g

Herba Menthae    9 g

Radix Scutellariae    12 g

Fructus Forsythiae    15 g

Herba Lophatheri    12 g.

The decoction of a dose is 200−300 ml. Take one half in the morning and the other half in the evening.

Proprietary: *Bing Peng San*. Apply a modicum of the medicine to the ulcerated parts of the buccal cavity by giving a puff, twice or thrice a day.

# 4. Pathologic Pregnancy

## 4.1 Abortion

If pregnancy terminates within 28 weeks and the weight of the fetus is less than 1000g, itis known as abortion. If the case happens within the first 12 weeks, it istermed early abortion; if it happens in the rest of the time, it is termedlate abortion. Artificial abortion refers to the termination of pregnancy by means of drugs, mechanical intervention or other artificial ways. Spontaneous abortion refers to the automatic isolation of the fetus or embryo from the maternal body by some cause. According to the different conditions of spontaneous abortion, it can be classified clinically into threatened abortion, inevitable abortion, incomplete abortion, complete abortion, missed abortion, septic abortion and habitual abortion. In TCM, threatened abortion belongs to the categories of "vaginal bleeding during menstruation "and "restless disturbance of the fetus". Early or late abortion and premature labour are discussed under the topics of "fallen fetus" and "premature birth". Habitual abortion is dealt with as "loose fetus".

### 4.1.1 Threatened Abortion

Threatened abortion occurs frequently in the first trimester of pregnancy, characterized by scarce vaginal bleeding and at times by slight lumbago and a pain in the lower abdomen bearing-down sensation. Morning sickness is apparent and gynecological examination finds that the cervical orifice is not open and the size of the uterus is much the same as that of the intermenstrual period. The result of pregnancy test is positive. In TCM, this illness falls into the categories of "vaginal bleeding during menstruation" and "restless disturbance of the fetus". The former refers to the scanty and intermittent vaginal bleeding without lumbago and abdominal pain; the latter refers to the distress of lumbago and abdominal pain which may be accompanied by the bearing-down sensation and distending pain in the lower abdomen or by scanty bleeding from the vagina. The illness may result from one of the following factors: destitution of the kidney-*Qi* in the maternal body, intemperance of sexual activity, the scarcity of *Qi* and blood, the attack of the fetus by heat-evil, leading to the derangement of *Qi* and blood in the *Chong* and *Ren* channels. Besides, it may be caused by the defect in the growth of the embryo due to the shortage of essence and *Qi* of the parents, leading to the insecure attachment of the embryo.

## Type and Treatment

### 1. Deficiency of the kidney

**Clinical manifestations:** Lumbago in the gestational period, bearing-down sensation in the lower abdomen, scanty vaginal bleeding which is dim in shade. In some cases it is accompanied by dizziness and tinnitus nocturia, frequent urination and even enuresis. The tongue is reddish pale with thin, whitish fur. The pulse is deep, slippery, weak ened, slow.

Therapeutic method: Reinforce the kidney and prevent miscarriage, supported by invigorating *Qi* .

Recipe: *Shou Tai Wan* (67), augmented.

Ingredients:Semen Cuscutae      18 g

Ramulus Taxilli      15 g

Radix Dipsaci      15 g

Colla Corii Asini (to be infused in hot deco

ction)      12 g

Cortex Eucommiae      12 g

Radix Codonopsis Pilosulae      15 g

Rhizoma Atractylodis Macrocephalae      9 g.

Decoct the above drugs in water to get 200—300ml of decoction. Take equal portions in the morning and evening.

Modification: In case of massive bleeding, add

Flium Artemisiae Argyi Carbonisatiote      9 g.

In case of frequent urination or urinary incontinence, add

Fructus Alpiniae Oxyphyllae      9 g.

In case of lumbago and abdominal pain with a bear –ing–down sensation,add

Rhizoma Cimicifugae Praeparata      6 g

Radix Astragali seu Hedysari      15 g.

**2. Scarcity of *Qi* and blood**

**Clinical manifestations:** Restless movement of the fetus in the gestational period, bearing—down sensation in the lower abdomen, scanty vaginal bleeding which is light in color. The patient has a pale complexion, weary limbs, and short breaths, accompanied by palpitation, lumbago and abdominalgia. The tongue is pale with thin, whitish coating. The pulse is either thready and slippery or deep and weak.

Therapeutic method: Invigorate *Qi* and enrich the blood; reinforce the kidney and prevent miscarriage.

Recipe: *Tai Yuan Yin* (80), modified.

Ingredients: Radix Codonopsis Pilosulae       15 g

Cortex Eucommiae       12 g

Rhizoma Atractylodis Macrocephalae       9 g

Radix Paeoniae Alba       9 g

Radix Rehmanniae Praeparata       12 g

Pericarpium Citri Reticulatae       9 g

Radix Astragali seu Hedysari Praeparata
15 g

Colla Corii Asini (to be infused in hot decoc
tion)       12 g

Radix Glycyrrhizae Praeparata       6 g.

The decoction of dose is 200—300ml. Take equal shares in the
morning and evening.

Modification: In case of severe abdominal pain, exchange 9g
of Radix Paeoniae Alba for 15 g.

In case of massive vaginal bleeding, add

Folium Artemisiae Argyi Carbonisatiote       9 g

Herba Agrimoniae       15 g

In case of whitish greasy fur, poor appetite and loose stools,
add

Fructus Amomi       6 g

Rhizoma Dioscoreae       12 g.

Proprietary: *Bao Tai Wan*. Take one bolus at a time, thrice a
day.

*Bazhen Yimu Wan*. Take one bolus at a time,
thrice a day.

### 3. Blood—heat

**Clinical manifestations:** Vaginal bleeding in the gestational period which is scarlet in color, or lumbago with a bearing—down sensation, accompanied by thirst, dysphoria and discomfort. The patient prefers cold drinks and has deep—colored urines and dry stools. The tongue is reddened with dry, yellowish coating. The pulse is rapid and slippery.

Therapeutic method: Nourish *Yin* and clear away the heat; replenish the blood and prevent miscarriage.

Recipe: *Bao Yin Jian* (5), augmented.

Ingredients: Radix Rehmanniae              12 g

                Radix Rehmanniae Praeparata         12 g

                Radix Paeoniae Alba        9 g

                Radix Dipsaci        15 g

                Rhizoma Dioscoreae praeparata        12 g

                Radix Scutellariae        9 g

                Cortex Phellodendri        6 g

                Radix Boehmeriae niveae        12 g

                Radix Glycyrrhizae        6 g.

The decoction of the above drugs is 200—300 ml. Take one half in the morning and the other half in the evening.

Modification: In case of copious bleeding, add

                Herba Ecliptae        15 g

                Receptaculum Nenumbinis Carbonisatiote

12g.

In case of severe *Yin* —deficiency, add

                Radix Ophiopogonis        9 g

                Herba Dendrobii        9 g.

In case of lumbago, add

                Semen Cuscutae        15 g

Cortex Eucommiae          12 g.

## 4. Traumatic injury

**Clinical manifestations:** After traumatic injury, sprain or contusion in the gestational period, the patient suffers from lumbago and abdominalgia with a bearing—down sensation, scarlet and sparse vaginal bleeding and a weak, slippery pulse.

Therapeutic method: Invigorate *Qi* and nourish the blood; reinforce the kidney and ensure gestation.

Recipe: *Sheng Yu Tang* (72) plus *Shou Tai Wan* (67).

Ingredient: Radix Angelicae Sinensis praeparata          9 g

Rhizoma Ligustici Chuanxiong          3 g

Radix Rehmanniae Praeparata          12 g

Radix Rehmanniae          12 g

Radix Codonopsis Pilosulae          18 g

Radix Astragali seu Hedysari          18 g

Semen Cuscutae          15 g

Radix Dipsaci          15 g

Ramulus Loranthi          15 g

Colla Corii Asini (to be infused in hot decoction)          12 g.

The decoction of a dose is 200—300 ml. Take equal shares in the morning and evening.

Modification: In case of copious bleeding, deduct

Radix Angelicae Sinensis praeparata

Rhizoma Ligustici Chuanxiong

but add

Folium  Artemisiae  Argyi  Carbonisatiote          9 g

Radix Boehmeriae niveae          12 g.

In case of dark red tongue and stabbing pain in the lower abdomen, add

> Pollen Typhae Praeparata       9 g
> Faeces Trogopterorum       9 g
> Powder of Radix Notoginseng       3 g (to infuse half of it each time).

The drugs should not be taken any longer as the symptoms of the disease have disappeared.

**Caution:**

The pregnant woman should have proper diet, work and rest, and keep fit and pleasant. She must be in bed when a successful gestation is to be ensured. Sexual activity is forbidden in the first trimester of pregnancy.

### 4.1.2    Inevitable Abortion

Inevitable abortion is derived from threatened abortion. It manifests itself by profuse bleeding, abdominalgia and wide—opening of the cervical orifice but the embryonic tissues are still kept in the uterus. It results from one of the following factors: shortage of nutrients due to the paucity of $Qi$ and blood, the loss of power to supply the embryo due to deficiency of the kidney, the impairment of the fetus by blood—heat or by traumatic injury, sprain and contusion. Since pregnancy cannot go on any longer, the best therapy is to protect the maternal body by removing the embryo.

**Clinical manifestations:** Copious vaginal bleeding in the gestational period which exceeds normal menses in volume and is mixed with blood clots or accompanied by liquid discharge and abdominal tenderness. Gynecological examination finds that the cervical orifice is wide open. The pulse is rapid and thready, or slippery, or uneven. The tongue is dim in shade or specked with ecchymoses.

Therapeutic method: Remove blood stasis and expel the dead fetus.

Recipe: *Tuo Hua Jian*(74), augmented.

Ingredients: Radix Angelicae Sinensis      15 g
                 Radix Cyathulae      15 g
                 Rhizoma Ligustici Chuanxiong      9 g
                 Flos Carthami      12 g
                 Semen Plantaginis(to be parcelled in gauze)
                 9 g
                 Ramulus Cinnamomi      6 g
                 Herba Leonuri      30 g.

Decoct the above drugs in water to get 200—300ml of decoction. Take one half of it in the morning and the other half in the evening.

Modification: In case of listlessness and lassitude with a pale complexion, add
                 Radix Codonopsis Pilosulae      30 g
                 Radix Astragali seu Hedysari Praeparata
                 30 g.

In case of abdominal cold—pain with a pale complexion and aversion to cold with cool limbs, add
                 Rhizoma Zingiberis      6 g
                 Fructus Foenicuii      9 g.

In case of severe distention of the chest and lower abdomen, add
                 Rhizoma Cyperi      12 g

Fructus Aurantii    9 g.

## 4.1.3    Incomplete Abortion

Incomplete abortion is a further development of inevitable abortion, It is characterized by continuous vaginal bleeding, abdominal pain, the wide opening of the cervical orifice and blockage of embryonic tissues at the threshold. In TCM, this case belongs to the category of "fallen fetus"    or "premature birth". Generally speaking, *Duo Tải*(fallen fetus) is defined as the abortion which occurs within 3 months of pregnancy when the fetus does not take shape; *Xiao Chan* (premature birth) refers to the abortion which occurs beyond 3 months of pregnancy during which the fetus has taken shape. The syndrome may result from one of the following factors: deficiency of the kidney— *Qi* , consumption of vital *Qi* due to repeated labours exposure to the cold or wind in abortion, disorder of *Qi* due to emotional depression, leading to the accumulation of blood stasis in the uterus.

### Type and Treatment

**1. Deficiency of *Qi* and blood stasis**

**Clinical manifestations:** Part of the fetus and placenta having been removed, there appears continuous vaginal bleeding which is mingled with blood clots and copious liquid discharge. The patient looks pale and weary and languid, accompanied by dizziness, palpitation and bearing—down abdominalgia. The tongue is pale and dull in color with teeth prints at its border or specked with ecchymoses. The fur is thin and whitish. The pulse is weak, taut and hesitant. Gynecological examination finds that the cervical orifice is wide open but the uterine contraction is not powerful enough so that the embryonic tissues are retained at the threshold.

Therapeutic treatment: Invigorate *Qi* and remove blood stasis.

Recipe: *Renshen Huangqi Tang*(56) plus *Shixiao San* (70),augmented

Ingredients:
| | | |
|---|---|---|
| Radix Ginseng | 6—9 g | |
| Radix Astragali seu Hedysari | 30 g | |
| Rhizoma Atractylodis Macrocephalae | 9 g | |
| Radix Angelicae Sinensis | 12 g | |
| Radix Paeoniae Alba | 9 g | |
| Folium Artemisiae Argyi | 4.5g | |
| Colla Corii Asini (to be infused in hot decoction) | 12 g | |
| Pollen Typhae | 12 g | |
| Faeces Trogopterorum | 12 g | |
| Radix Cyathulae | 15 g | |
| Herba Leonuri | 30 g. | |

Decoct the above drugs in water to get 200—300ml of decoction. Take one half of it in the morning and the other in the evening.

Modification:In case of distending pain in the hypochondia and lower abdomen, add

Fructus Aurantii　　9 g

Rhizoma Cyperi　　12 g.

## 2. Stagnancy of *Qi* and blood stasis

**Clinical manifestations:** After the removal of part of the fetus and placenta, there appears intermittent vaginal bleeding which is purplish dark in color or at times mixed with blood clots, accompanied by abdominal pain and tenderness which can be abated as the clots are dislodged. The tongue is dim in color with thin, whitish fur or dotted with ecchymoses. The pulse is taut and hesitant. Gynecological examination finds that the cervical orifice is wide open and in some cases the embryonic tissues are standing on the way.

Therapeutic method: Promote the flow of *Qi* and dislodge blood stasis.

Recipe: *Danggui Tang* (16), augmented.

Ingredients:Radix Angelicae Sinensis     15 g
Caulis Akebiae     6 g
Talcum     15 g
Radix Semiaquilegiae     12 g
Herba Dianthi     12 g
Radix Cyathulae     12 g
Fructus Aurantii     9 g.

The decoction of a dose is 200—300ml. Take equal shares in the morning and evening.

Modification: In case of cold—pain in the lower abdomen, add

Cortex Cinnamomi     6 g.

In case of copious vaginal bleeding, add

Powder of Radix Notoginseng     3 g (to be divided into two portions and taken after being infused in boiling water)

Pollen Typhae Praeparata     9 g
Herba Leonuri     30 g.

In case of *Qi* —deficiency such as short breaths and fatigue, add

Radix Codonopsis Pilosulae     30 g

Radix Astragali seu Hedysari Praeparata 30 g.

## 4.1.4 Complete Abortion

Complete abortion is a continuation of threatened and inevitable abortions. It is characterized by the complete evacuation of embryonic tissues out of the vagina, accompanied by gradual stoppage of vaginal bleeding and the receding abdominal pain. In TCM, it is discussed under the topic of "fallen fetus" or "premature birth".

### Type and Treatment

As for complete abortion, no special measures need to be taken, but if there is abdominal pain along with scanty blood stasis flowing out of the vagina, the case must be treated so as to promote the recovery of the uterus.

**Clinical manifestations:** After drastic abdominalgia, there appears profuse vaginal bleeding which is mixed with blood clots. Embryonic tissues are seen to have been evacuated and the abdominal pain is lessened as blood clots are removed and then gets mild and faint and even disappears. The vaginal bleeding is reduced or comes to an end. Gynecological examination finds that the cervical orifice has closed and the size of the uterus gets normal again.

Therapeutic method: Promote blood circulation and remove blood stasis, supported by invigorating $Qi$.

Recipe: *Shenghua Tang* (61) , augmented.

Ingredients:Radix Angelical Angelicae Sinensis    12 g

               Rhizoma Ligustici Chuanxiong    9 g

                    Semen Persicae        9 g
                    Rhizoma Zingiberis Carbonisatiote      3 g
                    Radix Glycyrrhizae Praeparata      3 g
                    Herba Leonuri      15 g
                    Radix Codonopsis Pilosulae      15 g.
The decoction of a dose is 200—300 ml. Add to it
                    millet wine      30 g
                    boy's urine    1 cup.
Take one half of the mixed decoction in the morning and the oth-
er half in the evening.

        Proprietary: *Yimucao Gao.* Take 10 ml at a time, twice a day.
                    *Shenghua Tang Wan.* Take one bolus at a time,
thrice a day.

## 4.1.5   Missed Abortion

This illness refers to the retention in the uterus of an abortus
that has been dead for more than 2 months. In traditional
Chinese medicine, it is termed "dead fetus" or "retention of the
dead fetus". It results from one of the following factors:
long—standing deficiency of the kidney—*Qi* of the pregnant woman, destitution of *Qi* and blood, intemperance of sexual activity,
traumatic injury which spoils the essence of the fetus,
undernourishment of the fetus leading to its developmental
arrest, and the failure of expulsion of the nonviable fetus due to
the uterine inertia or obstruction of blood stasis.

### Type and Treatment

**Clinical manifestations:** Intermittent vaginal bleeding occurs
during pregnancy, which is dark in color and mixed with blood

clots, but the symptoms of nausea, vomiting and fetal movement are no longer existent. The patienl is characterized by a dim complexion, foul breaths and cold sensation in the lower abdomen. The tongue is purplish dark, specked with ecchymoses. The pulse is deep and hesitant. Gynecological examination finds a smaller uterus than the normal in that month of pregnancy, and no heartbeat of the fetus is detectable by B—type ultrasonic examination or stethoscopy.

Therapeutic method: Promote the circulation of *Qi* and blood, remove blood stasis and expel the dead fetus.

Recipe: *Jiu Mu Dan* (34) plus *Tuo Hua Jian*(74), modified.

Ingredients:Radix Ginseng (to be decocted first)    9—15 g

Radix Angelicae Sinensis    12—18 g

Rhizoma Ligustici Chuanxiong    15 g

Herba Leonuri    30 g

Halloysitum Rubrum    6 g

Spica Schzonepetae Praeparata    9 g

Radix Cyathulae    15 g

Cortex Cinnamomi    6 g

Cortex Magnoliae Officinalis    9 g.

Modification: In case of swollen limbs, oppressed chest and thick, greasy fur, add

Rhizoma Alractylodis    12 g

Pericarpium Citri Reticulatae    12 g

Semen Plantaginis(to be packed in gauze)    12 g.

In case of distention in the chest, hypochondria and lower abdomen, add

Rhizoma Corydalis    9 g

Fructus Aurantii      9 g.

The decoction of a dose is 150ml. Take 2 doses daily, one in the morning, the other in the evening.

**Other therapies**

Intramuscular injection of *Tianhuafen Zhenji*

Directions: Give an injection *Tianhuajen Danbai Zherj i* 1.2—2.4 mg diluted by 2 ml of saline.i.m.

Caution: Have a skin test previous to the injection and observe for 20 minutes.

Observe after injection the reaction of the trial dosage for 2 hours.

The dosage of treatment is 1.2—2.4 mg.

After injection, the patienl should lie in bed for 48 hours. In the meantime, keep a constant watch on her body temperature, heart rate, blood pressure, etc. In order to prevent allergic reaction, the patient may be asked to take prednisone 10 mg at a time, thrice a day, for 2 days.

Phenergan, analgin, cortical hormone, hypertonic sugar and Vitamin C are commonly used for the treatment of side reactions.

Contraindication

Positive reaction to the trial dosage or skin test for *Tianhuafen*

Allergic constitution or allergic history to various drugs and foods.

Active hepatopathy and nephropathy, accompanied by insufficiency.

Caution must be taken when it is used in the case of hemorrhagic diseases or severe anemia.

In case of acute inflammation, the injection should be suspended.

## 4.1.6  Septic Abortion

If one is affected by pathogenic evil and toxic heat in the course of abortion or shortly after abortion, the syndrome is termed "septic abortion". This illness is characterized by fevers and chills, abdominal pain and stinking leukorrhea. It occurs most frequently in incomplete abortion though other kinds of abortion may also induce it. In TCM, septic abortion is treated under the topics of " puerperal fever" , " damp–heat and leukorrhea "and "invasion of the blood chamber by heat". As the blood chamber is wide open after abortion or delivery, the pathogenic evil takes advantage of this opportunity to invade; resulting in the accumulation of toxic heat in the uterus or the blockage of blood stasis which can also bring about heat over a long period.

### Type and Treatment

**Clinical manifestations:** The case manifests itself by fevers and chills, abdominal pain and tenderness, incessant lochiorrhea which is dark in color and mixed with blood clots, or stinking leukorrhea with reddish discharge. The tongue is dull in shade or dotted with ecchymoses. The fur is yellowish, rough or greasy. The pulse is wiry and rapid. Gynecological examination detects conspicuous tenderness on the uterus or its appendages. Blood examination reports the increase of white cell and neutrophil count.

Therapeutic method: Clear away pathogenic heat and toxic agent; promote blood circulation by removing blood stasis.

Recipe: *Wuwei Xiaodu Yin* (86) plus *Yinhua Jicai Yin*(97), augmented.

Ingredients: Flos Lonicerae     15 g

            Herba Taraxaci     15 g

            Herba Violae     15 g

            Herba Houttuyniae     15 g

            Rhizoma Smilacis Glabrae     30 g

            Flos Chrysanthemi Indici     12 g

            Radix Semiaquilegiae     9 g

            Cortex Moutan Radicis     15 g

            Radix Paeoniae Rubra     15 g

            Herba Schizonepetae     6 g

            Radix Glycyrrhizae     6 g.

The decoction of a dose is 200—300 ml. Divide it into two portions for the morning and evening.

Modification: In case of fatigue, lassitude and anorexia, add to the recipe

            Radix Codonopsis Pilosulae     18 g.

In case of profuse lochia with clots, add

            Radix Rubiae     15 g

            Os Sepiellae seu Sepiae     30 g.

## 4.1.7 Habitual Abortion

If spontaneous abortion occurs repeatedly more than 3 times to a single person, the case is known as "habitual abortion", namely "Huatai" as termed in traditional Chinese medicine. This case results from long—standing deficiency of both the spleen and the kidney and from the destitution of *Yin* —blood. Owing to the deficiency of the kidney and spleen—*Qi* , the fetus cannot be supplied with necessary nutrients while the destitution of *Yin* —blood gives rise to the interior heat which brings damage to uterine collaterals, and attacks the *Chong* and *Ren* channels, thus leading to successive abortions relative to frequent gestations.

## Type and Treatment

The chief method for treating this illness is to have drugs to strengthen the spleen and kidney before gestation and then keep on taking drugs to secure the fetus until the pregnant months of easy abortion have passed.

**1. Deficiency of both spleen and kidney.**

**Clinical manifestations:** The patient looks weary and languid, with dark orbits or dim speckles on the face. She is short of breath and lazy to speak and has poor appetite, sore loins, weak knees and loose stools, accompanied by dizziness, tinnitus and nocturia. The menses are always irregular, either preceded or delayed, either profuse or scanty. In some cases, conception is hard to achieve after habitual abortion. The tongue is pale and tender with thin coating. The pulse is deep and feeble.

Therapeutic method: Tonify the kidney, strengthen the spleen and reinforce the *Chong* and *Ren* channels.

Recipe: *Bushen Guchong Wan* (4)

Ingredients:Semen Cuscutae      240g

       Radix Dipsaci     90g

       Radix Morindae Officinalis     90g

       Cortex Eucommiae     90g

       Radix Angelicae Sinensis     90g

       Rhizoma Rehmanniae Praeparata     150g

       Cornu Cervi Degelatinatum     90g

Fructus Lycii        90g

Colla Corii Asini        120 g

Radix Codonopsis Pilosulae        120 g

Rhizoma Atracty lodis Macrocephalae        90 g

Fructus Ziziphi Jujubae (kernel removed) 50 dates

Fructus Amomi        15 g.

The above drugs are made into honeyed boluses. Take        6 g at a time, twice a day, starting in advance of conception but excluding the menstrual period. One course of treatment consists of 2 months.

Modification: In case of consistent debility, add

Placenta Hominis        90 g.

In case of aversion to cold and cold—pain in the lower abdomen with cool limbs, add

Herba Epimedii        120 g.

Proprietary: *Taichan Jindan* . Take one bolus at a time, twice a day.

## 2. Destitution of both *Qi* and blood

**Clinical manifestations:** The case is marked by a pale or sallow complexion, short breaths, feeble limbs, accompanied by dizziness, palpitation and lassitude; a pale tongue with thin, whitish fur; a small and feeble pulse.

Therapeutic method: Invigorate *Qi* and replenish the blood, supported by tonifying the kidney and preventing abortion.

Recipe: *Taishan Panshi San* (77)

Ingredients:Radix Codonopsis Pilosulae        15 g

Radix Astragali seu Hedysari        15 g

Radix Dipasaci        18 g

Rhizoma Rehmanniae Praeparata      12 g

Radix Angelicae Sinensis      9 g

Rhizoma Ligustici Chuanxiong      9 g

Rhizoma Atractylodis Macrocephalae      9 g

Radix Paeoniae Alba      9 g

Radix Scutellariae      9 g

Fructus Amomi      6 g

Radix Glycyrrhizae Praeparata      6 g

Glutinous rice a handful.

The decoction of a dose is 200—300 ml. Take one half in the morning and the other half in the evening.

Modification:In case of a hollow and bearing—down sensation in the lower abdomen, exchange both Radix Codonopsis Pilosulae and Radix Astragali seu Hedysari from 15g to 30g respectively, and add

Rhizoma Cimicifugae Praeparata      6g.

In case of heat due to deficiency of blood, add

Radix Rehmanniae      12 g.

In case of palpitation and insomnia, add

Semen Ziziphi Spinosae      30 g.

Proprietary:*Buzhong Yiqi Wan* . Take one bolus at a time, thrice a day, starting in advance of conception till the pregnant month of easy abortion has passed.

*Bao Tai Wan* . Take one bolus at a time, thrice a day.

**3. Blood—heat due to *Yin* —deficiency**

**Clinical manifestations:** The patient has flushed cheeks, a dry throat and a hot sensation in palms and soles, accompanied by magersucht and dysphoria. A reddened tongue with little coating. A thready and rapid pulse.

Therapeutic method: Replenish the vital essence and remove heat from the blood.

Recipe: *Bao Yin Jian* (5), augmented.

Ingredients:
| | |
|---|---|
| Radix Rehmanniae | 12 g |
| Rhizoma Rehmanniae Praeparata | 12 g |
| Radix Paeoniae Alba | 9 g |
| Radix Dipsaci | 15 g |
| Rhizoma Dioscoreae Praeparata | 12 g |
| Radix Scutellariae | 9 g |
| Cortex Phellodendri | 6 g |
| Radix Glycyrrhizae | 6 g |
| Radix Boehmeriae niveae | 12 g |
| Herba Ecliptae | 15 g. |

**Caution:**

In order to carry out effective treatment, multifold examinations must be carried out for both sexes, including blood groups, chromosomes, function of the uterine neck, etc.

The interval between two conceptions should be long euough. It is best to pass over one year or even more.

The female who has a history of habitual abortion should first of all free herself from mental tension and nervousness. In ordinary daily life, she should refrain from sexual activity. Especially in the first and last trimesters of pregnancy, sexual intercourse should be forbidden so as to prevent miscarriage and premature birth.

Habitual abortion caused by coldness of the uterus may be prevented by frequently eating eggs boiled with *Folium Artemisiae Argyi*.

Another way to prevent abortion is to use phoenix coat

which refers to the inner membrane of the egg shell as the chick has been hatched. Put a proper amount of phoenix coat on a clean tile and bake it slowly by soft fire till it turns yellowish. Infuse 10g of the drug into hot rice soup. Take the prepared mixture twice a day, for 5 successive days, starting in advance of the same month as that of the previous abortion.

## 4.2 Vomiting during Pregnancy

The early stage of pregnancy is often marked by a liking of sour food and other special diet, nausea or occasional vomiting in the early morning. All these reactions of pregnancy should not be regarded as morbid symptoms. If vomiting gets aggravated, and it occurs not only in the early morning and after meals, but also recurs many times everyday, this symptom is known as vomiting during pregnancy. If the case turns drastic and no food can enter, leading to electrolyte disturbance, metabolic disorder and positive reaction in the test of ketone in the urine, vomiting of this kind is called "hyperemesis gravidarum ." In TCM, pernicious vomiting is termed "ezu " which means morning sickness characterized by nausea and disorder in diet.

This syndrome is induced in most cases by long—standing debility of the spleen and stomach. After conception, the menses cease so that no more blood is evacuated from the uterus, thus leading to the storage of *Qi* and blood in the *Chong* and *Ren* channels. The blood assembles in the lower—*Jiao* to nourish the fetus. If the blood system is insufficient and *Qi* in the *Chong* channel which is subordinate to the *Yangming* channel (the stomach) is relatively plentiful, it will ascend adversely and attack the stomach or give rise to the incoordination between the liver and stomach, resulting in the failure in the descension of stomach—*Qi*

## Type and Treatment

### 1. Debility of the spleen and stomach

**Clinical manifestations:** Nausea and fluid vomiting in the first trimester of pregnancy, accompanied by lack of taste and appetite, listlessness and drowsiness. A pale tongue with moist, whitish coating. A slow, feeble and slippery pulse.

Therapeutic method: Strengthen the spleen and stomach, subdue the adverse flow of *Qi* and arrest vomiting.

Recipe: *Xiangsha liuj unzi Tang* (93)

Ingredients: Radix Codonopsis Pilosulae        12 g

Rhizoma Atractylodis Macrocephalae        9 g

Poria        9 g

Rhizoma Pinelliae Praeparata        9 g

Pericarpium Citri Reticulatae        9 g

Radix Aucklandiae        6 g

Fructus Amomi        6 g

Radix Glycyrrhizae        3 g

Rhizoma Zingiberis Recens 3 slices

Fructus Ziziphi Jujubae 3 pieces.

Decoct the above drugs in water to get 100—200 ml of decoction. Take it slowly, one dose per day.

Modification: In case of stomach—cold, add

Terra Flava Usta (to be packed in cloth) 18 g.

In case of hyperemesis and impairment of *Yin* —fluid, deduct Fructus Amomi

poria
Radix Aucklandiae
Rhizoma Zingiberis Recens

but add

Radix Ophiopogonis      9 g
Rhizoma Phragmitis      9 g
Rhizoma Polygonati Odorati      9 g.

## 2. Incoordination between the liver and stomach

**Clinical manifestations:** Vomiting sour or bitter fluid, distending pain in the chest, dizziness, bittler taste and extreme thirst. A reddened tongue with thin, yellowish fur. A taut and slippery pulse.

Therapeutic method: Soothe the liver and regulate the stomach; subdue the ascending *Qi* and arrest vomiting.

Recipe: *Suye Huanglian Tang* (71),augmented.

Ingredients:Folium Perillae      9 g
Rhizoma Coptidis      6 g
Rhizoma Pinelliae Praeparata      9 g
Caulis Bambusae in Taeniam      9 g
Rhizoma Phragmitis      15 g
Concha Haliotidis Praeparata      12 g
Pericarpium Citri Reticulatae      9 g.

The decoction of a dose is 100—200 ml. Take it slowly, one dose per day.

Modification:In case of a reddened tongue and dry mouth due to impairment of *Yin* —fluid, deduct

Rhizoma Pinelliae Praeparata
Pericarpium Citri Reticulatae

but add

Radix Adenophorae Strictae    12 g

Radix Ophiopogonis    9 g.

In case of severe dizziness, add

Flos Chrysanthemi    9 g

Ramulus Uncariae cum Uncis (to be added later)    12 g.

### 3. Stagnation of the phlegm

**Clinical manifestations:** Sialemesis, chest distress and epigastric distention, anorexia with a tasteless, sticky sensation in the mouth. A pale tongue with whitish, greasy fur. A taut and slippery pulse.

Therapeutic method: Strengthen the spleen and remove the phlegm; subdue the ascending *Qi* and prevent vomiting.

Recipe: *Xiao Banxia Tang* plus *Fuling Tang* (88), augmented.

Ingredients: Rhizoma Pinelliae Praeparata    12 g

poria    12 g

Rhizoma Zingiberis Recens    15 g

Rhizoma Atractylodis Macrocephalae    9 g

Pericarpium Citri Reticulatae    6 g

Fructus Amomi    6 g.

The decoction of a dose is 100–200 ml. Take it slowly, one dose per day.

Modification: In case of listlessness and lassitude accompanied by debility of the spleen and stomach, add

Radix Codonopsis Pilosulae    15 g.

In case of thick, yellowish fur, dark–colored urine and dry stools, add

Rhizoma Coptidis    6 g

Radix Scutellariae    9 g.

In case of palpitation and short breaths, add

> Fructus Perillae    9 g
>
> Semen Armeniacae Amarum    9 g.

## 4. Deficiency of both *Qi* and *Yin*

**Clinical manifestations:** Hyperemesis after meals or vomiting hemoid materials, fever and thirst, oliguria and constipation, magersucht and lassitude. A dry, reddened tongue with thin, yellowish coating or no coating at all. The pulse is rapid, thready and slippery.

Therapeutic method: Supplement *Qi* and replenish *Yin*, normalize the stomach and prevent vomiting.

Recipe: *Shengmai San* (64) plus *Zengye Tang* (111), augmented.

Ingredients: Radix Ginseng (to be decocted first)    6 g

> Radix Ophiopogonis    12 g
>
> Fructus Schisandrae    9 g
>
> Radix Rehmanniae    12 g
>
> Radix Scrophulariae    12 g
>
> Caulis Bambusae in Taeniam    9 g
>
> Radix Trichosanthis    9 g
>
> Pericarpium Citri Reticulatae    6 g
>
> Fructus Mume    9 g.

Decoct the above drugs in water to get 100—200 ml of decoction. Take it slowly, one dose per day.

Modification: In case of vomiting hemoid materials, add

> Nodus Nelumbinis Rhizomatis    9 g.

In case of distressed waist and abdomen or incessant vaginal bleeding, add

> Cortex Eucommiae    12 g

Radix Dipsaci          15 g
Radix Boehmeriae niveae      12 g.

**Other therapies**

The technique of negative pressure pot is applicable to one who vomits whatever she eats. Place a vacuum extractor or a small—sized teapot on the acupoint of *Zhongwan* , Connect one end of a rubber tube to the mouth of the pot or the vent of the extractor while the other end of the tube is joined with a 50 ml syringe. While forming negative pressure, the doctor encourages the patient to have some light, liquid diet. Caution: To prevent local effervescence of the skin, the application should never exceed 15—20 minutes.

Besides, one can rub the tongue with fresh ginger or its extract before meals.

**Prevention**

The diet for gravid women should be under control. Cold, raw and greasy foods should not be served up.

The patients should keep themselves in good humor.

# 4.3   Heterotopic Pregnancy

If the fertilized ovum nests outside the uterine cavity, it is known as "heterotopic pregnancy "or "extrauterine pregnancy". Clinically, it is chieflymarked by menolipsis (generally over 6 weeks), abdominal pain and tenderness ,irregular vaginal bleeding, faint or shock, one—sided appendicular tumefaction as discovered by gynecological examination, and positive reaction of the pregnancy test. In TCM, this illness is included in the topics of "gravid abdominal pain ","restless disturbance of the fetus", and "encysted mass in the abdomen". It is treated as an excess—syndrome of blood stasis in the lower abdomen. Heterotopic pregnancy may be caused by one of the following factors: as persistent and violent emotions give rise to the functional derangement of *Qi*, blood and *Zang—Fu* , the stagnation of the depressed liver—*Qi* leads to the disturbance of blood in its flowing; as *Qi* and blood are deficient in the menstrual or postpartum period, the damp—evil takes advantage of the oppportunity to invade and blocks the channels, resulting in *Qi* —stagnation and blood stasis; or owing to the congenital deficiency of the kidney— *Qi* , the *Chong* and *Ren* channels are feeble and obstructive, thus leading to the abnormal position of pregnancy. The most commonly seen heterotopic pregnancy is that of the oviduct. Clinically, this illness is divided into two types.

## 1. Unruptured type

**Clinical manifestations:** The patient may have morning sickness of different degrees or has dull pain and distention with a bearing—down sensation on one side of the lower abdomen. Gynecological examination finds that the oviduct is slightly expanded on one side or there exists a soft encysted mass that feels aching when pressed. The result of the urine pregnancy test is positive. The pulse is wiry and slippery.

Therapeutic method: Promote blood circulation by removing blood stasis, subside swelling and remove the embryo.

Recipe: Prescription No.2 for extrauterine pregnancy (46), augmented.

Ingredients: Radix Paeoniae Rubra    15 g

              Radix Salviae Miltiorrhizae    15 g

              Semen Persicae    9 g

Rhizoma Sparganii     6 g

Rhizoma Zedoariae     6 g

Radix Achyranthis Bidentatae     15 g

Scolopendra 3—6 in number.

The decoction of a dose is 200—300ml. Take one half in the morning and the other half in the evening.

To further the effect of removing the embryo, *Tianhuą en Zheŋ i* (Injectio Trichosanthis) can be used at the same time. See 4.1.5 for directions of *Tianhuą en Zheŋ i* (Injectio Trichosanthis) .

### 2. Ruptured type

(1)The shock type

**Clinical manifestations:** The patient may have morning sickness of different degrees, with or without a history of menolipsis. She feels abrupt pain and tenderness persistently or intermittently on one side of the lower abdomen which is colic or tearing—like. The case is marked by a pale complexion, cold sweat, cold limbs, nausea, vomiting, dysphoria and occasional syncope. The blood pressure is unsteady or falls. The pulse is either extremely weak, or rapid, feeble and thready. Gynecological examination finds that the posterior fornix is satiated, the neck of uterus feels conspicuous pain when hoisted or shaken, the womb is slightly enlarged and softened and may have a sense of levitation in the case of profuse internal hemorrhage. On one side of the womb there is an encysted mass having tenderness. The result of the urine pregnancy test is positive. Brown—colored, incoagulable blood can be obtained by way of culdocentesis.

Therapeutic method: Recuperate depleted *Yang* and rescue the patient from collapse. Activate the blood and remove blood stasis.

Recipe: *Shen Fu Tang* (59) plus *Shengmai San* (64)

Ingredients:Radix Ginseng        30 g

Radix Aconiti Praeparata        12 g

Radix Ophiopogonis        12 g

Fructus Schisandrae        12 g.

The above drugs are to be decocted on an intense fire into concentrated juice. Take it at a draught.

In case of acute disease and serious shock, such emergency
treatments as liquid or blood transfusion and oxygen therapy
should be adopted immediately.

When the oviduct is ruptured in extrauterine pregnancy, if
the systolic pressure of blood is kept at 80—90mm Hg and the
blood volume is sufficient, Prescription No.1 for extrauterine
pregnancy should be selected as early as possible so as to promote
the absorption of blood clots.

Recipe:   Prescription No.1 for extrauterine pregnancy  (45)

Ingredients:Radix Salviae Miltiorrhizae        15 g

Radix Paeoniae Rubra        15 g

Semen Persicae        9 g.

The decoction of a dose is 200—300 ml. Take one half in the
morning and the other half in the evening.

(2)The labile tpye

**Clinical manifestations:** Abdominal pain and tenderness
which is gradually lessened, encysted mass which has no distinct
boundaries, and at times scanty vaginal bleeding. The blood pressure is steady. The pulse is moderate and thready.

Therapeutic method: Promote blood circulation and remove
blood stasis, supported by invigorating *Qi* .

Recipe: Prescription No.1 for extrauterine pregnancy (45), augmented. Ingredients:Radix Salviae Miltiorrhizae    15 g

> Radix Paeoniae Rubra    15 g
>
> Semen Persicae    9 g
>
> Radix Codonopsis Pilosulae    18 g
>
> Radix Astragali seu Hedysari    15 g.

(3)Encysted mass type

**Clinical manifestations:** It is marked by the formation of hematoma or encysted mass after abortion or rupture due to extrauterine pregnancy, which can be detected in deep palpation and bimanual palpation,and by abdominal pain and tenderness which is gradually relieved and which is, in some cases, accompanied by bearing—down distention in the lower abdomen with the desire to defecate. The vaginal bleeding is abated by degrees. The pulse is uneven and thready.

Therapeutic method: Remove blood stasis and disintegrate the mass.

Recipe: Prescription No.2 for extrauterine pregnancy (46). See 4.3.A. Unruptured type.

Modification: In case of general asthenia, add

> Radix Codonopsis Pilosulae    18 g
>
> Radix Astragali seu Hedysari    15 g.

In case of hard encysted mass, add

> Carapax Trionycis Praeparata    12 g
>
> Squama Manitis    9 g.

In case of  low fever, add

> Radix Rehmanniae    12 g
>
> Cortex Moutan Radicis    9 g
>
> Herba Ecliptae    15 g.

In case of infection, add

> Flos Lonicerae    12 g
> Fructus Forsythiae    15 g
> Caulis Sargentodoxae    30 g
> Herba Patriniae    30 g.

## 3. Accompanying syndromes

In the process of non−operative treatment of extrauterine pregnancy, great importance must be attached to the accompanying syndromes. The most commonly seen are excess syndromes of *Fu*−organs, which are chiefly marked by stomach distress, abdominal distention and constipation. If the case gets severe, there appears abdominal pain and tenderness with the intestinal gurgling sound lowered or lost.

(1)Excess of heat: The case is marked by abdominal pain and tenderness, hectic fever and night sweating, thirst, dysphoria and constipation. The fur is yellowish, either thick or dry. The pulse is deep, full, rapid, slippery and forceful. The therapeutic method is to activate the blood and remove blood stasis,to clear away pathogenic heat and relieve constipation by purgation. Add to the recipe:

> Radix et Rhizoma Rhei (to be added later)
> 9 g
> Natrii Sulfas (to be infused into hot
> decoction)    6 g.

(2)Excess of cold: The case manifests itself by epigastric fullness, abdominal distention and megalgia, aversion to cold, preference for hot compress, constipation, a whitish and greasy fur,a deep, taut and tense pulse. The therapeutic method is to warm the channels, expel pathogenic cold, to alleviate pain and relieve constipation by purgation.

Recipe: *Dahuang Fuzi Xixin Tang*

Ingredients: Radix et Rhizoma Rhei (to be added later)
9 g

Radix Aconiti Praeparata     9 g

Herba Asari     3 g.

The decoction of a dose is 200–300 ml. Take equal shares in the morning and evening.

After expelling the cold, disintegrating the mass and relieving constipation, the method to be chosen is to activate the blood and remove the blood stasis, supported by warming the channels. Add to the recipe:

Rhizoma Zingibris Praeparata     1.5 g

Cortex Cinnamomi     1.5 g.

(3) In case of epigastric distention and abdominal megalgia, while purging the stomach and intestines, add to the recipe:

Fructus Aurantii Immaturus     9 g

Cortex Magnoliae Officinalis     9 g.

**Other therapies**

(1) Topical application of *Xiao Zheng San*

Ingredients: Folium Artemisiae Argyi     500g

Herba Speranskiae tuberculatae     250g

Ramulus Loranthi     120 g

Radix Angelicae Sinensis     120 g

Cortex Acanthopancis Radicis     120 g

Radix Dipsaci     120 g

Radix Angelicae Dahuricae     120 g

Radix Paeoniae Rubra     120 g

Cortex Schizophragmae integrifolii     60 g

Rhizoma Homalomenae     60 g

Pericarpium Zanthoxyli     60 g

Rhizoma seu Radix Notopterygii     60 g

Radix Angelicae Pubescentis     60 g

Resina Draconis     60 g

Resina Olibani     60 g

Myrrha     60 g.

Grind the above drugs into rough powder. Pack and seal in a gauze parcel 250 g of *Xiao Zheng San* and steam it for 15 minutes. Then apply the prepared parcel on the affected part as hot compress, once or twice a day. A course of treatment consists of 10 days. This therapy is fit for the encysted mass.

(2)Ingredients:Semen Persicae     15 g

Radix Salviae Miltiorrhizae     15 g

Radix Paeoniae Rubra     15 g

Rhizoma Corydalis     15 g

Rhizoma Sparganii     15 g

Rhizoma Zedoariae     15 g

Eupolyphaga seu Steleophaga     15 g

Resina Olibani Praeparata     15 g

Myrrha Praeparata     15 g.

Decoct the above drugs into 150—200ml of concentrated juice and use it for retention—enema, once a day. A course of treatment consists of 7 days. This therapy is also fit for the encysted mass.

(3)Ingredients:Semen Persicae     15 g

Radix Paeoniae Rubra     15 g

Radix Salviae Miltiorrhizae     15 g

Fructus Forsythiae     15 g

Herba Taraxaci        15 g
Caulis Sargentodoxae        30 g
Herba Patriniae        30 g.

Decoct the above drugs into concentrated juice of 150—200ml. add 10 ml of 1% procaine and use the mixture for retention—enema, once a day. 7 days form a course of treatment. Iontophoresis may also be used for inflammation.

(4) Add 10ml of Danshen injection ( Injectio Salviae miltiorrhizae) into 500ml of 10% glucose solution and use it for intravenous drips,once a day. 7 days form a course of treatment. This therapy is fit for the encysted mass.

**Caution:**

All through the period of treatment, the patient must lie quietly in bed without going outdoors. The diet should be strictly regulated. Avoid cold and raw foods. Eat as little fatty and sweet things as possible. Except for the case of old ectopic pregnancy, enema and unnecessary pelvioscopy should be forbidden. Try best to eliminate the factors that may heighten the abdominal pressure of the patient.

# 4.4   Hypertensive Syndrome of Pregnancy

This illness is characterized by syndromes of hypertension, hydrops and proteinuria that occur after 20 weeks of pregnancy. It is caused by spasms of systemic arterioles , which give rise to the stagnation of blood flow and insufficiency of blood supply for internal organs, resulting in tissue ischemia. In TCM , this syndrome is treated under the topics of "gravid edema", "gravid syncopy" and "eclampsia gravidarum". In most cases, this illness is induced by consistent Yin—deficiency of the liver and kidney. The gathering of blood to nourish the fetus results in the scarcity of essence and blood that fails to sustain the liver, thus leading to the hyperactivity of the liver—*Yang* and the up—stirring of the liver—wind. Besides, excessive heat due to *Yin*—deficiency transforms the body fluids into phlegm. Or the dysfunction of the spleen in digestion and transportation brings about the retention of dampness and water within the body which causes the formation of heat—phlegm and its upward invasion.

### 4.4.1 Gravid Edema

Gravid edema refers to facial and extremital hydrops after pregnancy. In TCM, different terms are used to denote the different positions and degrees of edema *Ziqi* refers to swollen legs along with clear, copious urines; the illness lies in dampness.*Zizhong* signifies facial and general edema along with scanty urines; the illness lies in water. *Cuijiao* designates puffy feet with thinned skin; the illness is caused by water. *Zhoujiao* stands for puffy feet with thickened skin; the illness is induced by dampness.

If the etiology lies in the retention of water, the skin of the patient is thinned, whitish and bright, and if pressed, pits will form and remain there in the puffy part. If the etiology lies in the stagnation of *Qi*, the patient's skin is thickened with its color unchanged and the puffy region will swell up directly after compression.

From the view of TCM, gravid edema is caused by consistent *yang*—deficiency of the spleen and kidney, the dysfunction of the spleen in digestion and transportation, and the insufficiency of the kidney—*Yang* that cannot provide enough warmth to the spleen—*Yang* and the urinary bladder, so that the disorder in water passages leads to the overwhelming of pathogenic water over the muscles and skin. Besides, edema may also be caused by the growth of the fetus that may obstruct the flow of original *Qi* of the fetus and disturb the functions of visceral organs, resulting in the retention of water and dampness within the body. Clinically, the sign "+ "is used to denote the degree of edema. (+)signifies the obvious pitting edema of the feet and shanks that does not subside after rest. (++) means that the edema has spread to the thighs and the skin looks like orange peel. (+++) indicates that edema is involved with the vulva and the abdomen, and the skin is thinned and looks bright. (++++)stands for general edema, at times accompanied by ascites.

## Type and Treatment

### 1. Deficiency of the spleen

**Clinical manifestations:** Facial and extremital hydrops after several months of pregnancy or general edema, thinned and bright and yellowish skin, poor appetite, loose stools, short breaths and general debility. A pale tongue with whitish, greasy fur. A weak, relaxed and slippery pulse.

Therapeutic method: Invigorate the spleen and induce diuresis.

Recipe: *Baizhu San* (6), augmented.

Ingredients: Rhizoma Atractylodis Macrocephalae     15 g
            Pericarpium Arecae     12 g
            Poria     30 g
            Cortex Zingiberis     9 g

Pericarpium Citri Reticulatae　　9 g

Semen Amomi　　6 g.

Decoct the above drugs in water to get 200—300ml of decoction. Take equal portions in the morning and evening.

Modification: In case of severe edema, add to the recipe

Radix Astragali seu Hedysari　　18 g

Radix Stephaniae Tetrandrae　　9 g.

In case of loose stools, add

Rhizoma Disoscoreae　　12 g

Semen Dolichoris　　18 g.

In case of abdominal distention, add

Caulis Perillae　　9 g

Cortex Magnoliae Officinalis　　9 g.

In case of accompanying dizziness, add

Ramulus Uncariae cum Uncis　　15 g

Flos Chrysanthemi Indici　　9 g.

## 2. Deficiency of the kidney

**Clinical manifestations:** Facial and extremital hydrops after several months of pregnancy, palpitation, dizziness, tinnitus, sore loins, cool feet, short breaths and general lassitude. A pale tongue with whitish, moist fur. A slow, deep and feeble pulse.

Therapeutic method: Warm the kidney and promote diuresis.

Recipe: *Zhen Wu Tang* (109)

Ingredients: Radix Aconiti Lateralis Praeparata　　6—9 g

Rhizoma Zingiberis Recens　　9 g

Poria　　18 g

Rhizoma Atractylodis Macrocephalae　　12 g

Radix Paeoniae Alba　　9 g.

The decoction of a dose is 200—300 ml. Take one half in the morning and the other half in the evening.

Modification: In case of severe hydrops,add

> Semen Plantaginis (to be packed in gauze)
> 9 g.

In case of lumbago, add

> Radix Dipsaci          15 g
> Cortex Eucommiae          12 g.

In case of dizziness, add

> Ramulus Uncariae cum Uncis (to be added later)          15 g
> Concha Haliotidis          30 g.

Proprietary: *Jinkui Shenqi Wan*. Take one bolus at a time, twice a day.

### 3. Stagnation of *Qi*

**Clinical manifestations:** Edema of lower limbs in the second and third trimesters of pregnancy or hyposarca in severe cases. The skin is unchanged in color and it swells up directly after compression. The patient has a depressed chest, distending hypochondria,accompanied by dizziness and anorexia. A thin, greasy fur. A wiry and slippery pulse.

Therapeutic method: Regulate the flow of *Qi* and remove its stagnation, strengthen the spleen and eliminate dampness.

Recipe: *Tianxianteng San*(78) plus *Si Ling San* (63).

Ingredients: Caulis Aristolochiae          15 g
Rhizoma Cyperi          12 g
Fructus Chaenomelis          12 g
Rhizoma Atractylodis Macrocephalae          12 g
Folium Perillae          9 g

Pericarpium Citri Reticulatae    9 g
Radix Linderae    9 g
Rhizoma Zingiberis Recens    9 g
Polyporus    9 g
Rhizoma Alismatis    9 g
Poria    18 g
Radix Glycyrrhizae    6 g.

The decoction of a dose is 200—300ml.Take equal shares in the morning and evening.

## 4.4.2  Gravid Hypertension

If the blood pressure of a pregnant woman who has not a history of hypertension is elevated to 130 / 90 mmHg after 20 weeks of pregnancy, if her systolic pressure is 30 mmHg higher and the diastolic pressure is 15 mmHg higher than the normal values, this symptom is known as gravid hypertension. In TCM, this illness is treated under the topic of " gravid syncope" . Clinically, when hypertension, edema and proteinuria . exist simultaneously and are accompanied by dizziness, dim eyesight, stomachache, nausea and vomiting, this syndrome can be diagnosed as preeclampsia. One must be vigilant against the occurrence of eclampsia gravidarum by accepting reliable treatment. In most cases, this disease results from the deficiency of the liver—*Yin* and the kidney—*Yin* and from the hyperactivity of the liver—*Yang*.

### Type and Treatment

1.  **Deficiency of liver**—*Yin* **and kidney**—*Yin*
**Clinical manifestations:** Dizziness, dysphoria, bitter taste,

poor sleep and dry stools. A reddened tongue with little fur. A wiry, rapid and slippery pulse. The blood pressure is over 130 / 90mmHg.

Therapeutic method: Tonify the kidney and replenish the liver.

Recipe: *Yiguan Jian* (95), augmented.

Ingredients: Radix Adenophorae          12 g
                Radix Ophiopogonis          12 g
                Fructus Lycii          12 g
                Radix Angelicae Sinensis          9 g
                Radix Rehmanniae          15 g
                Fructus Maliae Toosendan          6 g
                Concha Haliotidis          30 g
                Ramulus Uncariae cum Uncis (to be added
                      later)          18 g
                Radix Scutellariae          9 g.

Decoct the above drugs in water to get 200—300ml of decoction. Take one half of it in the morning and the other half in the evening.

Proprietary: *Qi Ju Dihuang Wan* . Take one bolus at a time, thrice a day.

**2. Hyperactivity of *Yang* due to *Yin*-deficiency**

**Clinical manifestations:** Flushed face, dry throat, depressed chest, dizziness, palpitation, insomnia, dysphoria, constipation and dark-colored urine. A reddened or crimson tongue. A wiry, rapid, thready and slippery pulse. The blood pressure is obviously elevated when measured. Protein is found in the urinoscopy. In some cases there exists mild hydrops.

Therapeutic method: Tonify the kidney and nourish the

liver, replenish the insufficient *Yang* and suppress the excessive *Yin*.

Recipe: *Lingjiao Gouteng Tang* (40).

Ingredients:Pulvis Cornu Saigae Tataricae 5g (to be infused in hot decoction)

Radix Rehmanniae 30 g

Ramulus Uncariae Cum Uncis (to be added later) 15 g

Radix Paeoniae Alba 9 g

Caulis Bambusae in Taeniam 9 g

Poria 9 g

Flos Chrysanthemi 9 g

Bulbus Fritillariae Cirrhosae 6 g

Folium Mori 6 g

Radix Glycyrrhizae 6 g.

The decoction of a dose is 200—300 ml. Take equal shares in the morning and evening.

Modification: In case of drastic headache, add

Concha Haliotidis 30 g

Spica Prunellae 15 g.

In case of obvious hydrops, add

Pericarpium Arecae 9 g

Polyporus 9 g.

In case of constipation,add

Radix et Rhizoma Rhei (to be added later) 9 g.

### 3. Debility of the spleen and hyperactivity of liver—*Yang*

**Clinical manifestations:** Facial and extremital hydrops in the second and third trimesters of pregnancy, dizziness, distending chest, poor appetite and loose stools. A thick, greasy fur. A taut and slippery pulse. Protein is found in the urinoscopy and the blood pressure is elevated.

Therapeutic method: Reinforce the spleen and promote diuresis, soothe the liver and subdue the exuberant liver–*Yang*.

Recipe: *Baizhu San* (6). See 4.4.1 for the recipe. Add to the recipe

| | |
|---|---|
| Ramulus Uncariae cum Uncis | 18 g |
| Concha Haliotidis | 30 g. |

The decoction of a dose is 200–300 ml. Take equal shares in the morning and evening.

Modification: In case of severe dizziness and headache with dim eyesight, add

| | |
|---|---|
| Rhizoma Gastrodiae | 9 g |
| Flos Chrysanthemi | 9 g |
| Concha Ostreae | 30 g. |

In case of morbid facial and extremital edema, add

| | |
|---|---|
| Rhizoma Alismatis | 9 g |
| Polyporus | 9 g |
| Semen Phaseoli | 30 g. |

In case of lassitude and fatigue, add

| | |
|---|---|
| Radix Codonopsis Pilosulae | 30 g |
| Radix Astragali | 30 g. |

Proprietary: *Renshen Jianpi Wan* . Take one bolus at a time, thrice a day.

### 4.4.3 Eclampsia Gravidarum

Eclampsia gravidarum is a further development of preeclampsia, which is accompanied by clonic convulsion and coma. It takes place most frequently in the third trimester of pregnancy or before labour, less frequently at the time of delivery and occasionally within 24 hours after labor. The life of the pregnant or parturient woman or the fetus may be in great danger if not rescued in time. Hence, attention should be paid to the prevention and treatment of this disease. In case it occurs, active measures must be taken by nasal feeding of the drugs for restoring life, removing phlegm and subduing spasms and convulsions.

## Type and Treatment

### 1. Up—stirring of the liver—wind

Clinical manifestations: The patient is characterized by a flushed face, palpitation and dysphoria in the third trimester of pregnancy, by sudden attack of extremital convulsion and even by loss of consciousness. The tongue is reddened with thin, yellowish fur. The pulse is taut, rapid and slippery.

Therapeutic method: Soothe the liver and put down the wind.

Recipe: *Lingjiao Gouteng Tang* (40), modified.

Ingredients:Pulvis Cornu Saigae Tataricae (to be infused in hot decoction)    5g

        Radix Rehmanniae    30 g

        Ramulus Uncariae cum Uncis (to be added later)    15 g

        Radix Paeoniae Alba    9 g

        Poria    9 g

        Plastrum Testudinis    30 g

        Concha Haliotidis    30 g

Flos Chrysanthemi Indici   9 g

Os Draconis   30 g

Concha Ostreae   30 g

Fructus Tribuli   12 g

Scorpio   6 g.

The decoction of a dose is 200—300ml. Feed 1 / 2 or 1 / 4 of the decoction at a time by way of the nose or mouth. Take 1 or 2 doses per day.

Modification: In case of a flushed face, blood—shot eyes, scanty and dark—colored urine, dysphoria and delirium,add

Rhizoma Coptidis   9 g

Radix Gentianae   9 g

Fructus Gardeniae   9 g.

In case of postpartum convulsion, add

Radix Pseudostellariae   30 g

Fructus Lycii   12 g.

In case of red threads in the abdomen and limbs,bluish purple lips and a tongue specked with ecchymoses, add

Radix Salviae Miltiorrhizae   30 g

Radix Paeoniae Rubra   12 g

Semen Persicae   9 g.

## 2. Upward invasion of heat—phlegm

Clinical manifestations: The patient is characterized by sudden attack of extremital convulsion and coma, accompanied by coarse breaths and rales. The tongue is reddened with yellowish, greasy fur. The pulse is taut and slippery.

Therapeutic method: Clear away the heat, disperse the phlegm and induce resuscitation.

Recipe: *Niuhuang Qingxin Wan* (44), augmented. It is composed of the following drugs:

> Calculus Bovis
> Succus Bambosae
> Rhizoma Coptidis
> Radix Scutellariae
> Fructus Gardeniae
> Cinnabaris
> Radix Curcumae

Mix the bolus with 60g bamboo juice. Feed 1 / 2 or 1 / 4 of the mixture at a time through a nasal–gastric tube. Take one or two boluses daily.

In recent years, there have been a lot of reports about the treatment of gravid hypertension syndrome by the method of invigorating the blood and removing blood stasis. The therapeutic method has gained good results in this aspect. For example, with

> Radix Salviae Miltiorrhizae
> Radix Paeoniae Rubra
> Rhizoma Chuanxiong
> Radix Angelicae Sinensis
> Semen Persicae
> Fructus Aurantii

as basic drugs of the prescription, drugs of tonifying the spleen, calming the liver and nourishing *Yin* may be added according to clinical differentiation of symptoms and signs. Another way of treatment is to use.

> Radix Salviae Miltiorrhizae
> Radix Paeoniae Rubra
> Herba Artemisiae Anomalae

Resina Olibani

Myrrha

Lignum Sappan

Radix Rubiae

as basic drugs of the prescription.

**other therapies**

**1. Emergency treatment of eclampsia**

(1)In case of coma, add 2—4 ampules of *Xingnaojing* into 500 ml of 5% glucose solution and use the mixed liquid for intravenous drips. Or give an intramuscular injection of *Xingnaojing* ,twice or thrice a day.

(2)In case of coma with convulsion, the alternate drugs are

① *Angong Niuhuang Wan* . Mix one bolus uniformly with boiled water and then feed 1 / 2 or 1 / 4 of the decoction at a time through a nasal—gastric tube. Take 2 boluses daily. This drug is fit for the case of profuse phlegm and excessive heat due to heart—fire and liver—fire.

② *Zixue Dan* . Mix 0.6—3g with boiled water and then feed 1 / 2 or 1 / 4 of the decoction at a time through a nasal—gastric tube. Take 3 doses daily. It is fit for the case of repeated attacks of spasms and convulsions.

③ *Zhibao Dan* . Mix one bolus with boiled water and then feed 1 / 2 or 1 / 4 of the decoction at a time through a nasal—gastric tube. Take 2 boluses daily. It is fit for deeper coma and unconsciousness.

**2. Dietetic therapy of gravid edema**

Dilute soybean milk or red phaseolus bean porridge should be taken frequently after pregnancy.

Decoct the waxgourd peel or water—melon peel in water and

drink the soup instead of tea.

**Prevention**

The prenatal examination should be made regularly with special attention to blood pressure, urinoscopy and the state of hydrops. If there is anything abnormal ,active measures must be taken timely to prevent the occurrence of eclampsia.

**Caution:** Those who are inflicted with primary hypertension, chronic nephritis or diabetic, are liabte to supervene this disease.

Remind the patient of proper rest and nutrition in the gestational period. The diet should be far from fatty and greasy but rich in nutrients of protein and vitamins, because the malnutrition of the maternal body, hypoproteinemia and severe anemia are easy to induce preeclampsia.

Advise the patient to keep herself in good humor.

Be cautions against the disease in advance by asking about the family history in detail.

## 4.5  Polyhydramnios

This illness manifests itself by the rapid expansion of the abdomen from the second or third trimester of pregnancy, by distending fullness in the chest and hypochondria, and by indistinct fetal position and distant fetal heart beat. The volume of amniotic fluid is often as much as 2000 ml and even more. Clinically, there are two types of polyhydramnios: acute and chronic. Acute polyhydramnios occurs mostly in the second trimester of pregnancy, marked by rapid increase of amniotic fluid and rapid expansion of the abdomen, accompanied by depressed chest and short breaths. Chronic polyhydramnios takes place mostly in the third trimester of pregnancy. It develops slowly, marked by gradual enlargement of the uterus and the accompanying fetal malformation. In TCM, this disease is discussed under the topics of "Ziman" (gestational edema) and "overabundance of amniotic fluid". In most cases, it is caused by consistent debility of the spleen or by the excessive consumption of cold and raw foods after conception, thus resulting in the impairment of the spleen—yang and accumulation of dampness in the uterus.

If fetal malformation is found , pregnancy should be put to an end as early as possible; if it is not found, the illness can be cured by traditional Chinese drugs.

## Type and Treatment

**Clinical manifestations:** Rapid expansion of the abdomen in the second and third trimesters of pregnancy which exceeds the normal size in a certain pregnant month, indistinct fetal position, distant fetal heart beat, accompanied by oppressed chest, rapid breaths, feeble limbs, abdominal pain, vulval and lower extremital edema. The tongue is pale and bulgy with whitish , greasy fur. The pulse is deep, feeble and slippery.

**Therapeutic method:** Invigorate the spleen and promote diuresis.

Recipe1: *Liyu Tang* (42), augmented.

Ingredients:Carp (with its scales and intestines removed)
$\qquad$ 250 g

$\qquad$ Rhizoma Atractylodis Macrocephalae $\quad$ 15 g

$\qquad$ Rhizoma Zingiberis Recens $\quad$ 9 g

$\qquad$ Radix Paeoniae Alba $\quad$ 9 g

$\qquad$ Radix Angelicae Sinensis $\quad$ 9 g

Poria          30 g

Pericarpium Citri Reticulatae          6 g.

First stew the carp in 1200ml of water. After removing the cooked fish, decoct the drugs in the fish soup. The decoction will be 200—300ml Eat the fish along with it before the meal, one dose a day. The other way is to decoct the drugs twice in advance. After removing the dregs, stew the carp in the decoction of 400—500 ml. Eat the fish and take one half of the decoction before lunch and the other half before supper. The recipe is fit for general asthenia.

Modification: In case of aversion to cold with cool limbs, add

Ramulus Cinnamomi          6—9 g.

In case of debility and lassitude with short breaths, add

Radix Codonopsis Pilosulae          18 g

Radix Astragali          15 g.

In case of severe edema and dysuria, add

Cortex Mori          9 g

Pericarpium Arecae          9 g.

Recipe 2: *Fuling Daoshui Tang* (23), augmented.

Ingredients:Poria          30 g

Rhizoma Atractylodis Macrocephalae          15 g

Fructus Chaenomelis          12 g

Pericarpium Citri Reticulatae          9 g

Polyporus          9 g

Rhizoma Alismatis          9 g

Caulis Perillae          9 g

Cortex Mori          9 g

Pericarpium Arecae          9 g

Semen Arecae       9 g

Semen Lepidii      9 g

Fructus Amomi      6 g

Radix Aucklandiae      6 g.

The decoction of a dose is 200—300 ml. Take equal shares in the morning and evening. It is fit for dyspnea due to distention in the chest.

## 4.6    Other Gravid Diseases

### 4.6.1    Embarrassment of the Fetus

This syndrome refers to abdominal pain during the gestational period, which is caused by the blockage of uterine collaterals and their loss of nutrition, or by the obstruction in the flow of *Qi* and blood. In TCM it is known as "Baozu" (embarrassment of the fetus). The disease can be induced by deficiency of the blood, by stagnation of *Qi* and by the cold due to deficiency.

### Type and Treatment

#### 1.  Deficiency of the blood

**Clinical manifestations:** Dull pain in the lower abdomen which may be lessened by compression, a sallow complexion and at times palpitation and insomnia. A pale tongue with thin, whitish coating. A weak, thready and slippery pulse.

Therapeutic method: Nourish the blood, prevent miscarriage and relieve the pain.

Recipe: *Danggui Shaoyao San* (15), modified.

Ingredients:Radix Angelicae Sinensis      9 g

Radix Paeoniae Alba        15 g

Rhizoma Ligustici Chuanxiong 4.5 g

Poria        12 g

Rhizoma Atractylodis Macrocephalae        12 g

Radix Polygoni Mutiflori Praeparata        15 g

Ramulus Taxilli        15 g.

The decoction of a dose is 200—300 ml. Take one half in the morning and the other half in the evening.

Modification: In case of cold pain in the lower abdomen, add

Folium Artemisiae Argyi        9 g.

In case of general debility and extremital lassitude, add

Radix Codonopsis Pilosulae        15 g

Radix Astragali        15 g.

In case of dysphoria and insomnia, add

Semen Ziziphi Spinosae        30 g

Caulis Polygoni Multiflori        30 g.

**2. Stagnation of** *Qi*

**Clinical manifestations:** Distending pain in the lower abdomen and hypochondria , accompanied by mental depression or by agitated irritation. The fur is thin and greasy. The pulse is wiry and slippery.

Therapeutic method: Soothe the liver and regulate the flow of *Qi,* prevent miscarriage and relieve the pain.

Recipe: *Xiaoyao San* (94), modified.

Ingredients:Radix Angelicae Sinensis        9 g

Radix Paeoniae Alba        12 g

Radix Bupleuri        9 g

Rhizoma Atractylodis Macrocephalae        9 g

Poria     12 g

Caulis Perillae    9 g

Radix Glycyrrhizae Praeparata    6 g.

Modification: In case of a dry throat with bitter taste in the mouth, a yellowish tongue with thin, yellowish fur, a rapid and slippery pulse, add

Fructus Gardeniae    9 g

Radix Scutellariae    9 g.

In case of poor appetite, feeble limbs and loose stools, add

Radix Codonopsis Pilosulae    18 g

Pericarpium Citri Reticulatae    9 g

Rhizoma Dioscoreae    15 g.

In case of sore loins, add

Radix Dipsaci    15 g

Ramulus Loranthi    15 g

Semen Cuscutae    15 g

Colla Corii Asini (to be infused in hot decoction)    12 g.

## 3. Cold due to deficiency

**Clinical manifestations:** Cold pain in the lower abdomen which may be alleviated by warmth and compression, aversion to cold with cool limbs and pale complexion, in some cases accompanied by poor appetite and loose stools. The tongue is palish with thin, whitish coating. The pulse is feeble and thready.

**Therapeutic method:** Warm the uterus and nourish the blood, prevent miscarriage and relieve the pain.

Recipe: *Jiao Ai Tang* (30), augmented.

Ingredients:Colla Corii Asini (to be infused)    12 g

Folium Artemisiae Argyi    9 g

Radix Angelicae Sinensis 9 g

Rhizoma Ligustici Chuanxiong 4.5 g

Radix Paeoniae Alba 9 g

Rhizoma Rehmanniae Praeparata 12 g

Radix Glycyrrhizae Praeparata 6 g

Radix Morindae Officinalis 9 g

Cortex Eucommiae 12 g

Rhizoma Atractylodis Macrocephalae 9 g.(fried)

The decoction of a dose is 200—300 ml. Take one half in the morning and the other half in the evening.

Modification: In case of abdominal cold—pain and cold limbs, add to the recipe

Radix Aconiti Lateralis Praeparata 6 g

In case of sore loins, add

Semen Cuscutae 15 g

Ramulus Loranthi 15 g.

## 4.6.2    Retarded Growth of the Fetus

If the abdomen is obviously less expanded than the normal size in the fourth or fifth month of pregnancy and the fetus is alive but grows slowly, the case is termed "retarded growth of the fetus" or "intrauterine growth retardation". In most cases, this illness results from scarcity of *Qi* and blood of the pregnant woman or from her consistent debility of the spleen and kidney, leading to the destitution of *Qi* and blood in *Zang* and *Fu*. Hence the fetus grows slowly as it gets little nutrition from the maternal body. It is highly necessary to distinguish it from the dead fetus by means of gynecological examination, auscultation of the fetal heart and

B—type ultrasonic inspection.

## Type and Treatment

### 1. Scarcity of *Qi* and blood

**Clinical manifestations:** The patient looks weak and frail with a pale or sallow complexion, also marked by dizziness and short breaths. The tongue is pale and tender with little coating. The pulse is feeble, thready and slippery.

Therapeutic method: Nourish the fetus by enriching blood and invigorating *Qi*.

Recipe: *Bazhen Tang* (8).

Ingredients: Radix Codonopsis Pilosulae    12 g

Poria    12 g

Rhizoma Atractylodis Macrocephalae    9 g

Radix Angelicae Sinensis    9 g

Radix Paeoniae Alba    9 g

Rhizoma Rehmanniae Praeparata    12 g

Rhizoma Ligustici Chuanxiong    4.5 g

Radix Glycyrrhizae Praeparata    6 g.

The decoction of a dose is 200—300ml. Take equal shares in the morning and evening.

Modification: In case of drastic dizziness, add to the recipe

Fructus Lycii    12 g.

In case of poor appetite, loose stools and whitish, greasy fur, add

Rhizoma Dioscoreae    12 g

Pericarpium Citri Reticulatae    9 g.

Proprietary: *Bazhen Yimu Wan*. Take one bolus at a time, thrice a day.

*Renshen Guipi Wan*. Take one bolus at a time, thrice a day.

**2. Debility of the spleen and kidney**

**Clinical manifestations:** Sore loins with a cold sensation, poor appetite and loose stools, at times aversion to the cold with cool limbs. A pale tongue with whitish coating. A deep and slow pulse.

Therapeutic method: Strengthen the spleen and warm the kidney.

Recipe: *Wentu Yulin Tang* (85), modified.

Ingredients: Radix Morindae Officinalis      9 g
Fructus Rubi      15 g
Rhizoma Atractylodis Macrocephalae      9 g
Radix Ginseng (to be decocted first)      6 g
Rhizoma Dioscoreae      12 g.

The decoction of a dose is 200—300 ml. Take one half in the morning and the other half in the evening.

Modification: In case of severe cold—pain in the loins, add
Cortex Eucommiae      12 g
Radix Dipsaci      18 g
Cornu Cervi      9 g
Semen Cuscutae      15 g.

Proprietary: *Shiquan Dabu Wan* . Take one bolus at a time, thrice a day.

# 4.6.3  Dysphoria during Pregnancy

If the pregnant woman feels unhappy, worried and restless, or is liable to be agitated and irritated, the case is termed *Zif an* which signifies dysphoria during the gestational period.

From the view of TCM, this disease is induced mostly by evil heat and morbid fire, leading to the disturbance of the heart and the dysfunction of mental activity. Different types are *Yin*—deficiency, phlegm—fire, stagnation of the liver—*Qi*

## Type and Treatment

### 1. *Yin* —deficiency

**Clinical manifestations:** mental vexation and restlessness, flushed cheeks and hectic fever, dry throat, dry cough without sputa, thirst but do not like to have much drink, scanty and dark—colored urines. The tongue is reddened with dry, thin and yellowish coating or no coating at all. The pulse is rapid, thready and slippery.

Therapeutic method: Clear away the heat and nourish *Yin*, tranquilize the mind and remove restlessness.

Recipe: *Renshen Maidong San* (57), modified.

Ingredients:Radix Ophiopogonis            9 g

Poria      9 g

Radix Scutellariae        9 g

Rhizoma Anemarrhenae          9 g

Radix Rehmanniae          12 g

Caulis Bambusae in Taeniam        9 g

Radix Glycyrrhizae Praeparata          6 g

Radix Glehniae        12 g

Plumula Nelumbinis        9 g.

Decoct the above drugs in water to get 200—300 ml of decoction. Take equal portions in morning and evening.

Modification:In case of palpitation and timidity, add

Dens Draconis        15 g

Poria cum Ligno Hospite      9 g.

In case of dry throat, dry cough without sputa, hectic fever and night sweat, add

Radix Asparagi      9 g

Bulbus Lilii      9 g

Rhizoma Anemrrhenae      9 g.

In case of dizziness, tinnitus, sore loins and weak knees, add

Plastrum Testudinis      9 g

Radix Scrophulariae      9 g

Fructus Ligustri Lucidi      12 g

Herba Ecliptae      15 g.

## 2. Phlegm—fire

**Clinical manifestations:** The type is characterized by dysphoria, dizziness, palpitation, chest distress, nausea and vomiting. The tongue has a greasy, yellowish fur. The pulse is rapid and slippery.

Therapeutic method: Clear away the heat and remove the phlegm.

Recipe: *Zhuli Tang*(107), augmented .

Ingredients:Succus Bambosae(to be put into hot decoction)

30 g

Radix Ophiopogonis      9 g

Radix Scutellariae      9 g

Poria      12 g

Radix Ledebouriellae      4.5 g

Bulbus Fritillariae Thunbergii      9 g.

The decoction of a dose is 200—300 ml. Take one half in the morning and the other half in the evening.

Modification: In case of copious, thick and yellowish sputa, add to the recipe

> Fructus Trichosanthis   15 g
>
> Rhizoma Coptidis   6 g
>
> Rhizoma Pinelliae   9 g.

In case of drastic vomiting and nausea, add

> Folium Eriobotryae   9 g
>
> Herba Agastachis   9 g.

### 3. Stagnation of the liver—*Qi*

**Clinical manifestations:** The type is characterized by dysphoria, mental depression, restlessness and irritability and hypochondriac pain or distention. The tongue is reddened with thin, whitish or yellowish coating. The pulse is taut and rapid.

Therapeutic method: Soothe the liver, clear away the heat and relieve mental depression and dysphoria.

Recipe: *Dan Zhi Xiaoyao San* (21), modified.

Ingredients:Radix Angelicae Sinensis   9 g

> Radix Paeoniae Alba   9 g
>
> Radix Bupleuri   9 g
>
> Poria   12 g
>
> Cortex Moutan Radicis   9 g
>
> Fructus Gardeniae   9 g
>
> Herba Menthae   6 g
>
> Rhizoma Atractylodis Macrocephalae   9 g
>
> Radix Glycyrrhizae   6 g.

The decoction of a dose is 200—300ml. Take equal shares in the morning and evening.

Modification: In case of dizziness, add

> Ramulus Uncariae cum Unicis (to be added later)   18 g

Flos Chrysanthemi          9 g

Spica Prunellae        12 g.

In case of severe pain or distention in the chest and hypochondria,add

Fructus Meliae Toosendan Praeparata        9 g

Radix Curcumae        9 g.

In case of serious dysphoria and chest distress,add

Rhizoma Anemarrhenae        9 g

Herba Lophatheri        9 g

Plumula Nelumbinis        9 g.

**Other therapies**

*Zhuru Tang* . Decoct 30 g of Caulis Bambusae in Taeniam in water and then drink it slowly. It is fit for the case of dysphoria in pregnancy caused by liver—depression and stomach—heat.

Pour 30 g of bamboo juice in boiled water for drinking. It is fit for the case of dysphoria in pregnancy caused by retention of phlegm—fire in the interior.

## 4.6.4    Upward Flow of Fetus—$Qi$

If the pregnant woman is characteried by chest fullness and abdominal distention, dysphoria and restlessness and in severe cases by dyspnea, it is termed *Zixuan* , which means the upward flow of fetus—$Qi$ . In most cases, this illness is induced by consistent *Yin* —deficiency and even more paucity of kidney—*Yin* after conception, leading to the loss of nourishment of the liver—channel and the domination of the spleen by the hyperactivity of the liver. As a result, the functional activity of $Qi$ is out of order in its rise and fall and so this illness results.

## Type and Treatment

**Clinical manifestations:** Chest fullness and abdominal distention, stuffiness and discomfort during pregnancy, accompanied by tachypnea, dysphoria and restlessness. The fur is thin and yellowish. The pulse is taut and slippery.

Therapeutic method: Soothe the liver and reinforce the spleen; regulate the flow of *Qi* and eliminate its stagnation.

Recipe: *Zisu Yin* (108), augmented.

Ingredients: Flium Perillae 6 g

Pericarpium Citri Reticulatae 9 g

Pericarpium Arecae 9 g

Radix Paeoniae Alba 9 g

Radix Angelicae Sinensis 9 g

Rhizoma Ligustici Chuanxiong 4.5 g

Radix Codonopsis Pilosulae 12 g

Radix Glycyrrhizae 6 g

Radix Scutellariae 9 g

Rhizoma Cyperi 12 g.

Decoct the above drugs in water to get 200—300ml of decoction. Prepare one dose for a day, take one half in the morning and the other half in the evening.

When the above symptoms have improved by *Zisu Yin,Ej iao Yangxue Tang* should be adopted instead, so as to nourish *Yin* , replenish the blood and cultivate the essence.

Colla Corii Asini (to be infused in hot decoction) 12 g

Radix Rehmanniae 15 g

Radix Glehniae 9 g

Radix Ophiopogonis 9 g

Fructus Ligustri Lucidi  9 g
Herba Ecliptae  12 g
Ramulus Taxilli  12 g.

The decoction of a dose is 200—300 ml. Take equal shares in the morning and evening.

## 4.6.5 Gestational Aphonia

If the patient's voice turns hoarse or gets utterly lost during pregnancy,it is termed Ziyin ,which means gestational aphonia.This illness chiefly results from insufficiency of the kidney—*Yin* . From the view of TCM, sounds coming from the lungs are rooted in the kidney and uttered by the tongue. If the-kidney—*Yin* is consistently deficient, and the condition gets more serious after conception as the blood has to gather and feed the fetus, the tongue will no longer have its necessary supply of nourishment and hence aphonia occurs, mostly in the third trimester of pregnancy.

### Type and Treatment

**Clinical manifestations:** The case is marked by a hoarse voice in the 8th and 9th months of pregnancy, dry throat and feverish sensation in palms, accompanied by dizziness, tinnitus, dysphoria, palpitation and constipation. The urine is scanty and dark in color. The tongue is reddened with exfoliative fur. The pulse is rapid and thready.

·Therapeutic method: Enrich the kidney and nourish *Yin*

Recipe: *Liuwei Dihuang Tang* (41), augmented.

Ingredients:Radix Rehmanniae Praeparata  12 g
Radix Rehmanniae  12 g

                Fructus Corni        12 g
                Rhizoma Dioscoreae        12 g
                Rhizoma Alismatis        9 g
                Cortex Moutan Radicis        9 g
                Poria        9 g
                Radix Glehniae        12 g
                Radix Ophiopogonis        12 g.

Decoct the drugs in water to get 200—300 ml of decoction. Take one half in the morning and the other half in the evening.

        Modification:In case of dry throat and thick sputa, deduct
                Rhizoma Alismatis
                Fructus Corni
but add
                Semen Trichosanthis        15 g
                Rhizoma Phragmitis        9 g
                Radix Platycodi        9 g
                Bulbus Fritillariae Cirrhosae        9 g.

**Simple Recipe and Proved Prescription**

(1) Put one fresh egg into boiling soybean milk of proper amount.having mixed it, take the soup early in the morning, once a day.

(2) Remove the kernel from the pear and place
                Semen Oroxyli        6 g
                crystallized sugar        6 g.

in its place. After steaming, take the pear with the soup.

## 4.6.6   Intractable Cough during Pregnancy

This illness is characterized by persistent and lingering coughing which in some cases is accompanied by dysphoria with a feverish sensation in palms, soles and the chest.TCM holds that *Zishou* which means intractable cough during pregnancy is caused by consistent *Yin* −deficiency which becomes more serious after conception as the blood has to gather and feed the fetus and also by the hyperactivity of fire whose heat invades upward and attacks the lungs and consumes its fluid. Besides, the illness may also be caused by inherent excess of *Yang* and exuberance of fetus− *Qi* after conception, both of which help the fire to attack the lungs and to make the fluid into sputa, thus leading to the blockage in the lung and impairment of its function of dispersion and descension.

### Type and Treatment

**1.** *Yin* −**deficiency and dryness of the lung**
**Clinical manifestations:** This type is marked by dry cough without sputa, but in severe cases blood−streaked sputa may be seen.The patient has a dry mouth and throat with a feverish sensation in palms and soles. The tongue is reddened with little fur. The pulse is rapid, thready and slippery.

Therapeutic method:Nourish *Yin* and moisten the lung; relieve cough and prevent abortion.

Recipe: *Baihe Guj in Tang* (3), modified.

Ingredients:Bulbus Lilii            12 g
          Radix Rehmanniae        12 g
          Radix Ophiopogonis      9 g
          Bulbus Fritillariae Cirrhosae    9 g
          Radix Paeoniae Alba     9 g
          Radix Scrophulariae     9 g
          Radix Platycodi         9 g

Radix Glycyrrhizae    6 g

Folium Mori    9 g

Radix Stemonae Praeparata    12 g

Semen Sesami    15 g.

Decoct the drugs in water to get 200—300 ml of decoction. Take equal shares in the morning and evening.

Modification: In case of hemoptysis and damage of pul monary vessels by heat, the following drugs may be added according to symptoms and signs,

Herba Ecliptae    15 g

Rhizoma Bletillae    9 g

Colla Corii Asini (to be infused in hot decoction)    12 g.

In case of flushed cheeks and hectic fever, accompanied by a hot sensation in palms and soles, add

Cortex Lycii    9 g

Radix Cynanchi Atrati    9 g

Rhizoma Polygonati    12 g.

In case of lassitude, listlessness and breathlessness, add

Radix Codonopsis Pilosulae    15 g

Radix Astragali seu Hedysari    15 g.

## 2. Attack of the lung by phlegm—fire

**Clinical manifestations:** This type is marked by thick, yellowish sputa that are hard to spit out. The patient has a yellowish complexion, a dry mouth, a reddened tongue with greasy, yellowish coating and a rapid, slippery pulse.

**Therapeutic method:**Remove the heat from the lung and dissolve the phlegm; stop coughing and prevent miscarriage.

**Recipe:** *Qing f ei Jianghuo Tang*(50), modified.

Ingredients: Radix Scutellariae        9 g

                Semen Armeniacae Amarum Praeparata        9 g

                Bulbus Fritillae Cirrhosae        9 g

                Radix Peucedani        9 g

                Semen Trichosanthis        15 g

                Pericarpium Citri Reticulatae        9 g

                Poria        12 g

                Rhizoma Pinelliae        9 g

                Radix Platycodi        9 g

                Fructus Aurantii        4.5 g

                Rhizoma Zingiberis Recens        3 slices

                Radix Glycyrrhizae        6 g

                Folium Mori        9 g

                Folium Eriobotryae        9 g.

The decoction of a dose is 200–300 ml. Take one half in the morning and the other half in the evening.

**Simple Recipe and Proved Prescription**

(1) Remove the kernel from a pear and place

                Bulbus Fritillariae Cirrhosae        3 g (powder)

                crystallized sugar        6 g

in the pear. After stewing on a gentle fire, eat the pear along with the soup.

(2) Put

                Bulbus Fritillariae Cirrhosae        3 g

                Extractum Folium Eriobotryae (proper amount)

in boiling water. After mixing it, drink the decoction.

(3) Decoct

                Flos Farfarae        9 g

crystallized sugar (proper amount) in water. Drink the docoction.

## 4.6.7 Stranguria during Pregnancy

If such symptoms as frequent micturition, urodynia, precipitant urination and urinary stuttering are shown during the gestational period, the illness is termed *Zilin* which means stranguria during pregnancy. From the view of TCM this disease is caused by one of the following factors: the flaring up of heart—fire, the downward flow of damp—heat and *Yin* —deficiency which results in the exuberance of fire. Hence the bladder fails to perform its normal function in regulating urination.

### Type and Treatment

**1. Flaring—up of heart—fire**

**Clinical manifestations:** The type is characterized by scanty, dark—colored urine, dysuria and urodynia. The patient has a flushed face and is worried and at times has canker and tongue sores. The tongue is reddened and lacks moisture with little or no coating. The pulse is rapid, thready and slippery.

Therapeutic method: Purge intense heat and promote micturition.

Recipe: *Daochi San* (14), augmented.

Ingredients:
| | |
|---|---|
| Radix Rehmanniae | 15 g |
| Caulis Akebiae | 6 g |
| Radix Glycyrrhizae | 9 g |
| Herba Lophatheri | 9 g |
| Radix Scrophulariae | 12 g |
| Radix Ophiopogonis | 9 g. |

Decoct the drugs in water to get 200–300 ml of decoction. Take one half of it in the morning and the other half in the evening.

Modification: In case of hot–pain during urination, add

|  |  |
|---|---|
| Fructus Gardeniae | 9 g |
| Herba Plantaginis | 12 g |

In case of dysphoria, add

|  |  |
|---|---|
| Plumula Nelumbinis | 9 g |
| Fructus Gardeniae | 9 g. |

In case of urination with blood

|  |  |
|---|---|
| Rhizoma Imperatae | 12 g |
| Nodus Nelumbinis Rhizomatis | 9 g. |

## 2. Damp–heat

**Clinical manifestations:** This type is characterized by frequent urination, precipitant urination, urinary stuttering, urodynia with burning and stabbing pain, and yellowish tawny–colored urines. The patient has a sallow complexion, poor appetite and chest distress. She is thirsty but does not like to have much drink. The tongue is reddened with greasy, yellowish fur. The pulse is rapid and slippery.

Therapeutic method: Clear away the heat, remove dampness and promote micturition

Recipe:*Jiawei Wulin San*(83), modified.

Ingredients:

|  |  |
|---|---|
| Fructus Gardeniae | 9 g |
| Poria Rubra | 12 g |
| Radix Angelicae Sinensis | 9 g |
| Radix Paeoniae Alba | 9 g |
| Radix Scutellariae | 9 g |
| Radix Glycyrrhizae | 6 g |
| Radix Rehmanniae | 12 g |

Rhizoma Alismatis        9 g

Semen Plantaginis (to be parcelled in gauze)
9 g

Caulis Aristolochiae Manshuriensis        6 g.

The decoction of a dose is 200—300 ml. Take equal shares in the morning and evening.

Modification: In case of damp—heat induced by exopathic causes, add

Flos Lonicerae        30 g

Herba Taraxaci        30 g.

In case of chest fullness and abdominal distention with thick, greasy, yellowish fur, add

Herba Agastachis        9 g

Herba Eupatorii        9 g.

3. *Yin* —deficiency

**Clinical manifestations:** This type is marked by frequent and dribbling urination, scanty in quantity and tawny in color, accompanied by burning and stabbing pain when micturating. The patient has flushed cheeks, a feverish sensation in palms and soles and symptoms of dysphoria, sleeplessness and constipation. The tongue is reddened, with thin, dry and yellowish coating. The pulse is rapid, thready and slippery.

Therapeutic method: Nourish *Yin* , moisten dryness, and induce diuresis.

Recipe: *Zhi Bai Dihuang Tang* (103), augmented.

Ingredients: Radix Rehmanniae Praeparata        12 g

Fructus Corni        12 g

Rhizoma Dioscoreae        12 g

Poria        9 g

Cortex Moutan Radicis 9 g

Rhizoma Alismatis 9 g

Rhizoma Anemarrhenae 9 g

Cortex Phellodendri 9 g

Radix Ophiopogonis 9 g

Fructus Schisandrae 9 g

Herba Plantaginis 12 g.

The decoction of a dose is 200—300 ml. Take one half in the morning and the other half in the evening.

Modification: In case of conspicuous hectic fever and night sweating, add

Radix Scrophulariae 12 g

Cortex Lycii 9 g

Radix Cynanchi Atrati 9 g.

In case of urination with blood, add

Fructus Ligustri Lucidi 15 g

Herba Ecliptae 18 g

Rhizoma Imperatae 15 g.

In case of constipation due to dryness of the intestines, add

Radix Angelicae Sinensis 9 g

Fructus Cannabis 9 g.

### 4.6.8 Gravid Anuresis

If uroschesis occurs during the gestational period, which in some cases may give rise to dysphoria and restlessness with drastic distention and pain in the lower abdomen, this case is known as gravid anuresis or *Zhuanbao* as termed in TCM , meaning dysuria due to the pressure of the fetus. This illness is caused either by consistent insufficiency of *Qi* in the middle–*Jiao* or by scarcity of the kidney–$Qi$ so that the fetus cannot be raised to a proper position after conception. The other etiology is the debility of the kidney which links with the fetus in an impotent way due to the debility of the kidney, so that the fetus as it is growing heavier, sinks down and oppresses the urinary bladder, thus leading to its dysfunction and the obstruction of the waterway. As a result, it is hard to void the urine.

## Type and Treatment

### 1. Deficiency of $Qi$

**Clinical manifestations:** This case is marked by incapability to void the urine or by scanty and frequent urination, accompanied by abdominal distention and pain. The patient is weary and restless with a pale complexion and short breaths. She is dizzy, heavy–headed, reserved in speech and has distress in defecation. The tongue is pale with thin, whitish coating. The pulse is feeble and slippery.

Therapeutic method:Replenish $Qi$ and elevate the sinking fetus.

Recipe: *Yiqi Daoniao Tang* (100).

Ingredients:Radix Codonopsis Pilosulae      30 g

             Rhizoma Atractylodis Macrocephalae      9 g

             Semen Dolichoris      15 g

             Poria      12 g

             Ramulus Cinnamomi      6 g

             Rhizoma Cimicifugae praeparata      6 g

             Radix Platycodi      9 g

             Medulla Tetrapanacis      9 g

             Radix Linderae      9 g.

Decoct the above drugs in water to get 200–300ml of decoction.

Take one half in the morning and the other half in the evening.

Modification: In case of a sallow complexion, add
Colla Corii Asini (to be infused in hot
decoction)    12 g
Radix  Polygoni  Multiflori  Praeparata
15 g.

In case of dizziness, short breaths and tenesmus and dis
—tention in the lower abdomen, add
Radix Astragali seu Hedysari    30 g.

In case of poor appetite with whitish fur, add
Pericarpium Citri Reticulatae    9 g
Herba Agastachis    9 g
Fructus Amomi    6 g.

**2. Deficiency of the kidney**

**Clinical manifestations:** This type is marked by frequent
micturition and dysuria followed by anuresis, with a fuil, distending and painful sensation in the lower abdomen. The patient
is fidgety, restless and avers to cold with cool limbs, sore loins
and weak knees. The tongue is pale with thin, moist coating. The
pulse is deep, feeble and slippery.

Therapeutic method: Warm the kidney and reinforce its vital
function; promote the flow of *Qi* and alleviate water retention.

Recipe: *Shenqi Wan* (66), modified.

Ingredients: Radix Rehmanniae Praeparata    15 g
Rhizoma Dioscoreae    12 g
Fructus Corni    12 g
Rhizoma Alismatis    9 g
Poria    12 g
Ramulus Cinnamomi    6 g

Herba Epimedii     9 g.

The decoction of a dose is 200—300 ml. Take equal shares in the morning and evening.

Modification: In case of lassitude and listlessness, short breaths and general debility, add

> Radix Codonopsis Pilosulae seu Hedysari
> 18 g
> Radix Astragali     15 g
> Rhizoma Atractylodis Macrocephalae Praeparata     9 g.

In case of sore loins and weak knees, add

> Cortex Eucommiae     12 g
> Ramulus Taxilli     15 g
> Semen Cuscutae     12 g.

**Other therapies**

( 1 )    Acupuncture and moxibustion: needle the points of Qihai, Pangkuangyu (pair) and Yinlingquan (pair). Apply an ignited moxa—stick over the point of *Kuanyuan* .

(2)    Hot medicated compress

① Compress a hot towel over the suprasymphysary vesical region.

② Stalks and roots of Chinese green scallion 500 g

Get them washed clean, cut short by hand, pounded and fried hot in a pan. At first, pack half of the prepared drug, i.e. 250g in a piece of cloth or in a towel, apply the newly—made hot pack on the lower abdomen, moving it slowly from the umbilical part down to the pubic region. Then repeat the same procedure with the other half of the drug. The hot compress lasts for about 30 minutes, once a day.

# 5. Perverse Labor and Abnormal Puerperium

## 5.1  Abnormality of the Force of Labor

The force of labor refers to the motive force by which the fetus is pushed out of the uterus. It depends chiefly on uterine contraction. When the birth canal and the fetal conditions are normal, the uterine contraction plays a decisive role in the dilatation of the cervical orifice and the progress of birth process. If its rhythmicity, symmetry and activeness are damaged, or its intensity and frequency are changed, this symptom is termed "abnormality of uterine contraction". Clinically two sorts of abnormality must be distinguished: metratonia and metrypercinesia. In TCM, this illness is treated under the topic of dystocia. This illness is caused by one of the following factors: insufficiency of vital-$Qi$ due to consistent debility of the pregnant woman, over-consumption of and strength due to untimely exertion of force during child-bearing or exhaustion of the fluid due to premature rupture of the amniotic membrane. Besides, dystocia may also be caused by excessive stress and anxiety during labor, extravagant ease and comfort during pregnancy, or the invasion of exopathic cold, leading to the stagnation and delicacy of $Qi$ and blood. The deficiency of $Qi$ fails to push the fetus out while blood stasis will hinder the delivery of the child.

## Type and Treatment

### 1. Deficiency of *Qi* and blood

**Clinical manifestations:** The case is characterized by weak labor pain in childbearing, shortened uterotonic time with prolonged pause, sluggish progress of birth process, and in some cases by profuse and light—colored bleeding. The patient looks weary and languid with a pale complexion, rapid heart beat and short breaths. The tongue is pale with thin, whitish coating. The pulse is either empty and large, or deep, weak and thready. Obstetric examination finds that the myometrium is not stiff at the time of uterine contraction, something like a pit is perceivable at the fundus of the uterus, the cervical orifice is unable to dilate regularly and the presentation of the fetus cannot drop out as expected.

Therapeutic method: Nourish *Qi* and replenish the blood in an effective way.

Recipe: *Caisongting's Nanchan Fang*(11).

Ingredients:Radix Astragali seu Hedysari Praeparata     30 g

Radix Angelicae Sinensis     12 g

Poria     9 g

Radix Codonopsis Pilosulae     30 g

Plastrum Testudinis     15 g

Rhizoma Ligustici Chuanxiong     9 g

Radix Paeoniae Alba     12 g

Fructus Lycii     12 g.

Decoct the drugs in water to get 200—300 ml of decoction. Take it at a time.

Modification: In case of uterine atony, profuse perspiration on the head, weak and thready pulse, substitute Radix Codonopsis Pilosulae for

Radix Ginseng        3—6 g

which should be decocted separately and then added into the decoction of the above drugs. Take it at a time and if necessary have another dose 2 hours later.

**2. *Qi*—Stagnation and blood stasis**

**Clinical manifestations:** The case is marked by drastic pain in the loins and abdomen at the time of child bearing, powerful uterine contraction yet with irregular pause, sluggish progress of birth process, and in some causes by scanty, reddish dark bleeding. The patient looks tense and nervous with a purplish dark complexion, chest distention and epigastric distress, intermittent nausea and vomiting. The tongue is dark—red with normal or greasy coating. The pulse is taut and large, sometimes cacorhythmic. Obstetric examination finds that the uterus is in a hypertonic state even with tenderness when touched, that the position of the fetus is hard to judge, and that the fetal heart beats cacorhythmically.

Therapeutic method: Regulate the flow of *Qi* and activate the blood; remove blood stasis and strengthen the force of labor.

Recipe: *Cuisheng Yin*(12).

Ingredients: Radix Angelicae Sinensis        12 g

Rhizoma Ligustici Chuanxiong        9 g

Pericarpium Arecae        12 g

Fructus Aurantii        12 g

Radix Angelicae Dahuricae        12g.

The decoction of a dose is 200—300ml. Take it at a time and if necessary have another dose 4 hours later.

Modification: In case of prolonged birth process due to Qi–deficiency and asthenia, add

Radix Ginseng        3–6 g

which should be made separately into concentrated decoction and then mixed with the decoction of the above drugs.

In case of dysphoria and severe abdominal pain, add

Poria cum Ligno Hospite        12 g
Semen Ziziphi Spinosae        15 g
Ramulus Uncariae cum Uncis        12 g
Radix Achyranthis Bidentatae        15 g
Herba Leonuri        30g.

**Other therapies**

Acupuncture: After eliminating the abnormality of the birth canal and the fetus,needle the acupoints of Hoku, Sanyinjiao and Taichung with strong stimulation and prolonged retention.

**Caution:**

Prenatal examination should be carried out regularly so as to treat abnormality in time.

Sedative and uterotonic agents must not be used before labor lest they induce the uterine atony, metryperceinesia and dysrhythmia.

During the period from pregnancy to labor, the parturient should be quiet and peaceful, free from alarm, fear and anxiety. She should take part in some proper activities. Don't sleep too much nor eat too much. Avoid liquors, wines and miscellaneous drugs.

## 5.2 Abnormal Fetal Position

Except that the occipitoanterior position is normal, all other positions are abnormal, which may lead to dystocia. Among them the persistent occipitoposterior position, occipitotransverse position, face presentation, brow presentation, breech presentation and scapular presentation are commonly seen. In TCM, abnormal fetal position is discussed in various topics such as "transverse presentation", "umbilical dystocia", "oblique presentation" and "sitting position labor". So long as there exists no abnormality in birth canal and the fetus, the abnormal fetal position can be corrected by making use of traditional Chinese drugs.

**Rectification:** The abnormal fetal position should be corrected in time when discovered in the 28th week of pregnancy.

Recipe: *Baochan Wuyou San*(2)

Ingredients:Radix Angelicae Sinensis          9 g

                 Rhizoma Ligustici Chuanxiong          6 g

                 Radix Paeoniae Alba          9 g

                 Radix Astragali seu Hedysari          15 g

                 Cortex Magnoliae Officinalis          6 g

                 Rhizoma seu Radix Notopterygii          6 g

                 Semen Cuscutae          9 g

                 Bulbus Fritillariae Cirrhosae          6 g

                 Fructus Aurantii          9 g

                 Spica Schizonepetae          6 g

                 Folium Artemisiae Argyi          3 g

                 Rhizoma Zingiberis Recens          3 slices.

The decoction of a dose is 200—300 ml. Take equal shares in the morning and evening.

Moxibustion: The pregnant woman is lying in the supine position with her knees bent and her girdle loosened. Apply an ignited moxa—stick over the acupoints of *Zhiyin* on both feet, 15 minutes at a time, once or twice a day. A course of treatment consists of 7 days. The moxibustion should end at the time of rectification.

Based on clinical observations and exploration of the mechanism, we have found that moxibustion on the acupoint of Zhiyin can promote the secretion of adrenocortical hormone (ACH), favor the activities of the womb and the fetus and is therefore beneficial to the rectification of the fetal position.

Laser radiation: Apply it over the acupoint of *Zhiyin* on both feet, 15 minutes at a time, once or twice a day. A course of treatment consists of 7 days. The treatment will end at the time of rectification.

Physical posture: After micturition, the pregnant woman should loose her dresses and belts first, kneel down on the bed, lower her chest to the level of the bed and raise her buttock in a high position. This physical posture should be kept for 10—15 minutes at a time, twice or thrice a day.

**Caution**

Dresses should be soft, loose and comfortable without using broad, stiff belts. The parturient woman should keep from bending or crouching for a long time.

Prenatal examination should be made regularly so that the abnormality of fetal position, once discovered, can be corrected in time.

## 5.3  Puerperal Infection

The disease caused by the infection of the reproductive system after labor is called puerperal infection or puerperal fever. The patient has a history of prolonged birth process, premature rupture of amniotic membrane and operative delivery, and the disease is marked by postpartum fever, local pain, profuse and stinking lochiorrhea (except the case of hemolytic streptococcus). Obstetric examination finds either red swelling and pain in the local region or tenderness in the uterus with thickened appendages. In TCM , puerperal infection is dealt with under the topic of "postpartum fever". It is considered to be a result of birth trauma and bleeding in labor which lead to the consumption of vital-$Qi$, or an outcome of careless nursing by which the toxic evil takes the opportunity to invade the uterus.

### Type and Treatment

#### 1. Domination of the toxic evil

**Clinical manifestations:** The case is characterized by chills and high fevers which may occur 24 hours to 10 days after labor and then persist without recession, or by pyrexia from the very beginning (The body temperature reaches 38.5℃ or even higher), by abdominal pain and tenderness profuse or scanty lochia which is purplish dark in color and purulent with foul odor, dysphoria, thirst, scarce and dark urines and dry stools. The tongue is reddened with yellowish coating. The pulse is rapid and forceful.

Therapeutic method: Clear away the toxic heat, cool the blood and remove blood stasis.

Recipe: *Wuwei Xiaodu Yin*(86),modified.

Ingredients:Flos Lonicerae    12 g

                Fructus Forsythiae    12 g

                Herba Taraxaci    12 g

                Herba Violae    9 g

                Herba Patriniae    12 g

                Caulis Sargentodoxae    12 g

                Radix Salviae Miltiorrhizae    30 g

                Radix Angelicae Sinensis    12 g

                Rhizoma Ligustici Chuanxiong    9 g

                Radix Paeoniae Rubra    15 g

                Olibanum Praeparata    9 g

                Myrrha Praeparata    9 g

                Radix Scrophulariae    12 g

                Rhizoma Corydalis    9 g

                Radix Glycyrrhizae    6 g

Decoct the above drugs in water to get 200—300 ml of decotion. Take one half of it in the morning and the other half in the evening.

Modification: In case of purulent lochia or reddish purulent leukorrhea, add

                Herba Houttuyniae    12 g

                Semen Coicis    30g.

The decoction of a dose is 200—300 ml. Take two doses daily.

### 2. Retention of toxic—heat in the uterus

**Clinical manifestations:** Severe pain in the lower abdomen, impeded lochia with foul odor, pyrexia and constipation. The tongue is purplish dark. The pulse is taut, rapid and uneven.

Therapeutic method: Clear away the toxic—heat and expel

the retention of pathogen by purgation.

Recipe: *Qingre Zhuyu Fang*

Ingredients:Radix Salviae Miltiorrhizae    30 g

Semen Persicae    9 g

Flos Carthami    9 g

Radix Angelicae Sinensis    12 g

Cortex Moutan Radicis    12 g

Radix Paeoniae Rubra    15 g

Fructus Aurantii    12 g

Pollen Typhae    15 g

Radix Sanguisorbae    12 g

Flos Lonicerae    12 g

Herba Taraxaci    9 g

Radix et Rhizoma Rhei    9 g

The decoction of a dose is 200—300 ml. Take two doses daily.

**3. Invasion of** *Ying Fen* **and** *Xue Fen* **by heat**

**Clinical manifestations:** High fever with perspiration, dysphoria and vague macular eruptions. The tongue is crimson with dry, yellowish fur. The pulse is taut, rapid and thready.

Therapeutic method: Expel the heat and toxic materials, cool the blood and replenish *Yin*

Recipe: *Qingying Tang*(55)

Ingredients:Radix Scrophulariae    12 g

Radix Rehmanniae    12 g

Radix Ophiopogonis    9 g

Flos Lonicerae    12 g

Fructus Forsythiae    12 g

Herba Lophatheri    9 g

Radix Salviae Miltiorrhizae    30 g

Rhizoma Coptidis     3 g

Cornu Rhinoceri (to be ground into powder and infused in the hot decoction)     1.5 g.

Cornu Rhinoceri can be replaced by Cornu Antelopis of the same amount. The decoction of a dose is 200 ml. Take it when cooled, 2 doses a day.

### 4. Invasion of the pericardium by heat

**Clinical manifestations:** Continuous high fever, stupor, delirium and in some cases even coma and unconsciousness. The patient has a pale complexion and cold limbs and a rapid pulse.

**Therapeutic method:** Remove the heat, replenish *Yin* and induce resuscitation with aromatics.

Recipe: *Qingying Tang*(55). See 5.3. The decoction of a dose is 200 ml. Take it at a time along with one bolus of *Angong Niuhuang Wan*(to be infused) or 3g of *Zixue Dan*.

**Other therapies**

(1)Infra-red radiation. It is applied to the infection of perineal wound.

(2)Incision and drainage. It is fit for the case of suppurative wound.

(3)*ShengjiGao*. It can be applied to the affected part where the pus has been removed from the wound. It helps to remove necrotic tissues and promote granulation. The wound will be healed quickly.

**Caution:**

Pay attention to antenatal care and prenatal hygiene. Sitz bath and sexual intercourses are forbidden in the third trimester of pregnancy.

Strict aseptic manipulation must be carried out in the course of delivery.

Antibiotic treatment must be offered to one who has premature rupture of amniotic membrane.

Avoid or reduce possible injuries to a small extent. In case it happens, the wound must be sutured timely, correctly and carefully.

Be mindful of puerperal care and keep the vulva clean and dry.

## 5.4    Late Puerperal Hemorrhage

If massive bleeding of the uterus occurs 24 hours after labor or during the puerperal period, the case is known as "late puerperal hemorrhage". In TCM, it is dealt with under the topics of "puerperal fainting" and "postpartum lochiorrhea". Detailed examination should be made to ascertain whether there are remnants of the placenta or fetal membranes. If the operative suture is conducted improperly, it should be rectified at once.

### Type and Treatment

#### 1. Exhaustion of *Qi* due to hemorrhea

**Clinical manifestations:** The case is marked by excessive blood loss after delivery and abrupt fainting. The patient has a pale complexion, rapid heart beat, chest and epigastric distress. She may gradually fall into coma with eyes closed and mouth open, and in some cases even with cold limbs and cold sweat. The tongue is pale with no coating. The pulse is either extremely faint or floating and empty. Obstetric examination finds that the womb is not well—recovered as the body of the uterus is large and soft with cervical relaxation and in some cases with perceivable remnants of the placenta and fetal membranes.

Therapeutic method: Supplement *Qi*, recuperate depleted *Yang* and rescue the patient from collapse.

Recipe:*Dushen Tang*(20)

Radix Ginseng     3—6 g.

Take the condensed decoction at a time.

Modification: In case of cold limbs and cold sweat, *Shen Fu Tang* should be adopted.

Radix Ginseng     3 g
Radix Aconiti Lateralis Praeparata     9 g

Boil the drugs into 100 ml of decoction, and take it at a time.

In case of persistent vaginal bleeding, the following drugs should be added to *Shen Fu Tang*:

Rhizoma Zingiberi Praeparata     9 g
Folium Artemisiae Argyi     9 g

**2. Blood stasis**

**Clinical manifestations:** The type is characterized by incessant bleeding after delivery, either massive or scarce, or by abrupt, voluminous discharge which is purplish dark in color and mixed with blood clots and in some cases with small pieces of tissues. The patient is characterized by abdominal pain and tenderness, a purplish dark face, lips and tongue and an uneven pulse. Obstetric examination finds that the body of the uterus is large and stiff with tenderness and the remnants of the placenta and fetal membranes are perceivable.

Therapeutic method: Promote blood circulation, eliminate blood stasis and arrest bleeding.

Recipe: *Shenghua Tang*(61) plus *Duoming San*(19)

Ingredients:  Radix Angelicae Sinensis     12 g

Rhizoma Ligustici Chuanxiong     9 g

Semen Persicae     9 g

Rhizoma Zingiberi Praeparata     6 g

Radix Glycyrrhizae Praeparata     6 g

Myrrha     9 g

Resina Draconis     3 g.

The decoction of a dose is 200 ml. Take it at a time, one dose a day.

Modification: In case of accompanying deficiency of *Qi*, add

Radix Codonopsis Pilosulae     30 g

Radix Astragali seu Hedysari     30 g.

In case of a reddened tongue with yellowish coating and a rapid pulse, deduct

Rhizoma Zingiberi Praeparata

but add

Radix Salviae Miltiorrhizae     30 g

Radix Scutellariae     9 g

Radix Sanguisorbae     12 g.

Proprietary

*Yunnan Baiyao*. Take one small tube of the powdered medicine at a time, twice a day. It is fit for the case of massive bleeding.

*Sanqi Pian*(Tabellae Radix Notoginsheng). Take 6−10 pills at a time, thrice a day. It is fit for profuse bleeding accompanied by abdominal pain and blood clots.

*Yimucao Gao*(Extractum Leonuri). Take 10 ml at a time, thrice a day.

**Caution**

After the removal of the placenta, examine carefully if there are remnants left. If any, it must be taken out timely. In the cesarean section, when a transverse incision is made in the lower uterine segment, if obviously active hemorrhagic spots are seen on both sides of the section, the appropriate treatment is to ligate them by operating forceps and silk sutures. Caution: Don't suture in bulks nor stitch too compactly, otherwise hematoma and necrosis may occur after the operation, preventing the wound from healing. Besides, anemia should be cured by improving the nutriture and infection should also be prevented.

## 5.5   Puerperal Heat-stroke

This is an acute febrile disease which results from the central thermotactic dysfunction due to the influences of the hot, humid environment on the parturient woman who has not recovered from postpartum debility yet. As a rule, this syndrome occurs in mid-summer, with early symptoms of general asthenia, dizziness, chest distress, nausea, thirst, profuse sweat and frequent micturition. If not treated in time, the patient will have a higher body temperature with a flushed face and dry skin and in severe cases she may even fall into coma, delirium and collapse. In TCM , this illness is discussed under the topic of "puerperal fever". By taking advantage of the postpartum asthenia of the lying-in wom-an, the morbid summer-heat invades into the body and consumes large quantities of *Qi* and fluid, thus leading to the exhaustion of *Yin*, abrupt stagnation of *Yang* and blockage of the channels. As a result, puerperal heat-stroke occurs.

## Type and Treatment

### 1. Early development of heat-stroke

**Clinical manifestations:** Dizziness, palpitation, chest distress, nausea, thirst, profuse sweat and general asthenia. The tongue is reddened with little coating. The pulse is rapid and thready.

Therapeutic method: Remove summer heat, replenish the vital-*Yin* and promote the secretion of body fluid.

Recipe: *Qingluo Ying*(52)

Ingredients:Exocarpium Citrulli 50 g

Flos Dolichoris Recens 30 g

Flos Lonicerae Recens 30 g

Herba Lophatheri Recens 9 g

Folium Nelumbinis Recens 9 g

Retinervus Luffae Fructus 12 g

Decoct the drugs in water to get 200-300 ml of decoction. Take it at a time, once a day.

Simple Recipes:

Eat a watermelon with a spoon

Mung bean 250 g

Decoct the beans in water and drink the soup at times.

### 2. Sudden attack of heat-evil

**Clinical manifestations:** High fever, flushed face, profuse sweat, thirst, dizziness and dysphoria. The longue is reddened. The pulse is either full and large, or rapid and slippery.

Therapeutic method: Remove summer heat from the body.

Recipe: *Qushu Fang*

Ingredients:Gypsum Fibrosum (to be decocted

first)      30 g

> Rhizoma Anemarrhenae      9 g
> Rhizoma Coptidis      6 g
> Talcum (to be ground into powder)      9 g
> Radix Scrophulariae      12 g
> Herba Agastachis      12 g
> Herba Eupatorii      9 g
> Folium Nelumbinis      6 g.

The decoction of a dose is 200—300 ml. Take half of it at a time, 2 doses a day.

For the case of stupor and delirium, *Angong Niuhuang Wan* plus *Shenxi Dan* should be given.

### 3. Impairment of *Yin* by heat—evil

**Clinical manifestations:** Feverish sensation, copious sweat, deep—colored urine, vexation, thirst, and debility. The tongue is reddened with little saliva. The pulse is either large and empty, or rapid and thready.

Therapeutic method: Expel summer—heat and reinforce *Qi*, replenish the vital essence and promote the production of body fluid.

Recipe: *Qingshu Yiqi Tang* (54)

Ingredients:Radix Panacis Quinquefolii      3 g
> (or Radix Pseudostellariae      15 g)
> Herba Dendrobil      9 g
> Radix Ophiopogonis      9 g
> Rhizoma Coptidis      3 g
> Herba Lophatheri      9 g
> Petiolus Nelumbinis      9 g
> Rhizoma Anemarrhernae      6 g

Semen Oxyzae Sativae     9 g

Exocarpium Citrulli     9 g

Radix Glycyrrhizae     6 g

The decoction of one dose for a day is 200—300ml. Take one half in the morning and the other half in the evening.

Modification: In case of dizziness, chest distress and a greasy fur, add

Herba Agastachis     9 g

Herba Eupatorii     9 g

Fructus Amomi     6 g

In case of pale complexion, rapid and thready pulse, add the following drugs to reinforce *Qi* and promote the production of body fluid:

*Shengmai San*(64)

Radix Ginseng

Radix Ophiopogonis

Fructus Schisandrae

In case of feverish convulsion, add *Qingying Tang* plus the drugs below to relieve spasms and alleviate the endogenous wind:

Ramulus Uncariae cum Uncis     9 g

Cornu Antelopis     3 g

Lumbricus     12 g

Bombyx Batryticatus     12 g

**Other therapies**

Acupuncture: For mild cases, needle the acupoints of Tazhui, Fengchi and zusanli. In emergency treatment, prick the fingers directly at *Shixuan* for blood—letting, accompanied by acupuncture at Renzhong and *Yongquan*.

Proprietaries

*Zhibao Dan.* Take one bolus (3g) with boiled water.

*Zixue Dan.* Take 1.5–3g at a time, with cooled boiled water once or twice a day. It is fit for the case of coma, convulsion and delirium.

*Huoxiang Zhengqi Shui.* Take 1–2 bottles at a time. It is fit for the mild case of heat–stroke.

**Caution**

Pay enough attention to personal hygiene during the puerperal stage. The living room should be ventilated, and the dressings and beddings appropriately provided in summer.

Once the symptom of heliosis occurs , the parturient must be shifted as quickly as possible to the fresh air. Provide her with enough drinks such as diluted saline waler, watermelon juice and mung–bean soup, and control the development of the disease in an effective way.

# 5.6  Other Postpartum Diseases

## 5.6.1 Lochiorrhea

If lochia persists in dripping for more than 20 days after labor, the case is known as "lochiorrhea". It may be caused by one of the following factors: the deficiency and hypofunction of *Qi* due to its excessive consumption and the loss of blood in the process of labor; the accumulation of damp–heat due to the blockage of blood stasis, the endogenous heat due to *Yin*–deficiency or stagnation of liver–*Qi*, leading to the asthenia of the *Chong* and *Ren* channels and their disturbance by heat–evil; the invasion of pathogenic cold into the uterus and its struggle with the blood, leading to blood stasis in the interior, or the remnants of the placenta influences the *Chong* and *Ren* channels, making the blood go astray. Hence, lochiorrhea results.

## Type and Treatment

### 1. *Qi*–Deficiency
**Clinical manifestations:** Lochia, pinkish, dilute and odorless, persisting longer than the normal date, copious or with incessant drippings. The patient looks weary and reserved, and has a pale complexion and a hollow sensation and tenesmus in the lower abdomen. The tongue is palish red with thin, whitish coating. The pulse is feeble and relaxed.

Therapeutic method: Tonify *Qi* and arrest bleeding.

Recipe: *Yiqi Shexue Tang*

Ingredients: Radix Pseudostellariae          30 g

Radix Astragali seu Hedysari          30 g

Rhizoma Atractylodis Macrocephalae          9 g

Rhizoma Dioscoreae          12 g

Radix Polygoni Multiflori          12 g

Fruclus Schisandrae          9 g

Radix Paeoniae Alba          15 g

Os Draconis Praeparata          30 g

Concha Os treae Praeparata          30 g

Herba Leonuri          30 g

Radix Glycyrrhizae Praeparata          9 g

Decoct the above drugs in water to get 200–300 ml of decoction. Prepare one dose for a day Take one half of it in the morning and the other half in the evening.

Modification: In case of accompanying lumbago and lassitude, add to the recipe

> Radix Dipsaci Praeparata　　30 g
>
> Colla Cornus Cervi (to be melt first and mixed into the decoction)　　12 g
>
> Folium Artemisiae Argyi Carbonisatiotis　　9 g

Proprietary: *Renshen Guipi Wan*. Take one bolus at a time, thrice a day.

### 2. Blood heat

**Clinical manifestations:** Lochia, crimson, viscid and thickened with foul odor, persisting longer than the normal date. The patient has a flushed face, dry throat, reddened tongue and rapid, thready pulse.

Therapeutic method: Remove the heat, nourish the kidney—*Yin* and arrest bleeding.

Recipe: *Baoyin Jian*(5), modified.

Ingredients:Radix Rehmanniae　　12 g

> Rhizoma Dioscoreae　　12 g
>
> Radix Paeoniae Alba　　12 g
>
> Radix Scutellariae　　9 g
>
> Radix Dipsaci　　15 g
>
> Herba Ecliptae　　12 g
>
> Cortex Moutan Radicis　　12 g
>
> Radix Glycyrrhizae　　6 g

The decoction of a dose is 200—300 ml. Take equal shares in the morning and evening.

Modification: In case of chest distress, dysphoria,a yellowish fur and taut, rapid pulse, *Dan Zhi Xiaoyao San* is applicable to soothe the depressed liver and to dispel heat from the blood, but the following drugs should be added to it:

Herba Ecliptae    12 g

Fructus Ligustri Lucidi    9 g

Radix Rubiae    12 g

Radix Rehmanniae    12 g

The decoction of a dose is 200—300 ml. Take one half in the morning and the other half in the evening.

### 3.Blood stasis

**Clinical manifestations:** Impeded lochia, incessant but scanty, purplish dark in color and mixed with blood clots. The patient feels fierce pain and tenderness in the lower abdomen . The tongue is purplish dark or dotted with ecchymoses on its margin. The pulse is taut, rough and forceful.

Therapeutic method: Invigorate the blood, remove blood stasis and arrest hemorrhage.

Recipe: *Shenghua Tang*(61)

Ingredients:  Radix Angelicae Sinensis    12 g

             Rhizoma Chuanxiong Ligustici    9 g

             Semen Persicae    9 g

             Rhizoma Zingiberi Praeparata    6 g

             Radix Glycyrrhizae Praeparata    6 g

The decoction of a dose is 200—300 ml. Take equal shares in the morning and evening.

Modification: In case of massive bleeding and drastic pain in the lower abdomen, add

Herba Leonuri    30 g

Pollen Typhae    12 g

Pollen Typhae Praeparata    12 g

Faeces Trogopterorum Praeparata    9 g

In case of abdominal tenesmus and pain, lassitude and listlessness, add

          Radix Codonopsis Pilosulae     30 g

          Radix Astragali seu Hedysari    30 g

In case of foul−odored lochia, add

          Herba Taraxaci     12 g

          Flos Lonicerae     12 g

          Cortex Moutan Radicis     12 g

          Fructus Forsythiae     12 g

Proprietaries

*Yimucao Gao.* Take 10 ml at a time after it is infused in water, thrice a day.

*Shenghua Tang Wan.* Take one bolus at a time, thrice a day.

## 5.6.2　Postpartum Constipation

If the parturient woman has difficulty and distress in defecation after labor or has no stools for several days, the symptom is known as　"postpartum constipation". It is caused either by the loss of blood in the sudden consumption of the *Ying*−blood and body fluid, or by the deficiency of *Yin* leading to the flaring−up of endogenous fire that exhausts the body fluid. As a result, the intestines cease to be moistened and nourished, and so the task of transportation is poorly carried out.

### Type and Treatment

**Clinical manifestations:** The case is characterized by troubles in defecation after childbirth with dry or no stools for several days. The patient is normal in appetite and has no abdominal distention or pain, but her face is sallow and her skin unmoistened. The tongue is pale with thin, whitish coating. The pulse is feeble and uneven.

Therapeutic method: Nourish the blood and promote the production of body fluid; moisten the bowels and relieve constipation.

Recipe: *Siwu Tang*(69), Augmented

Ingredients:Radix Angelicae Sinensis           12 g

Rhizoma Ligustici Chuanxiong           9 g

Radix Rehmanniae       12 g

Radix Rehmanniae Praeparata       12 g

Radix Paeoniae Alba       9 g

Semen Persicae       9 g

Semen Armeniacae Amarum       9 g

Fructus Cannabis       9 g

Fructus Trichosanthis       30 g

Radix Ophiopogonis       12 g

Rhizoma Polygonati       12 g

Radix Platycodi       9 g

Decoct the above drugs in water to get 200—300 ml of decoction. Prepare one dose for a day. Take one half of it in the morning and the other half in the evening.

Modification: In case of dyspnea, spontaneous perspiration, dizziness and listlessness, add

Radix Codonopsis Pilosulae       30 g

Radix Astragali seu Hedysari       30 g

In case of a dry throat, reddened and unmoistened tongue, rapid and thready pulse, add

Radix Scrophulariae     12 g

Herba Dendrobii     9 g

In case of chest fullness and abdominal distention, add

Fructus Aurantii     9 g

Cortex Magnoliae Officinalis     9 g

Fruc tus Crataegi     12 g

**Simple Recipe and Proved Prescription**

(1) Take proper amounts of white honey and sesame oil and mix them into 200 ml boiled water. Drink the prepared water before breakfast everyday till the defecation gets regular.

(2) *Ma Su Zhou*

Fructus Perillae     9 g

Semen Sesami     30 g

Crush them into pieces and cook them with glutinous rice into porridge.

(3) Infuse  3 g of Folium cassiae in heated water and drink it for tea.

**Caution**

Have some physical activities after labor to promote the intestinal peristalsis.

Take more vegetable, fruit and water.

## 5.6.3  Postpartum Pyrexia

If persistent fever is the main symptom accompanied by other symptoms emerging in the puerperal period, the symptom is termed "postpartum pyrexia". This illness may be caused by following factors: the retention of blood stasis after childbirth obstructs the flow of *Qi*, leading to the disharmony between *Ying* and *Wei*; by taking advantage of the time when blood channels are exhausted after labor and the striae of skin, muscles and viscera are not yet compact , external evils attack, resulting in the dysfunction of *Ying* and *Wei*; the excessive loss of blood in or after the process of delivery leads to the extreme scarcity of *Yin*—blood, which is so scarce that *Yang* has no place to abode and so it floats up to the exterior; owing to the injury and trauma at the time of delivery or as a result of careless nursing, the morbid toxics invade the uterus directly and spread over the whole body, giving rise to a fierce conflict between good and evil. Hence, postpartum pyrexia occurs. Clinically this illness must be carefully diagnosed and treated.

## Type and Treatment

### 1. Affection by exo—pathogenic factors
(1)Affected by wind—cold

**Clinical manifestations:** It is characterized by puerperal fevers with aversion to cold, headache, extremital pain, anhidrosis, and in some cases, also by cough and nasal watery discharge. The fur is thin and whitish. The pulse is floating.

Therapeutic method: Tonify the blood, dispel the wind—cold and get rid of exterior syndromes.

Recipe: *Jingfang Siwu Tang* (33)

Ingredients:Herba Schizonepetae          9 g
    Radix Ledebouriellae          9 g
    Radix Angelicae Dahuricae          12 g
    Radix Peucedani          9 g
    Rhizoma seu Radix Notopterygii          9 g

Radix Angelicae Sinensis     9 g

Rhizoma Ligustici Chuanxiong     6 g

Radix Paeoniae Alba     9 g

Radix Rehmanniae     9 g

Herba Menthae     6 g

Radix Platycodin     9 g

Decoct the above drugs in water to get 200—300 ml of decoction. Prepare one dose for a day. Take one half of it in the morning and the other half in the evening.

(2)  Affected by wind—heat

**Clinical manifestatons:** The case is marked by puerperal fever, slight aversion to wind—cold, headache, cough, thirst, slight perspiration or anhidrosis. The tip and margin of the tongue are reddened, with thin fur, either whitish or yellowish. The pulse is rapid and floating.

Therapeutic method: Dispel wind—heat and get rid of exterior syndromes by using cool—natured, pungent drugs.

Recipe: *Yinqiao San*(101)

Ingredients: Flos Lonicerae     12 g

Fructus Forsythiae     9 g

Herba Lophatheri     9 g

Spica Schizonepetae     9 g

Fructus Arctii     9 g

Herba Menthae     6 g

Radix Platycodi     9 g

Semen Sojae Preparatum     9 g

Rhizoma Phragmitis     9 g

Radix Glycyrrhizae     6 g

The decoction of one dose for a day is 300 ml. Take equal shares in the morning and evening.

(3)External evils dwelling in the *Shaoyang* channel

**Clinical manifestataions:** The case is marked by alternate attacks of chills and fever after labor, a dry throat with bitter taste, a whitish, moist fur and a taut pulse.

Therapeutic method: Compromise the exterior and interior and treat the syndrome in Shaoyang.

Recipe: *Xiao Chaihu Tang* (89)

Ingredients:Radix Bupleuri        9 g

Radix Scutellariae        9 g

Radix Codonopsis Pilosulae        12 g

Radix Glycyrrhizae        6 g

Rhizoma Zingiberis Recens        3 slices

Rhizoma Pinelliae Praeparata        12 g

Fructus Ziziphi Jujubae        5 dates

Decoct the drugs in water to get 200—300 ml of decoction. Prepare one does for a day . Take one half of it in the morning and the other half in the evening.

**2. Scarcity of blood**

**Clinical manifestations:** Excessive loss of blood after labor, mild fever, spontaneous sweating, dizziness, palpitation, insomnia, persistent abdominal pain and extremital numbness. The tongue is palish red, with thin, whitish fur. The pulse is feeble and slightly rapid.

Therapeutic method: Invigorate *Qi* and replenish the blood.

Recipe: *Yiqi Yangxue Qingre Fang*

Ingredients:Radix Pseudostellariae        15 g

Radix Astragali seu Hedysari        15 g

Rhizoma Polygonati        12 g

> Colla Corii Asini (to be infused)　　12 g
>
> Radix Angelicae Sinensis　　9 g
>
> Rhizoma Ligustici Chuanxiong　　6 g
>
> Radix Paeoniae Alba　　12 g
>
> Radix Rehmanniae　　12 g
>
> Radix Ophiopogonis　　9 g
>
> Herba Ecliptae　　12 g

The decoction of one dose for a day is 200—300 ml. Take equal shares in the morning and evening.

Modification: In case of hectic fever with flushed cheeks, thirst with preference for cold drinks, dry stools and deep—colored urines, a reddened tongue with thin, dry and yellowish coating, a rapid and thready pulse, add to the recipe.

> Radix Scrophulariae　　12 g
>
> Rhizoma Anemarrhenae　　6 g
>
> Cortex Lycii Radicis　　12 g
>
> Semen Biotae　　12 g

## 3.　Blood stasis

**Clinical manifestations:** Scanty or no lochia in purplish dark color and mixed with blood clots, abdominal pain and tenderness, thirst but no desire for drinks, a dark tongue specked or dotted with ecchymoses, a taut and uneven pulse.

Therpeutic method: Promote the blood flow and eliminate blood stasis.

Recipe: *Shenghua Tang*(61), augmented.

Ingredients:Radix Angelicae Sinensis　　15 g

> Rhizoma Ligustici Chuanxiong　　12 g
>
> Semen Persicae　　12 g
>
> Rhizoma Zingiberis Praeparata　　6 g

Radix Glycyrrhizae Praeparata     9 g
Herba Leonuri     30 g
Radix Salviae Miltiorrhizae     15 g
Cortex Moutan Radicis     9 g

4. Infection of morbid toxics (Same as puerperal infection, see 5.3).

## 5.6.4  Postpartum Pantalgia

If in the puerperal period the female feels sore, painful or numb in the body with weary limbs, the case is termed "postpartum pantalgia". The illness is chiefly caused by the destitution of blood after delivery which fails to nourish muscles and joints, so numbness or pain is felt. Besides, it may result from the invasion of wind—cold, leading to the obstruction of the flow of *Qi* and blood, or it is induced by consistent debility of the kidney, resulting in the impairment of the uterine collaterals.

### Type and Treatment

**1. Destitution of blood**

**Clinical manifestations:** Pantalgia with extremital soreness and numbness, dizziness and palpitation. The patient has a sallow complexion and unmoistened skin; she is short of breath and reserved in speaking. The pulse is feeble and thready.

Therapeutic method: Enrich the blood and replenish *Qi*, warm the channels, promote the flow of *Qi* and blood and relieve the pain.

Recipe:*Huangqi Guizhi Wuwu Tang*(29), modified

Ingredients:Radix Astragali seu Hedysari     15 g

Ramulus Cinnamomi        9 g

Radix Paeoniae Alba        12 g

Rhizoma Zingiberis Recens        3 slices

Fructus Ziziphi Jujubae        5 dates

Radix Angelicae Sinensis        12 g

Rhizoma Ligustici Chuanxiong        9 g

Caulis Spatholobi        12 g

Fructus Trichosanthis        12 g

Radix Gentianae Macrophyllae        9 g

Decoct the drugs in water to get 200—300 ml of decoction. Prepare one dose for a day. Take one half of it in the morning and the other half in the evening.

Modification: In case of severe lumbago, add to the recipe

Ramulus Loranthi        15 g

Radix Dipsaci        30 g

Fructus Psoraleae        12 g

In case of poor appetite and loose stools, add

Rhizoma Dioscoreae        12 g

Semen Dolichoris Album        12 g

Semen Coicis        30 g

In case of constipation, add

Herba Cistanchis        12 g

Fructus Cannabis        12 g

## 2. Invasion of wind—cold

**Clinical manifestations:** The case is characterized by general arthralgia and articular dyskinesia. The patient feels the articular pain shifting without fixed spots, sometimes so drastic as being pierced by an awl. In other cases, the patient is characterized by extremital swelling and numbness, dull sensation and difficult gait. The syndrome can be lessened by warmth. The tongue is light in color with thin, whitish fur. The pulse is thready and relaxed.

Therapeutic method: Nourish the blood, dispel the wind—cold and promote diuresis.

Recipe: *Duhuo Jisheng Tang*(18)

Ingredients:Radix Angelicae Pubescentis     9 g

           Ramulus Loranthi     15 g

           Radix Gentianae Macrophyllae    9 g

           Radix Ledebouriellae    9 g

           Herba Asari    3 g

           Rhizoma Angelicae Sinensis    12 g

           Radix Paeoniae Alba    12 g

           Rhizoma Ligustici Chuanxiong    6 g

           Radix Rehmanniae    9 g

           Cortex Eucommiae    12 g

           Radix Achyranthis Bidentatae    12 g

           Radix Codonopsis Pilosulae    15 g

           Poria    12 g

           Radix Glycyrrhizae    6 g

           Cortex Cinnamomi    6 g

The decoction of one dose for a day is 200—300 ml. Take one half in the morning and the other half in the evening.

Modification: In case of conspicuous dullness of limbs, deduct

           Radix Glycyrrhizae

           Radix Paeoniae Alba

           Radix Rehmanniae

but add

Rhizoma Atractylodis        9 g
Poria        12 g
Fructus Chaenomelis        12 g

## 3. Debility of the kidney

**Clinical manifestations:** The patient has sore loins, weak knees and aching heels after labor. The tongue is reddish, with thin, whitish coating. The pulse is deep and thready.

Therapeutic method: Tonify the kidney and strengthen the loins and knees.

Recipe: *Bushen Huoluo Fang*

Ingredients: Radix Aconiti Praeparata        6 g
Radix Dipsaci        30 g
Cortex Eucommiae        12 g
Fructus Psoraleae        15 g
Radix Rehmanniae Praeparata        12 g
Fructus Corni        9 g
Fructus Lycii        12 g
Fructus Chaenomelis        12 g
Radix Gentianae Macrophyllae        15 g
Herba Asari        3 g
Radix Glycyrrhizae Praeparata        9 g

The decoction of one dose for a day is 200—300 ml. Take equal shares in the morning and evening.

Modification: In case of cold pain in the loins and knees and watery leukorrhea, add

Cornu Cervi Degelatinatum        12 g

## 4. Blood stasis

**Clinical manifestations:** Postpartum general aching, articular dyskinesia, and in some cases accompanied by abdominal pain and impeded lochia. The tongue is dark in color or dotted with ecchymoses. The pulse is deep and uneven.

Therapeutic method: Promote blood flow in the channels, eliminate blood stasis and relieve the pain.

Recipe: *Shentong Zhuyu Tang*(68)

Ingredients:Semen Persicae        9 g

Flos Carthami        9 g

Radix Angelicae Sinensis        12 g

Rhizoma Ligustici Chuanxiong        6 g

Radix Gentianae Macrophyllae        12 g

Rhizoma seu Radix Notopterygii        9 g

Myrrha        9 g

Faeces Trogopterorum        9 g

Rhizoma Cyperi        12 g

Radix Achyranthis Bidentatae        15 g

Lumbricus        9 g

Radix Glycyrrhizae        6 g

The decoction of one dose for a day is 200−300 ml. Take one half in the morning and the other half in the evening.

**Caution**

The parturient woman should have sufficient nutrition and rest after delivery to recover the vital *Qi*, keep away from the wind and cold so as to prevent the invasion of external evils. Even in hot summer days, don't stay long in the cold environment lest the cold and dampness attack at the weakened body. One who has no operative injury should get out of bed 2−3 days after labor and have some physical activities to prevent the formation of blood stasis in the collaterals.

## 5.6.5    Agalactia

If the mother has little or no milk after labor, the symptom is termed "agalactia". In TCM , it is also known as insufficient lactation or no secretion of milk. As milk is transformed from blood, its flow depends on $Qi$ and both blood and $Qi$ are derived from food essence, so this illness is chiefly caused by the deficiency of $Qi$ and blood which results from the poor health and insufficiency of the source. Thus no milk is produced for feeding the infant. In other cases, the illness may be caused by the stagnation of the liver-$Qi$ and the resultant blockage of collaterals. So the mother's milk is unable to flow out. Clinically the deficiency syndrome is marked by soft breasts while the excess syndrome by hard breasts with distending pain.

### Type and treatment

#### 1. Deficiency of $Qi$ and blood
**Clinical manifestations:** The patient has only little, watery milk or no milk at all. She looks weary and gloomy, with soft breasts and poor appetite. The tongue is light in color, with little fur. The pulse is feeble and thready.

Therapeutic method: Enrich $Qi$ and replenish the blood, supported by promoting lactation.

Recipe: *Tongru Dan* (76)

Ingredients: Radix Codonopsis Pilosulae      15 g
            Radix Astragali seu Hedysari      15 g
            Radix Angelicae Sinensis      9 g
            Radix Ophiopogonis      12 g

Caulis Akebiae      6 g
(or Medulla Tetrapanacis      6 g
Radix Platycodi      9 g
Pig's foot 1 trotter

First cook the trotter in water and then decoct the drugs in the consomme. The decoction of one dose for a day is 200—300 ml. Take one half in the morning and the other half in the evening.

Modification: In case of obvious debility of the parturient, exchange Radix Codonopsis Pilosulae for Radix Ginseng in 3g. Decoct Ginseng separately and then mix the extract into the decoction.

In case of poor appetite and loose stools, add

Poria      12 g
Rhizoma Dioscoreae      12 g
Semen Dolichoris Album      15 g

### 2. Stagnation of the liver—$Qi$

Clinical manifestations: Little or no secretion of milk after child birth, hard and distending breasts, chest distress with mental depression and in some cases hard lumps are detectable. The patient may have mild fever and poor appetite. The tongue has a thin, yellowish fur. The pulse is either rapid or taut and thready.

Therapeutic method: Soothe the liver and relieve the depression; put through the collaterals and promote lactation.

Recipe:*Xiaru Yongquan San*(92)

Ingredients:Radix Angelicae Sinensis      12 g
Rhizoma Ligustici Chuanxiong      9 g
Radix Rehmanniae      12 g
Radix Paeoniae Alba      12 g
Radix Bupleuri      9 g

Pericarpium Citri Reticulatae Viride    9 g

Radix Trichosanthis    12 g

Semen Vaccariae    9 g

Squama Manitis Praeparata    15 g

Radix Rhapontici seu Echinopsis    9 g

Radix Platycodi    9 g

Caulis Akebiae    6 g

Medulla Tetrapanacis    6 g

Radix Angelicae Dahuricae    12 g

The decoction of the drugs for a day is 200—300 ml. take equal shares in the morning and evening.

Modification: In case of obvious chest distress and poor appetite, deduct

Radix Rehmanniae

Radix Trichosanthis

but add

Pericarpium Citri Reticulatae    9 g

Fructus Citri Sarcodactylis    9 g

In case of distending breasts with hard masses, deduct

Radix Rehmanniae

Radix Glycyrrhizae

but add

Spica Prunellae    12 g

Fructus Forsythiae    12 g

Retinervus Citri Reticulatae Fructus    12 g

Rhizoma Cyperi    12 g

In case of mild fever or a hot sensation in the breasts, add

Herba Taraxaci    9 g

Fructus Tribuli    12 g

Radix Scutellariae     9 g

Proprietary: *Xiaru Yongquan San* . Cook one parcel of drugs in water for a day's use to get 300ml of decoction. Take one half in the morning and the other half in the evening.

**Other therapies**

(1)Acupuncture: Take *Shanzhong* and *Rugen* as main acupoints and *Shaoze, Tianzong* and *Heka* as adjunct acupoints. (For details, see the volume on acupuncture).

(2)Dietotherapy: In case of deficiency of qi and blood, decoct

Caulis Spatholobi     30 g

Fructus Ziziphi Jujubae     10 dates

Ramulus Loranthi     12 g

in water. Drink 300 ml of decoction for tea. In the meantime, eat 30g of raw black sesame seeds.

(3)External treatment: Simmer a certain amount of tangerine peel in water and use the decoction for hot compress on the breasts. At the same time, scrape the breasts toward the nipples with a hair comb. This action will help the flow of *Qi* and blood and promote the secretion of milk.

**Caution**

The nipples should be kept clean and rhagades should be treated timely by applying vegetable oil to the affected region.

Lactation may start from the 12th hour after childbirth and is to be conducted regularly, 15–20 minutes at a time with the time interval of 3–4 hours. It is best to have the breast milk sucked up every time.

Be pleasant with ease at heart

Enjoy liquid diets of high nutrition and high calories and reject fried or pungent foods so as to secure the smooth flow of abundant milk supply.

## Appendix

1.Delactation:Fructus Hordei Germinatus Praeparata 100 g Fructus Crataegi 60 g are simmered in water and made into 200 ml of decoction. Take one dose daily. In addition, fill 500g of Natrii Sulfas equally into two cloth bags and use them as external compresses on both breasts after fixing them in position by broad strips of cloth.

2.In case of the acute mastitis which is marked by fevers with aversion to cold and breasts swollen with tenderness, the following recipe can be adopted.

Flos Lonicerae            12 g

Fructus Forsythiae        9 g

Fructus Arctii            12 g

Fructus Trichosanthis     15 g

Radix Trichosanthis       12 g

Radix Scutellariae        9 g

Pericarpium Citri Reticulatae Viride      9 g

Pericarpium Citri Reticulatae     9 g

Fructus Gardeniae         6 g

Spina Gleditsiae          9 g

Radix Bupleuri            9 g

Radix Glycyrrhizae        6 g

The decoction of a dose is 200 ml. Take one dose daily as it gets cool.

If there is no pus yet, apply crushed cactus on the affected region after removing its spines. If pus is already there, incise the affected part immediately for pus drainage.

3.Galactorrhea

If breast milk flows out spontaneously without the sucks of the infant, the case is termed 'galactorrhea'. This illness may be induced by the deficiency of $Qi$ and blood which manifests itself by scarce, watery milk and soft breasts without distention.

Therapeutic method: Invigorate $Qi$,enrich the blood and astringe the flow of milk.

Ingredients:Radix Pseudostellariae     15 g

                 Radix Astragali seu Hedysari     15 g

                 Rhizoma Dioscoreae Praeparata     12 g

                 Semen Euryales     12 g

                 Semen Nelumbinis     12 g

                 Fructus Corni     9 g

                 Fructus Schisandrae     9 g

                 Poria     12 g

                 Radix Glycyrrhizae Praeparata     6 g

The decoction of the drugs is 200 ml. Take one dose daily when it is still warm.

This illness may also result from the stagnation of the liver−$Qi$ which manifests itself by condensed milk, distending breasts, dysphoria and irritability, a reddened tongue with thin, yellowish fur and a taut, rapid pulse.

Therapeutic method: Soothe the liver and clear away pathogenic heat.

Ingredients: Radix Bupleuri     9 g

                 Radix Scutellariae     9 g

                 Radix Curcumae     9 g

                 Cortex Moutan Radicis     12 g

Fructus Gardeniae        9 g

Spica Prunellae        12 g

Concha Ostreae        30 g

Radix Scrophulariae        12 g

Herba Lophatheri        9 g

Radix Paeoniae Rubra        15 g

Caulis Akebiae        6 g

The decoction of the drugs is 200 ml. Take one dose daily as it gets cool.


## 5.6.6   Postpartum Paruria

The inability to urinate after labor, the frequent micturition and urinary incontinence are generally termed   "postpartum paruria". This illness is, in most cases, caused by consistent asthenia and the insufficiency of the lung—$Qi$ which becomes even more exhausted after delivery, thus leading to the hypofunction of the bladder. Besides, it may also be caused by deficiency of the kidney—$Qi$ that results in the dysfunction of the bladder in maintaining its normal water metabolism, or caused by injuries of the bladder in the operation of delivery.


### Type and Treatment

**1. Insufficiency of the lung—$Qi$**

**Clinical manifestations:** The cause is marked by inability to urinate with urgent distention in the lower abdomen, or by frequent micturition or urinary incontinence. The patient looks gloomy and reserved with short breaths and weak knees. The tongue is light in color with little fur. The pulse is feeble and relaxed.

Therapeutic method: Replenish *Qi* and promote diuresis.

Recipe: *Yiqi TongPao Ying*

|  |  |
| --- | --- |
| Radix Pseudostellariae | 30 g |
| Radix Astragali seu Hedysari | 30 g |
| Rhizoma Atractylodis Macrocephalae | 9 g |
| Rhizoma Dioscoreae | 12 g |
| Radix Aucklandiae | 9 g |
| Fructus Aurantii | 12 g |
| Radix Platycodi | 9 g |
| Poria | 12 g |
| Medulla Tetrapanacis | 6 g |
| Herba Plantaginis | 9 g |

Decoct the drugs in water to get 200—300 ml of decoction. Take one half of it in the mornig and the other half in the evening.

Modification: In case of frequent micturition and urinary incontinence, add

|  |  |
| --- | --- |
| Fructus Alpiniae Oxyphyllae | 9 g |
| Fructus Rosae Laevigatae | 9 g |
| Fructus Schisandrae | 9 g |

## 2. Deficiency of the kidney—*Qi*

**Clinical manifestations:** The case is characterized by inability to urinate with distending pain in the lower abdomen, or by frequent micturition or enuresis . The patient looks dim with sore loins and weak knees. The tongue is light in color with moist fur. The pulse is deep, slow and thready.

Therapeutic method:Tonify the kidney and warm *Yang*,activate vital energy and promote diuresis.

Recipe: *Shenqi Wan*(66)

Ingredients:Radix Rehmanniae          12 g

Rhizoma Dioscoreae          12 g

Fructus Corni          9 g

Poria          12 g

Cortex Moutan Radicis          9 g

Rhizoma Alismatis          9 g

Cortex Cinnamomi          6 g

Radix Aconiti Lateralis          9 g

The decoction of one dose for a day is 200—300 ml. Take one half in the morning and the other half in the evening.

Modification: In case of frequent micturition or urinary incontinence, add

Oötheca Mantidis          12 g

Fructus Rubi          12 g

Fructus Psoraleae          15 g

Os Draconis          30 g

Concha Ostreae Praeparata          30 g

### 3. Injury of the bladder

**Clinical manifestations:** The case is characterized by uncontrollable enuresis or urinary drippings mixed with blood threads. The fur is normal .The pulse is slow.

Therapeutic method: Invigorate $\hat{Q}i$ and cure the bladder.

Recipe: *Huangqi Danggui San* (28), augmented.

Ingredients:Radix Astragali seu Hedysari          30 g

Radix Angelicae Sinensis          12 g

Radix Ginseng          15 g

Rhizoma Atractylodis Macrocephalae          15 g

Radix Paeoniae Alba          15 g

Radix Glycyrrhizae     9 g
Rhizoma Zingiberis Recens     6 g
Fructus Ziziphi Jujubae 3 dates
Pig's Bladder 1 bladder
Rhizoma Bletillae     12 g

The decoction of a dose is 200—300 ml. Take one dose daily.

The patient should lie in bed for the whole period of treatment. In case of protracted enuresis and resultant urnary fistula, careful examination must be made so as to carry on operative repair of the bladder properly.

**Other therapies**

(1)Acupuncture and moxibustion. Select the acupoints of *Kuanyuan, Qihai, Sanyinjiao, Yinling Quan* and *Shuidao*.

(2) Induction of urination: Fumigate and wash the vulva with hot water, or douche the surroundings of the orifice of urethra to induce urination.

(3) Hot compress: Place a hot—water bag on the lower abdomen to promote the contraction of the bladder and the excretion of the urine.

# 6.  Miscellaneous Gynecopathy

## 6.1  Hysteromyoma

This illness is a sort of benign tumors which are commonly seen in the female reproductive system. It is characterized by profuse menstruation, prolonged menstrual cycle and abdominal distention with a sensation of tenesmus. In some cases, no signs can be found except in time of bodily examination.In TCM, hysteromyoma falls into the category of *Zhengj i a*,which means "abdominal mass". Its formation is concerned with the asthenia of vital *Qi* and its derangement with the blood. In most cases,it results from the stagnation of *Qi* or the retention of blood stasis or the accumulation of phlegm—dampness. The longer the pathogenic factor persists, the larger the mass will be.

### Type and Treatment

#### 1. *Qi*–Stagnation
**Clinical manifestations:** Abdominal mass which can be moved by pushing, with changing, unsettled pain, accompanied by distending distress in the lower abdomen. The fur is thin and moist, the pulse is deep and taut. Gynecological examination finds that the uterus is expanded, stiff in texture and rugged on its surface.

Therapeutic method:Promote the flow of *Qi*  and get rid of its stagnation; activate the blood and eliminate the mass.

Recipe: *Xiang Leng Wan*(91)

Ingredients: Radix Aucklandiae      9g

     Flos Caryophylli      6g

     Rhizoma Sparganii      9g

     Fructus Aurantii      12g

     Pericarpium Citri Reticulatae Viride      9g

     Fructus Foeniculi      6g

     Rhizoma Zedoariae      9g

     Fructus Meliae Toosendan Praeparata      12g

Decoct the drugs in water to get 200—300 ml of decoction. Prepare one does for a day .Take one half in the morning and the other half in the evening.

Modification: In case of scanty or delayed menstruation, add

     Radix Angelicae Sinensis      12g

     Rhizoma Ligustici Chuanxiong      9g

In case of severe abdominal pain which can be abated by the discharge of blood clots, add

     Herba Leonuri      30g

     Pollen Typhae      12g

     Faeces Trogopterorum Praeparata      9g

## 2. Blood Stasis

**Clinical manifestations:** Abdominal mass which is solid in texture and fixed in position, accompanied by abdominal pain and tenerness. The patient has a gloomy complexion or her face is marked by chloasma. Her skin is dry and unmoistened. She is thirsty but has little desire to drink. The case may also manifest itself by massive or delayed menses, or by incessant drippings of vaginal bleeding which looks purplish dark and is mixed with blood clots. The patient feels abdominal pain in the menstrual period which can be lessened by discharging of blood stasis. The tongue is purplish dark, with ecchymoses on its margin. The pulse is deep and uneven. Gynecological examination has the same discovery as that in the case of *Qi*-stagnation.

Therapeutic method:Promote the circulation of blood, expel blood stasis, and resolve the hard mass.

Recipe: *Huoyu Sanjie Fang*

Ingredients:Ramulus Cinnamomi     9g

           Semen Persicae     9g

           Radix Angelicae Sinensis     12g

           Rhizoma Ligustici Chuanxiong     9g

           Radix Paeoniae Rubra     12g

           Fructus Aurantii.     15g

           Radix Cyathulae     15g

           Radix Salviae Miltiorrhizae     30g

           Rhizoma Sparganii     9g

           Rhizoma Zedoariae     12g

           Spica Prunellae     12g

           Concha Ostreae     30g

The decoction of one dose for a day is 200—300 ml. Take equal shares in the morning and evening.

Modification: In case of copious menses mixed with blood clots and accompanying abdominal pain, deduct

           Spica Prunellae

           Concha Ostreae

but add

           Pollen Typhae     12g

           Faeces Trogopterum Praeparata     9g

In case of pesistent metrorrhagia, deduct

Rhizoma Sparganii

Rhizoma Zedoariae

but add

Radix Pseudostellariae    15g

Radix Notoginseng (to be infused in hot
decoction)    3 g

In case of delayed menstruation or amenorrhea with abdominal pain, add

Sanguis Draconis (to be infused)    3 g

Herba Lycopi    12 g

### 3. Phlegm—dampness

**Clinical manifestations:** Abdominal mass which is not so hard in texture, scarce and delayed menses or amenorrhea, fairly massive leukorrhea which is whitish and viscid, chest distress and aversion to cold. The tongue is purplish dark with whitish, greasy fur. The pulse is either soft and thready or deep and slippery.

Therapeutic method: Regulate the flow of *Qi*, dispel phlegm—dampness and resolve the abdominal mass.

Recipe:*Kaiyu Erchen Tang*(36)

Ingredients:Pericarpium Citri Reticulatae Viride    9 g

Pericarpium Citri Reticulatae    9 g

Rhizoma Cyperi    12 g

Rhizoma Ligustici Chuanxiong    6 g

Radix Aucklandiae    9 g

Semen Arecae    12 g

Rhizoma Pinelliae Praeparata    12 g

Rhizoma Atractylodis    12 g

Radix Glycyrrhizae    6 g

Rhizoma Zingiberis Recens    3 slices

                    Poria      12 g
                    Rhizoma Zedoariae    12 g
The decoction of one dose for a day is 200—300 ml. Take equal
shares in the morning and evening.
        Modification: In case of scarce menses or amenorrhea, add
                    Radix Salviae Miltiorrhizae    30 g
                    Radix Cyathulae    15 g
    In case of chest distress, nausea and anorexia, add
                    Endothelium Corneum Gigeriae Galli    12 g
                    Massa Medicata Fermentata    30 g
                    Fructus Crataegi    30 g
but deduct Rhizoma Zedoariae from the recipe
        In case of yellowish, viscid and foul—odored leukorrhea, de-
duct
                    Rhizoma Pinelliae Praeparata
but add
                    Radix Sophorae Flavescentis    30 g
                    Radix Gentianae    12 g
    Proprietaries:
    *Qizhi Xiangfu Wan*, Take one bolus at a time, thrice a day. It
is fit for the stagnation of *Qi* and blood stasis.
    *Daihuang Zhechong Wan*. Take one bolus at a time, thrice a
day. It is fit for blood stasis caused by exaberant pathogens.

## 6.2    Endometriosis

    If endometrial tissues emerge outside the uterine cavity, the
symptom is termed "Endometriosis". It is characterized by secondary,progressive dysmenorrhea, irregular menstruation and

sterility. In TCM, it is discussed under the topics of *Tong jing* (dysmenorrhea), *Beng Lou* (metrorrhagia and metrostaxis), *Zhengjia* (abdominal mass) and *Bu Yun* (sterility). This illness is caused by impeded flow of *Qi* and blood, leading to the obstruction of the *Chong* and *Ren* channels and dysfunction of the uterus.

## Type and Treatment

This disease is commonly caused by the stagnation of *Qi* and blood stasis.

**Clinical manifestations:** Abdominal pain starting from 1-2 days preceding the menstrual cycle, drastic pain on the first day of menstruation which is aggravated progressively year by year; the pain in the lower abdomen and lumbo-sacral region which radiates to the perineum, the anus or the thighs; copious menses or prolonged menstrual cycle with incessant drippings of bleeding; a case history of sterility. The tongue is purplish dark with thin, either whitish or yellowish fur. The pulse is either deep and taut or uneven.

Gynecological examination finds purplish blue nodes in the posterior fornix of the vagina or in the uterine cervix, with the uterus retroversed, adhered and fixed, and with its activity restricted. On the posterior uterine wall, in the retrouterine excavation and uterosacral ligament, bean-like, hard-textured nodes can be touched with obvious tenderness; in the appendicular region in active cystic mass is perceivable with mild tenderness when pressed.

Therapeutic method: Promote blood circulation and get rid

of blood stasis.

Recipe: *Gexia Zhuyu Tang*(25)

Ingredients:
| | |
|---|---|
| Radix Angelicae Sinensis | 12 g |
| Faeces Trogopterorum Praeparata | 9 g |
| Rhizoma Ligustici Chuanxiong | 9 g |
| Radix Paeoniae Rubra | 12 g |
| Semen Persicae | 9 g |
| Flos Carthami | 9 g |
| Fructus Aurantii | 12 g |
| Rhizoma Corydalis | 9 g |
| Cortex Moutan Radicis | 12 g |
| Rhizoma Cyperi | 12 g |
| Radix Linderae | 12 g |
| Radix Glycyrrhizae | 6 g |

Decoct the drugs in water to get 200—300 ml of decoction for a day's dose. Take one half of it in the morning and the other half in the evening.

Modification: In case of listlessness and poor appetite, deduct Faeces Trogopterorum Praeparata but add to the recipe

| | |
|---|---|
| Radix Codonopsis Pilosulae | 30 g |
| Radix Astragali seu Hedysari | 30 g |

In case of cold pain in the lower abdomen which can be relieved by warmth, deduct.

Cortex Moutan Radicis

Radix Paeoniae Rubra

but add

| | |
|---|---|
| Fructus Foeniculi | 9 g |
| Fructus Evodiae | 9 g |

In case of sterility due to obstruction of the oviduct, add

>           Herba Speranskiae Tuberculatae        12 g
>           Squama Manitis        15 g
>           Spina Gleditsiae        9 g

**Other therapies**

Medicated enema by using traditional Chinese drugs:

>           Radix Salviae Miltiorrhizae        30 g
>           Rhizoma Ligustici Chuanxiong        9 g
>           Rhizoma Sparganii        9 g
>           Rhizoma Zedoariae        9 g
>           Resina Olibani Praeparata        12 g
>           Myrrha        12 g
>           Flos Carthami        9 g
>           Sanguis Draconis        3 g

Decoct the above drugs into 150—200 ml of decoction. Inject the liquid into the colon through the anus as its temperature drops to 37℃. The operation is done before night sleep.

**Caution**

The stricture of the cervix and the excessive retroflexion of the uterus must be rectified so as to prevent the countercurrent of the menses caused by blood stasis.

Avoid unnecessary pelvioscopy during the menstrual period. Avoid the implantation of endometria caused by manipulations in the surgical operation.

# 6.3   Sterility

If a newly—married couple live together for 2 years, and the reproductive function of the husband is normal and no contraceptive means is taken, the female should have become pregnant. If it is not the case, primary sterility should be considered. If the female is no more conceived over 2 years after labor or abortion, it is known as secondary sterility.

This section does not deal with the congenital deformity of the female reproductive organs such as *Wubunu( Luo, Wun, Gu, Jiao and Mai)*. In ancient Chinese classics of medicine, there were five types of female sterility, i.e. the spiral stria of the vulva, the stricture of the vagina, imperforate hymen, elongated clitoris, amenorrhea or menoxenia.

As the kidney controls reproduction, so sterility is most closely connected with it. Clinically, this illness is in most cases caused by the congenital deficiency of the kidney—*Qi*, the destitution of the vital essence and the blood. In some other cases,it may be induced by stagnation of the liver—*Qi*, leading to its abnormal flow, or by the derangement between *Qi* and blood and the paucity of the *Chong* and *Ren* channels. Besides,the retention of excessive dampness in the uterus due to the hypofunction of the spleen—*Yang*, and the blood stasis caused by pathogenic cold from the external world may also result in sterility.

## Type and Treatment

### 1. Deficiency of the kidney
(1)*Yang*—deficiency

**Clinical manifestations:** This type is characterized by acyesis long after marriage, delayed menstruation which is scanty and light—colored, or occasional and in severe cases even reduced to amenorrhea. The patient has a gloomy complexion, sore loins and weak knees, and is indifferent to sexual activity. The leukorrhea is cold, watery and incessant, either profuse or scarce with a dry sensation in the vulva and a cold sensation in the lower abdomen. This type is also manifested by loose stools, and copious, clear urines especially in the night. The tongue is light in color with thin, whitish fur. The pulse is deep, either slow or thready.

Gynecological examination frequently discovers the maldevelopment of the uterus.

Therapeutic method: Warm *Yang* and tonify the kidney; nourish the blood and regulate menstruation.

Recipe: *Yishen Yangxue Tiaochong Fang*

Ingredients:Herba Epimedii    12 g

           Fluoritum    30 g

           Radix Morindae Officinalis    9 g

           Radix Dipsaci    15 g

           Cornu Cervi Degelatinatum    12 g

           Pericarpium Zanthoxyli    1.5 g

           Fructus Lycii    12 g

           Radix Angelicae Sinensis    12 g

           Rhizoma Ligustici Chuanxiong    9 g

           Radix Paeoniae Alba    12 g

           Radix Rehmanniae Praeparata    9 g

           Radix Aucklandiae    9 g

Decoct the drugs in water to get 200—300 ml of decoetion. Take one half of it in the morning and the other half in the evening but not in the menstrual period.Prepare one dose for a day.

Modification: In case of short breath and listlessness with a sensation of tenesmus in the lower abdomen, add

                Radix Codonopsis Pilosulae        30 g
                Radix Astragali seu Hedysari       30 g
In case of cold and incessant discharges from the vagina, add
                Semen Euryales         12 g
                Fructus Rosae Laevigatae        9 g
In case of copious urines and nocturia, add
                Fructus Alpiniae Oxyphyllae        9 g
                Oötheca Mantidis        12 g
                Os Draconis         30 g

(2) Yin—deficiency

**Clinical manifestations:** The type is manifested by acyesis long after marriage, preceded menstruation which is scanty and crimson without blood clots. The patient looks lean and meager, with sore loins and weak knees. The illness is also characterized by dizziness palpitation, insomnia, thirst and low fever in the afternoon. dysphoria with a feverish sensation in the chest, palms and soles. The tongue is reddened with little coating. The pulse is rapid and thready.

Therapeutic method: Enrich *Yin* and nourish the blood, clear away the heat and regulate menstruation.

Recipe: *Liuwei Dihuang Tang,*(41) modified

Ingredients: Radix Rehmanniae        15 g
                Fructus Corni        9 g
                Rhizoma Dioscoreae         12 g
                Cortex Moutan Radicis        12 g
                Rhizoma Alismatis        9 g
                Cortex Lycii Radicis        9 g
                Radix Angelicae Sinensis        9 g
                Radix Paeoniae Alba        15 g

Herba Ecliptae          24 g
Fructus Ligustri Lucidi      9 g
Flos Carthami      9 g
Radix Dipsaci      30 g

The decoction of one dose for a day is 200—300 ml. Take equal shares in the morning and evening.

Modification: In case of thirst and unmoistened fur, add

Radix Scrophulariae      12 g
Rhizoma Anemarrhenae      6 g
Radix Ophiopogonis      9 g

In case of dysphoria and sleeplessness, add

Semen Biotae      9 g
Fructus Schisandrae      9 g
Semen Ziziphi Spinosae Praeparata      30 g

Proprietary: *Liuwei Dihuang Wan*,Take one bolus at a time, twice a day.

**2. Stagnation of the liver—*Qi***

**Clinical manifestations:** Acyesis long after marriage, irregular menstrual cycle, abdominal pain in the premenstrual and menstrual periods, and impeded flow of the menses. The bleeding is scarce, dark in color and mixed with clots. The illness also manifests itself by mental depression, restlessness and irritability and distending pain in the chest and breasts prior to the menstruation. The tongue is normal or dark red with thin, whitish fur. The pulse is taut.

Therapeutic method: Relieve the depressed liver to enrich the blood and regulate menstruation.

Recipe: *Shuyu Tiaojing   Tang*

Ingredients:Radix Bupleuri      9 g

Radix Curcumae    9 g

Fructus Meliae Toosendan    12 g

Rhizoma Cyperi    12 g

Radix Angelicae Sinensis    9 g

Rhizoma Ligustici Chuanxiong    6 g

Radix Paeoniae Alba    9 g

Radix Rehmanniae    12 g

Fructus Mori    12 g

Fructus Aurantii    12 g

Herba Leonuri    15 g

The decoction of one dose for a day is 200—300 ml. Take equal shares in the morning and evening.

Modification: In case of breast pain and distention in the premenstrual period and gelosis in the breasts, add

Spica Prunellae    12 g

Semen Citri Reticulatae    9 g

Fructus Liquidambaris    9 g

Concha Ostreae    30 g

In case of scanty menstruation which is hard to dislodge and accompanied by severe abdominal pain, add

Rhizoma Zedoariae    12 g

Rhizoma Corydalis    9 g

Pollen Typhae    15 g

but deduct Radix Rehmanniae and Fructus Mori.

In case of a reddened tongue with yellowish fur and a taut, rapid pulse, deduct Fructus Mori but add

Cortex Moutan Radicis    12 g

Fructus Gardeniae    9 g

Radix Scrophulariae    12 g

Proprietary:

　　*Xiaoyao Wan.*Take 6—9g at a time, twice a day.

　　*Qizhi Xiangfu Wan,*Take one bolus at a time, twice a day.

## 3. Retention of phlegm—dampness

**Clinical manifestations:** Acyesis long after marriage, delayed menstruation which is scanty and in severe cases even reduced to amenorrhea, profuse and viscid leukorrhea. The patient looks pale and plump, accompanied by dizziness, palpitation, chest distress and nausea. The fur is whitish and greasy. The pulse is slippery.

Therapeutic method: Dispel phlegm—dampness, regulate the flow of *Qi* and readjust menstruation.

Recipe: *Zaoshi Huotan Fang*

Ingredients: Rhizoma Atractylodis Praeparata　　9 g

　　　　　　Rhizoma Atractylodis Macrocephalae

　　　　　　Praeparata　　9 g

　　　　　　Concretio Silicea Bambusae　　9 g

　　　　　　Rhizoma Pinelliae Praeparata　　12 g

　　　　　　Relinervus Citri Fructus　　9 g

　　　　　　Pollen Typhae　　12 g

　　　　　　Rhizoma Zedoariae　　9 g

　　　　　　Rhizoma Acori Graminei　　9 g

　　　　　　Arisaema cum Bile Praeparata　　9 g

　　　　　　Fructus Aurantii　　9 g

　　　　　　Caulis Bambusae in Taeniam　　9 g

　　　　　　Poria　　12 g

The decoction of one dose for a day is 200—300 ml. Take equal shares in the morning and evening.

Modification: In case of short breaths and profuse leukorrhea, add

           Radix Codonopsis Pilosulae       15 g
           Radix Astragali seu Hedysari      15 g
           Radix Paeoniae Alba Praeparata     15 g
In case of scarce, delayed menses, add
           Herba Epimedii        12 g
           Radix Dipsaci          30 g
           Radix Angelicae Sinensis     12 g

### 4. Blood stasis

**Clinical manifestations:** Acyesis long after marriage, delayed menstruation which is scarce, purplish dark in color and mixed with blood clots, accompanied by abdominal pain and tenderness which can be alleviated after discharge of blood clots. The tongue is purplish dark in color or specked with ecchymoses on its margin. The pulse is taut and uneven. Pelvic inflammation is often found in gynecological examination.

Therapeutic method: Promote blood circulation, eliminate blood stasis and regulate menstruation.

Recipe: *Tao Hong Siwu Tang*,(75) modified

Ingredients: Semen Persicae        9 g
           Flos Carthami          9 g
           Radix Angelicae Sinensis      12 g
           Rhizoma Ligustici Chuanxiong      9 g
           Radix Paeoniae Rubra       15 g
           Radix Paeoniae Alba        15 g
           Rhizoma Zedoariae        12 g
           Rhizoma Corydalis         6 g
           Radix Linderae          12 g

Rhizoma Cyperi          12 g

Radix Salviae Miltiorrhizae          30 g

The decoction of one dose for a day is 200–300 ml. Take equal shares in the morning and evening.

Modification: In case of abdominal pain which can be abated by warmth, add

Fructus Foeniculi          9 g

Folium Artemisiae Argyi          9 g

In case of obstructed oviduct, add

Spina Gleditsiae          9 g

Herba Speranskiae Tuberculatae          12 g

Squama Manitis Praeparata          15 g

In case of pelvic inflammation and resultant frequent abdominal pain, add

Caulis Spatholobi          15 g

Fructus Forsythiae          12 g

Rhizoma Sparganii          9 g

## 5. Paucity of *Qi* and blood

**Clinical manifestations:** Acyesis long after marriage, delayed menstruation which is scanty, watery and light in color, and in some cases amenorrhea. The patient has a sallow complexion, dry and sapless eyes, poor appetite, and is also marked by dizziness, palpitation, lassitude and listlessness. The tongue is light in color with thin, whitish coating. The pulse is feeble and thready. The maldevelopment of the uterus is often found in gynecological examination.

Therapeutic method: Replenish *Qi*, enrich the blood and readjust menstruation.

Recipe: *Yulin Zhu*, (98) modified

Ingredients:Radix Codonopsis Pilosulae      15 g

Radix Astragali seu Hedysari      15 g

Rhizoma Atractylodis Macrocephalae

Praeparata      9 g

Poria      9 g

Radix Angelicae Sinensis      9 g

Rhizoma Ligustici Chuanxiong      9 g

Radix Rehmanniae Praeparata      12 g

Radix Paeoniae Alba      12 g

Colla Corii Asini (to be infused in hot decoction)

12 g

Semen Cuscutae      12 g

Pericarpium Zonthoxyli      1.5 g

Herba Epimedii      12 g

The decoction of a dose is 200—300 ml. Take equal shares in the morning and evening.

Modification: In case of scanty leukorrhea, unmoistened vulva and indifference to sexual activity, add to the recipe

Placenta Hominis      30 g

Cornu Cervi Degelatinatum      12 g

In case of dull pain in the lower abdomen during the menstrual cycle , add

Caulis Spatholobi      12 g

Herba Leonuri      15 g

Proprietary: *Shiquan Dabu Wan*. Take one bolus at a time, twice a day.

**Other therapies**

(1)Add 4 ml injection of ligustrazine into 10 ml sterilized water for injection and drive the liquid slowly into the uterine cavity every other day, starting from 3–5 days after the end of menstruation up to the preovulatory phase. One course of treatment consists of 3–4 injections. It is fit for the blockage of the oviduct.

(2)For the treatment of sterility caused by pelvic inflammation and obstructed oviduct, use 10 ml injection of Radix Salviae Miltiorrhizae for intravenous drips everyday after mixing it with 500 ml glucose injection. One course of treatment lasts for 10 days.

(3)Decoction of Chinese drugs used for retention–enema.

Radix Salviae Miltiorrhizae     30 g
Flos Carthami     12 g
Ramulus Cinnamomi     9 g
Herba Speranskiae tuberculatae     15 g
Caulis Spatholobi     15 g
Olibanum     9 g
Myrrha     9 g

The decoction of a dose is 100 ml. Apply the liquid for enema before night sleep, except in the menstrual period. One course of treatment lasts for 10 day. It is fit for all sorts of obstruction and pain.


## 6.4 Prolapse of the Uterus

If the female's uterus slips out of place or the vaginal wall expands out, the illness is generally termed *Yin Ting*(Prolapse of the uterus) in TCM, metroptosis is diagnosed according to the extent that the uterus falls down from its normal position and sinks along the vagina: whether the external cervical orifice descends lower than the spines of ischium or in severe cases the whole uterus drops out of the vaginal orifice. The pathogenesis of the illness is chiefly due to the fact that birth trauma has not been repaired in time or the parturient takes part in heavy physical work immediately after labor, thus resulting in the sinking of *Qi* and the deficiency of the kidney and consequently impairing the uterine collaterals which fail to keep the uterus high in its normal position. The illness may be caused by various elements: spending strength too early for delivery, dystocia, prolonged process of labor, spending too much strength in labor, taking part in physical work too early or too vigorously, or lingering cough, constipation, consistent debility, intemperance in sexual activity, multiparity, etc.

## Type and Treatment

### 1.*Qi*—Deficiency

**Clinical manifestations:** It is chiefly marked by metroptosis which may be aggravated by fatiguing work. The patient has a sensation of tenesmus in the lower abdomen. She looks weary and reserved, with short breaths and weak limbs, having frequent urines and copious leukorrhea which is whitish and watery. The tongue is light in color with thin fur. The pulse is feeble and thready.

Therapeutic method: Replenish *Qi* and elevate the uterus.

Recipe: *Buzhong Yiqi Tang* (7) See 5.6.1 for the prescription.

Modification: In case of sore loins and copious, watery leukorrhea, add

                Radix Dipsaci        30 g
                Fructus Rosae Laevigatae        12 g
                Semen Euryales        9 g

## 2. Debility of the kidney

**Clinical manifestations:** Metroptosis, sore loins, weak knees, frequent urines, nocturia, dizziness and tinnitus, a palish red tongue and a deep, feeble pulse.

Therapeutic method: Tonify the kidney and strengthen the channels of the uterus.

Recipe: *Dabuyuan Jian*, (13) modified

Ingredients: Radix Rehmanniae Praeparata        12 g

                Rhizoma Dioscoreae        12 g

                Fructus Corni        12 g

                Poria        9 g

                Fructus Lycii        12 g

                Cortex Eucommiae        12 g

                Radix Dipsaci        15 g

                Fructus Rosae Laevigatae        12 g

                Colla Cornus Cervi (to be infused in hot
                decoction)        12 g

                Semen Euryales        9 g

                Radix Astragali seu Hedysari        15 g

The decoction of one dose for a day is 200—300 ml. Take one half in the morning and the other half in the evening.

## 3. Damp—heat

**Clinical manifestations:** Part of the uterus that has slipped out of the vaginal orifice is reddened, swollen and ulcerated with incessant drippings of yellowish fluid. The leukorrhea is profuse, yellowish in color or mixed with pus and blood and stinking in odor, accompanied by fever and thirst, deep—colored urines and local burning pain. The tongue is reddened with yellowish, greasy coating. The pulse is rapid.

Therapeutic method: Dispel damp—heat.

Recipe:*Longdan Xiegan Tang* (38)

Ingredients:Radix Gentianae          9 g

Fructus Gardeniae          9 g

Radix Scutellariae          9 g

Semen Plantaginis (to be parcelled in gause)          9 g

Caulis Clematidis Armandii          6 g

Rhizoma Alismatis          9 g

Radix Rehmanniae          9 g

Radix Angelicae Sinensis          12 g

Radix Bupleuri          9 g

Radix Glycyrrhizae          6 g

The decoction of one dose for a day is 200—300 ml. Take equal shares in the morning and evening.

Modification: In case of with aversion to cold high fevers, frequent urination with burning pain, add

Folium Pyrrosiae          15 g

Herba Taraxaci          15 g

Flos Lonicerae          15 g

Rhizoma Corydalis          9 g

**Other therapies**

(1)Simple recipe:

Ingredients:Radix Gossypii herbaci          60 g

Fructus Aurantii   -   30 g

(Or Fructus Rosae Laevigatae          60 g)

Decoct the drugs to get 200 ml of decoction. Take one dose daily.

(2)Acupuncture: Select *Weibao*(6 *Chun* beside *Kuanyuan*), *Zigong, Sanyinjiao* as main acupoints and take *Zhangqiang, Baihui* and *Yinlingquan* as adjunct acupoints. Accept the treatment two or three times a week. One course of treatment lasts 2—3 weeks.

(3)External treatment: Decoct the following drugs for fumigation which lasts 10—15 minutes at a time, once or twice a day.

Ingredients:Calla Chinensis     15 g
Fructus Aurantii     30 g
Fructus Chebulae     9 g
Cortex Phellodendri     15 g
Caulis Clematidis Armandii     9 g
Borneolum Syntheticum (to be added later in hot decoction of 1000 ml)     1.5 g

(4)The pessulum is applicable to noninfected metroptosis of the first or second degree, and it should be done under the instruction of the doctor.

(5)The operative treatment should be considered in case all the above therapies are invalid.


# 6.5    Flatus Vaginalis

If there is air escaping at times from the vagina which sounds like the wind from the bowels, the illness is termed *Yin Chui* which means flatus vaginalis. But it should not be regarded as a disease if it is not accompanied by other malaises.

Generally, this case is caused by the stagnation of *Qi* in the

Fu—organs as the fluid in the stomach and intestines has dried up, or by the destitution of $Qi$ in the middle—$Jiao$ due to consistent debility of the spleen and stomach, or by the retention of excessive fluid in the middle—$jiao$, leading to stagnation of the essence derived from food. But in the view of modern medical science, the illness results from the vaginal trauma at the time of delivery, and from the laxation of tissues.

## Type and Treatment

### 1. Aridity of the intestines

(1)Accumulation of heat in the intestines

**Clinical manifestations:** Air emitted at times from the vagina with loud sounds, difficult defecation with dry stools, thirst with the desire for cold drinks. The tongue is reddened with rough, yellowish coating. The pulse is rapid.

Therapeutic method: Clear away the heat and moisten the dryness; regulate the flow of $Qi$ and remove its stagnation.

Recipe: *YunüJian*(99)

Ingredients:Gypsum Fibrosum      30 g
          Rhizoma Anemarrhenae     9 g
          Radix Rehmanniae Preparata     12 g
          Radix Ophiopogonis     12 g
          Radix Cyathulae     15 g

Decoct the drugs in water to get 200—300ml of decoction. Take one half of it with warm water in the morning and the other half in the evening.

Modification: In case of excessive heat and obvious stagnation of $Qi$ and dryness of the intestines, add

> Radix Rehmanniae    12 g
>
> Fructus Trichosanthis    30 g
>
> Semen Biotae    9 g
>
> Herba Dendrobii    9 g
>
> Semen Armeniacae Amarum    9 g
>
> Pericarpium Citri Reticulatae    9 g

(2) *Yin*—deficiency and fluid exhaustion

**Clinical manifestations:** Air emitted at times from the vagina, emaciation with withered complexion and dried skin, thirst or dysphoria with a feverish sensation in the chest, palms and soles, hectic fever, constipation with dry stools and scanty, yellow urines. The tongue is reddened with unmoistened fur. The pulse is thready and slightly rapid.

Therapeutic method: Nourish *Yin* and replenish the body fluid; moisten the dried intestines and relieve constipation.

Recipe: *Wuren Wan*(84)

Ingredients:Semen Armeniacae Amarum    9 g

> Semen Persicae    9 g
>
> Semen Biotae    9 g
>
> Semen Pruni    12 g
>
> Semen Pini    12 g

The decoction of a dose is 200—300 ml. Take equal shares in the morning and evening.

Modification: In case of lack of fluid but having no abdominal distention and no stagnation of *Qi*, deduct Semen Pruni, but add

> Fructus Trichosanthis    30 g
>
> Rhizoma Polygonati    12 g
>
> Radix Rehmanniae    12 g

## 2. Qi-Destitution

**Clinical manifestations:** Air emitted from the vagina with a low, deep sound, accompanied by pale complexion, short breath, low voice, palpitation, lassitude, tenesmus in the lower abdomen, frequent urination, dry or loose stools. The leukorrhea is profuse and watery. The tongue is palish red with thin, whitish fur. The pulse is feeble and relaxed.

Therapeutic method: Invigorate *Qi* and tonify the vital essence.

Recipe: *Buzhong Yiqi Tang* (7). See 5.6.1 for the prescription.

Modification: In case of constipation, add

Herba Cistanchis      12 g

Radix Rehmanniae Praeparata      12 g

## 3. Retention of excessive fluid

**Clinical manifestations:** Air emitted from the vagina, obesity with a pale, swollen face, chest oppression, poor appetite, sialemesis, palpitation, insomnia, dizziness, dry or viscid stools. The tongue is flabby and light in color with whitish, greasy fur. The pulse is taut, either slow or slippery.

Therapeutic method: Promote diuresis and dispel the phlegm-dampness, with the help of strengthening the spleen.

Recipe: *Ju Ban Gui Ling Zhi Jang Tang*(31)

Ingredients:Pericarpium Citri Reticulatae      9 g

Rhizoma Pinelliae      12 g

Ramulus Cinnamomi      9 g

Poria      12 g

Fructus Aurantii Immaturus      9 g

Rhizoma Zingiberis Recens 3 slices

The decoction of one dose for a day is 200-300 ml. Take equal shares in the morning and evening.

Modification: In case of difficult defecation with dry stools, deduct Rhizoma Zingiberis but add

Fractus Trichosanthis　　30 g

Natrii Sulfas　　3 g

### 4. Stagnation of the liver—*Qi*

**Clinical manifestations:** Air emitted intermittently from the vagina, distending pain in the chest and lower abdomen, mental depression, dysphoria, irritability, poor appetite, belching and sighing at times, and dry stools. The menstruation is irregular and indefinite in quantity. The fur of the tongue is thin and whitish. The pulse is taut, or taut and uneven.

Therapeutic method: Soothe the liver, regulate the flow of *Qi* and relieve the mental depression.

Recipe: *Sini San*(65)

Ingredients:Radix Bupleuri　　9 g

Radix Paeoniae Alba　　12 g

Fructus Aurantii Immaturus　　12 g

Radix Glycyrrhizae　　6 g

Decoct the drugs to get 200—300 ml of decoction for a day's does. Take one half of it in the morning and the other half in the evening.

Modification: In case of abdominal distention and dry stools, add

Semen Trichosanthis　　30 g

Semen Persicae　　9 g

Semen Pruni　　12 g

# Index of Prescriptions （方剂索引）

**1.** *Ai Fu Nuangong Wan* 艾附暖宫丸                  **115,386**

Ingredients:

Radix Angelicae Sinensis 当归

Radix Rehmanniae 生地

Radix Paeoniae Alba 白芍

Rhizoma Ligustici Chuanxiong 川芎

Radix Astragali seu Hedysari 黄芪

Cortex Cinnamomi 肉桂

Folium Artemisiae Argyi 艾叶

Fructus Euodiae 吴茱萸

Rhizoma Cyperi 香附

Radix Dipsaci 续断

(From *Sheshi Zunsheng Shu*《沈氏尊生书》,"Shen's Work on the Importance of Life Preservation")

**2.** *Baochan Wuyou San* 保产无忧散                  **213,430**

Ingredients:

Radix Angelicae Sinensis 当归

Rhizoma Ligustici Chuanxiong 川芎

Spica Schizonepetae 荆芥穗

Radix Astragali seu Hedysari Praeparata 炙黄芪

Folium Artemisiae Argyi 艾叶

Cortex Magnoliae Officinalis 厚朴

Fructus Aurantii 枳壳

Semen Cuscutae 菟丝子

Bulbus Fritillariae Cirrhosae 川贝母

Radix Paeoniae Alba　白芍

Rhizoma seu Radix Notopterygii　羌活

Radix Glycyrrhizae　甘草

Rhizoma Zingiberis Recens　生姜

(From *Fu Qingzhu Nüke*《傅青主女科》,"Fu Qingzhu's Obstetrics and Gynecology")

### 3. *Baihe Gujin Tang*　百合固金汤　　　　　199,423

Ingredients:

Radix Rehmanniae　生地

Radix Rehmanniae Praeparata　熟地

Radix Ophiopogonis　麦冬

Bulbus Lilii　百合

Radix Scrophulariae　玄参

Radix Platycodi　桔梗

Bulbus Fritillariae Thunbergii　浙贝母

Radix Angelicae Sinensis　当归

Radix Paeoniae Alba　白芍

Radix Glycyrrhizae　甘草

(From *Yifang Jijie*《医方集解》, "Collection of Prescriptions with Notes")

### 4. *Bushen Guchong Wan*　补肾固冲丸　　　　153,403

Ingredients:

Semen Cuscutae　菟丝子

Radix Rehmanniae Praeparata　熟地

Colla Corii Asini　阿胶

Cornu Cervi Degelatinatum　鹿角霜

Rhizoma Atractylodis Macrocephalae Praeparata　炒白术

Fructus Lycii 枸杞子

Radix Morindae Officinalis 巴戟

Cortex Eucommiae 杜仲

Radix Dipsaci 续断

Radix Angelicae Sinensis 当归

Fructus Amomi 砂仁

Fructus Ziziphi Jujubae 大枣

(From "New Edition of Traditional Chinese Medicine")

5. *Bao Yin Jian* 保阴煎        71,123,140,158,
                               228,367,389,
Ingredients:                   397,404,437

Radix Rehmanniae 生地

Radix Rehmanniae Praeparata 熟地

Rhizoma Dioscoreae 山药

Radix Paeoniae Alba 白芍

Radix Dipsaci 续断

Radix Scutellariae 黄芩

Cortex Phellodendri 黄柏

Radix Glycyrrhizae 甘草

(From *Jingyue Quanshu* 《景岳全书》, "Jing Yue's Complete
  Works")

6. *Baizhu San* 白术散        172,180,411,
                             414

Ingredients:

Rhizoma Atractylodis Macrocephalae 白术

Poria 茯苓

Pericarpium Arecae 大腹皮

Cortex Zingiberis 生姜皮

Pericarpium Citri Reticulatae 陈皮

(From *Quansheng Zhimi Fang*《全生指迷方》,"Quansheng's
Guidebook of Prescriptions")

## 7. *Buzhong Yiqi Tang*　补中益气汤　　　　108,270,276,
　　　　　　　　　　　　　　　　　　　　　　　383,455,457
Ingredients:

　　Radix Ginseng　人参

　　Radix Astragali seu Hedysari　黄芪

　　Radix Glycyrrhizae　甘草

　　Radix Angelicae Sinensis　当归

　　Pericarpium Citri Reticulata　陈皮

　　Rhizoma Cimicifugae　升麻

　　Radix Bupleuri　柴胡

　　Rhizoma Atractylodis Macrocephalae　白术

　　(From *Pi Wei Lun*《脾胃论》,"Treatise on the Spleen and the
　　　Stomach")

## 8. *Bazhen Tang*　八珍汤　　　　　　　　190,419,

Ingredients:

　　Radix Angelicae Sinensis　当归

　　Radix Rehmanniae Praeparata　熟地

　　Radix Paeoniae Alba　白芍

　　Rhizoma Ligustici Chuanxiong　川芎

　　Radix Codonopsis Pilosulae　党参

　　Rhizoma Atractylodis Macrocephalae　白术

　　Poria　茯苓

　　Radix Glycyrrhizae　甘草

　　(From *Zhengti Leiyao*《正体类要》,"Classification and Treatment
　　　of Traumatic Diseases")

## 9. *Chaihu Shugan San* 柴胡疏肝散      99,379

Ingredients:

Radix Bupleuri 柴胡

Radix Paeoniae Alba 白芍

Fructus Aurantii 枳壳

Rhizoma Ligustici Chuanxiong 川芎

Rhizoma Cyperi 香附

Pericarpium Citri Reticulatae 陈皮

Radix Glycyrrhizae 甘草

(From *Jingyue Quanshu*《景岳全书》,"Jing Yue's Complete Works")

## 10. *Cang Fu Daotang Wan* 苍附导痰丸      129,391

Ingredients:

Poria 茯苓

Rhizoma Pinelliae 半夏

Pericarpium Citri Reticulatae 陈皮

Radix Glycyrrhizae 甘草

Rhizoma Atractylodis 苍术

Rhizoma Cyperi 香附

Arisaema cum Bile 胆南星

Fructus Aurantii 枳壳

Rhizoma Zingiberis Recens 生姜

Massa Fermentata Medicinalis 神曲

(From *Ye Tianshi Nüke Zhenzhi Mifang*《叶天士女科诊治秘方》, "Ye Tianshi's Secret Records of Internal Medicine")

**11.** *Caisongting's Nanchan Fang*　蔡松汀难产方　　210,428

Ingredients:

Radix Astragali seu Hedysari　黄芪

Radix Angelicae Sinensis　当归

Poria cum Ligno Hospite　茯神

Radix Codonopsis Pilosulae　党参

Plastrum Testudinis　龟板

Radix Paeoniae Alba　白芍

Fructus Lycii　枸杞

Rhizoma Ligustici Chuanxiong　川芎

(From *Jingyan Fang*《经验方》,"Classical Proved Prescriptions")

**12.** *Cuisheng Yin*　催生饮　　211,429

Ingredients:

Radix Angelicae Sinensis　当归

Rhizoma Ligustici Chuanxiong　川芎

Pericarpium Arecae　大腹皮

Fructus Aurantii　枳壳

Radix Angelicae Dahuricae　白芷

(From *Ji Yin Gangmu*《济阴纲目》,"Synopsis of Treating
Women's Diseases")

**13.** *Dabuyuan Jian*　大补元煎　　271,455

Ingredients:

Radix Ginseng　人参

Rhizoma Dioscoreae　山药

Radix Rehmanniae Praeparata　熟地

Cortex Eucommiae　杜仲

Radix Angelicae Sinensis  当归

Fructus Corni  山茱萸

Fructus Lycii  枸杞

Radix Glycyrrhizae Praeparatae  甘草

(From *Jingyue Quanshu*《景岳全书》, "Jing Yue's Complete Works")

## 14. *Daochi San*  导赤散  202,425

Ingredients:

Radix Rehmanniae  生地

Caulis Clematidis Armandii  川木通

Herba Lophatheri  淡竹叶

Radix Glycyrrhizae  甘草梢

(From *Xiaoer Yaozheng Zhijue*《小儿药证直诀》, "Key to Therapeutics of Childen's diseases")

## 15. *Danggui Shaoyao San*  当归芍药散  186,418

Ingredients:

Radix Angelicae Sinensis  当归

Rhizoma Ligustici Chuanxiong  川芎

Radix Paeoniae Alba  白芍

Poria  茯苓

Rhizoma Atractylodis Macrocephalae  白术

Rhizoma Alismatis  泽泻

(From *Jinkui Yaolüe*《金匮要略》, "Synopsis of Prescriptions of the Golden Chamber")

## 16. *Danggui Tang*  当归汤  146,399

Ingredients:

Radix Angelicae Sinensis  当归

Radix Achyranthis Bidentatae  牛膝

Caulis Clematidis Armandii  川木通

Talcum  滑石

Fructus Malvae Vertillatae  冬葵子

Herba Dianthi Praeparata  黑瞿麦

(From *Ji Yin Gangmu*《济阴纲目》, "Synopsis of Treating
Women's Diseases")

## 17. *DangGui YinZi*  当归饮子 66,365

Ingredients:

Radix Angelicae Sinensis  当归

Rhizoma Ligustici Chuanxiong  川芎

Radix Paeoniae Alba  白芍

Radix Rehmanniae  生地

Radix Ledebouriellae  防风

Herba Schizonepetae  荆芥

Radix Astragali seu Hedysari  黄芪

Fructus Tribuli  白蒺藜

Radix Polygoni Multiflori  何首乌

Radix Glycyrrhizae  甘草

(From *Zhengzhi Zhunsheng*《证治准绳》, "Standards of Diagnosis
and Treatment")

## 18. *Duhuo Jisheng Tang*  独活寄生汤 239,441

Ingredients:

Radix Angelicae Pubescentis  独活

Ramulus Loranthi  桑寄生

Cortex Cinnamomi  桂心

Radix Ledebouriellae  防风

Rhizoma Ligustici Chuanxiong  川芎

Radix Ginseng  人参

Radix Glycyrrhizae  甘草

Rhizoma Angelicae Sinensis  当归

Radix Paeoniae  芍药

Radix Rehmanniae  干地黄

Cortex Eucommiae  杜仲

Radix Achyranthis Bidentatae  牛膝

Radix Gentianae Macrophyllae  秦艽

Poria  茯苓

(From *Beiji Qianjin Yaofang*《千金要方》, "Prescriptions Worth a
Thousand Gold for Emergencies")

## 19. *Duoming San*  夺命散                                220,433

Ingredients

Myrrha  没药

Resina Draconis  血竭

(From *Zhengzhi Zhunsheng*《证治准绳》, "Standards of Diagnosis
and Treatment")

## 20. *Dushen Tang*  独参汤                                220,433

Ingredients:

Radix Ginseng  人参

(From *Shi Yao Shenshu*《十药神书》, "A Miraculous Book of Ten
Prescriptions")

## 21. *Dan Zhi Xiaoyao San*  丹栀逍遥散                    111,194,
                                                          384,421

Ingredients:

Cortex Moutan Radicis　丹皮

Fructus Gardeniae　栀子

Radix Angelicae Sinensis　当归

Radix Paeoniae Alba　芍药

Radix Bupleuri　柴胡

Rhizoma Atractylodis Macrocephalae　白术

Poria　茯苓

Radix Glycyrrhizae Praeparata　甘草

(From *Neike Cuoyao*《内科撮要》, "Essentials of Internal Medicine")

## 22. *Erzhi Wan*　二至丸 75,369

Ingredients:

Herba Ecliptae　旱莲草

Fructus Ligustri Lucidi　女贞子

(From *Yifang Jijie*《医方集解》, "Collection of Prescriptions with Notes")

## 23. *Fuling Daoshui Tang*　茯苓导水汤 185,147

Ingredients:

Poria　茯苓

Polyporus Umbellatus　猪苓

Semen Arecae　槟榔

Fructus Amomi　砂仁

Radix Aucklandiae　木香

Pericarpium Citri Reticulatae　陈皮

Rhizoma Alismatis　泽泻

Rhizoma Atractylodis Macrocephalae　白术

Fructus Chaenomelis　木瓜

Cortex Mori Radicis　桑白皮

Folium Perillae　苏叶

Pericarpium Arecae　大腹皮

(From *Yi Zong Jin Jian*《医宗金鉴》,"The Golden Mirror of
　Medicine")

## 24. *Guben Zhibeng Tang*　固本止崩汤　　　　　　74,366

Ingredients:

　Radix Rehmanniae Praeparata　熟地

　Rhizoma Atractylodis Macrocephalae　白术

　Radix Astragali seu Hedysari　黄芪

　Radix Angelicae Sinensis　当归

　Rhizoma Zingiberis Recens Praeparatae　黑姜

　Radix Ginseng　人参

　(From *Fu Qingzhu Nuke*《傅青主女科》,"Fu Qingzhu's Obstetrics
　　and Gynecology")

## 25. *Gexia Zhuyu Tang*　膈下逐瘀汤　　　　　　83,258,
　　　　　　　　　　　　　　　　　　　　　　　　　　372,449

Ingredients:

　Radix Angelicae Sinensis　当归

　Rhizoma Ligustici Chuanxiong　川芎

　Radix Paeoniae Rubra　赤芍

　Semen Persicae　桃仁

　Flos Carthami　红花

　Fructus Aurantii　枳壳

　Rhizoma Corydalis　延胡索

　Faeces Trogopterorum　五灵脂

　Cortex Moutan Radicis　丹皮

　Radix Linderae　乌药

Rhizoma Cyperi Praeparata　制香附

Radix Glycyrrhizae　甘草

(From *Yilin Gaicuo*《医林改错》,"Corrections on the Errors of
Medical Works")

## 26. *Gui Shen Wan*　归肾丸　　　　　　　　　　90,127,375,390

Ingredients:

Radix Rehmanniae Praeparata　熟地

Rhizoma Dioscoreae　山药

Fructus Corni　山茱萸

Poria　茯苓

Radix Angelicae Sinensis　当归

Fructus Lycii　枸杞

Cortex Eucommiae　杜仲

Semen Cuscutae　菟丝子

(From *Jingyue Quanshu*《景岳全书》.,"Jing Yue's Complete
Works")

## 27. *Gu Yin Jian*　固阴煎　　　　　　　　　　120,388

Ingredients:

Radix Ginseng　人参

Radix Rehmanniae Praeparata　熟地

Rhizoma Dioscoreae　山药

Fructus Corni　山茱萸

Radix Polygalae　远志

Semen Cuscutae　菟丝子

Fructus Schisandrae　五味子

Radix Glycyrrhizae Praeparata　　甘草

(From *Jingyue Quanshu*《景岳全书》,"Jing Yue's Complete

Works")

**28.** *Huangqi Danggui San*  黄芪当归散　　　　250,446

Ingredients:

Radix Astragali seu Hedysari　黄芪

Radix Angelicae Sinensis　当归

Radix Ginseng　人参

Rhizoma Atractylodis Macrocephalae　白术

Radix Paeoniae Alba　白芍

Radix Glycyrrhizae　甘草

Rhizoma Zingiberis Recens　生姜

Fructus Ziziphi Jujubae　大枣

Sus Scrofa Domestica Brisson　猪尿脬

(From *Yi Zong Jin Jian*《医宗金鉴》, "The Gold Mirror of
Medicine")

**29.** *Huangqi Guizhi Wuwu Tang*  黄芪桂枝五物汤　237,441

Ingredients:

Radix Astragali seu Hedysari　黄芪

Ramulus Cinnamomi　桂枝

Radix Paeoniae Alba　白芍

Rhizoma Zingiberis Recens　生姜

Fructus Ziziphi Jujubae　大枣

(From *Jinkui Yaolue*《金匮要略》, "Synopsis of Prescriptions of
the Golden Chamber")

**30.** *Jiao Ai Tang*  胶艾汤　　　　　　　　188,419

Ingredients:

Radix Angelicae Sinensis　当归

Rhizoma Ligustici Chuanxiong　川芎

Radix Rehmanniae　干地黄

Radix Paeoniae Alba　白芍

Folium Artemisiae Argyi　艾叶

Colla Corii Asini　阿胶

Radix Glycyrrhizae　甘草

(From *Jinkui Yaolùe*《金匮要略》,"Synopsis of Prescriptions of the Golden Chamber")

## 31. *Ju Ban Gui Ling Zhi Jang Tang*　橘半桂苓枳姜汤　　276,457

Ingredients:

Rhizoma Pinelliae　半夏

Fructus Aurantii Lmmaturus　枳实

Pericarpium Citri Reticulatae　橘皮

Ramulus Cinnamomi　桂枝

Poria　茯苓

Rhizoma Zingiberis Recens　生姜

(From *Wenbing Tiaobian*《温病条辨》,"Treatise on Differentiation and Treatment of Epidemic Febrile Diseases")

## 32. *Jian Gu Tang*　健固汤　　　　　　　101,380

Ingredients:

Radix Codonopsis Pilosulae　党参

Rhizoma Atractylodis Macrocephalae　白术

Poria　茯苓

Semen Coicis　薏苡仁

Radix Morindae Officinalis　巴戟天

(From *Fu Qingzhu Nüke*《傅青主女科》,"Fu Qingzhu's Obstetrics and Gynecology")

### 33. *Jingfang Siwu Tang* 荆防四物汤　　　　233,439

Ingredients:

Radix Paeoniae Alba　白芍

Radix Angelicae Sinensis　当归

Rhizoma Ligustici Chuanxiong　川芎

Radix Rehmanniae Praeparata　熟地

Herba Schizonepetae　荆芥

Radix Ledebouriellae　防风

(From *Yi Zong Jin Jian*《医宗金鉴》,"The Golden Mirror of Medicine")

### 34. *Jiu Mu Dan* 救母丹　　　　149,401

Ingredients:

Radix Ginseng　人参

Radix Angelicae Sinensis　当归

Rhizoma Ligustici Chuanxiong　川芎

Herba Leonuri　益母草

Halloysitum Rubrum　赤石脂

Spica Schizonepetae Praeparata　炒芥穗

(From *Fu Qingzhu's Nüke*《傅青主女科》,"Fu Qingzhu's Obstetrics and Gynecology")

### 35. *Ju Yuan Jian* 举元煎　　　　122,388

Ingredients:

Radix Ginseng　人参

Radix Astragali seu Hedysari　黄芪

Rhizoma Cimicifugae　升麻

Rhizoma Atractylodis Macrocephalae　白术

Radix Glycyrrhizae Praeparata 炙甘草

(From *Jingyue Quanshu*《景岳全书》,"Jing Yue's Complete Works")

## 36. *Kaiyu Erchen Tang* 开郁二陈汤 255,448

Ingredients:

Pericarpium Citri Reticulatae 陈皮

Rhizoma Pinelliae Praeparata 制半夏

Poria 茯苓

Pericarpium Citri Reticulatae Viride 青皮

Rhizoma Cyperi 香附

Rhizoma Ligustici Chuanxiong 川芎

Rhizoma Zedoariae 莪术

Radix Aucklandiae 木香

Semen Arecae 槟榔

Radix Glycyrrhizae 甘草

Rhizome Atractylodis 苍术

Rhizoma Zingiberis Recens 生姜

(From *Wanshi Furen Ke*《万氏妇人科》,"Wan's Obstetrics and Gynecology")

## 37. *Liang Di Tang* 两地汤 112,384

Ingredients:

Radix Rehmanniae 生地

Radix Scrophulariae 玄参

Radix Paeoniae Alba 白芍

Radix Ophiopogonis 麦冬

Colla Corii Asini 阿胶

Cortex Lycii Radicis 地骨皮

(From *Fu Qingzhu Nüke*《傅青主女科》, "Fu Qingzhu's Obstetrics and Gynecology")

**38.** *Longdan Xiegan Tang*　龙胆泻肝汤　　　　　33,43,271

351,355,455

Ingredients:

Radix Gentianae　龙胆草

Fructus Gardeniae　山栀子

Radix Scutellariae　黄芩

Semen Plantaginis　车前子

Caulis Clematidis Armandii　川木通

Rhizoma Alismatis　泽泻

Radix Rehmanniae　生地

Radix Angelicae Sinensis　当归

Radix Bupleuri　柴胡

Radix Glycyrrhizae　甘草

(From *Yi Zong Jin Jian*《医宗金鉴》, "The Golden Mirror of Medicine")

**39.** *Liang ge San*　凉膈散　　　　　　　　　135,393

Ingredients:

Radix et Rhizoma Rhei　大黄

Natrii Sulfas　朴硝

Fructus Gardeniae　山栀

Herba Menthae　薄荷叶

Radix Sculellariae　黄芩

Fructus Forsythiae　连翘

Herba Lophatheri　竹叶

Radix Glycyrrhizae　甘草

(From *He Ji Ju Fang*《和剂局方》, "Formularies")

## 40. *Lingjiao Gouteng Tang*　羚角钩藤汤

176,179, 413,415

Ingredients:

Ramulus Uncariae cum Uncis　钩藤

Cornu Saigae Tataricae　羚羊角

Folium Mori　桑叶

Bulbus Fritillariae Cirrhosae　川贝

Radix Rehmanniae　生地

Flos Chrysanthemi　菊花

Radix Paeoniae Alba　白芍

Poria cum Ligno Hospite　茯神

Caulis Bambusae in Taeniam　竹茹

Radix Glycyrrhizae　甘草

(From "Revised Popular Treatise on Febrile Diseases")

## 41. *Liuwei Dihuang Tang*　六味地黄汤

197,262, 423.451

Ingredients:

Radix Rehmanniae Praeparata　熟地

Rhizoma Dioscoreae　山药

Fructus Corni　山茱萸

Poria　茯苓

Rhizoma Alismatis　泽泻

Cortex Moutan Radicis　丹皮

(From *Xiaoer Yaozheng Zhijue*《小儿药证直诀》, "Key to Therapeutics of Children's Diseases")

## 42. *Liyu Tang*　鲤鱼汤

184,417

Ingredients:

Cyprinus Carpio　鲤鱼

Rhizoma Atractylodis Macrocephalae  白术

Rhizoma Zingiberis Recens  生姜

Radix Paeoniae Alba  白芍

Radix Angelicae Sinensis  当归

Poria  茯苓

(From *Beiji Qianjin Yaofang* 《千金要方》, "Prescriptions Worth a
   Thousand Gold for Emergencies")

## 43. *Nei Bu Wan*  内补丸                                         46,357

Ingredients:

Cornu Cervi Pantotrichum  鹿茸

Cortex Cinnamomi  肉桂

Semen Cuscutae  菟丝子

Radix Astragali seu Hedysari  黄芪

Fructus Tribuli  白蒺藜

Herba Cistanchis  肉苁蓉

Ootheca Mantidis  桑螵蛸

Radix Aconiti Praeparata  熟附子

Radix Asteris  紫菀茸

Semen Astragali Complanati  沙苑蒺藜

(From *Nüke Qie Yao* 《女科切要》, "Essentials of Obstetrics and
   Gynecology")

## 44. *Niuhuang Qingxin Wan*  牛黄清心丸                          180,413

Ingredients:

Calculus Bovis  牛黄

Cinnabaris  朱砂

Rhizoma Coptidis  黄连

Radix Scutellariae  黄芩

Radix Curcumae    郁金

Fructus Gardeniae    山栀

(From *Dou Zhen Shiyi Xin Fa*《痘疹世医心法》, "Personal Insight
of Smallpox and Rash Diseases")

## 45. Prescription No.1 for Extrauterine Pregnancy    宫外孕
### Ⅰ号方                                            165,408

Ingredients:

Radix Paeoniae Rubra    赤芍

Radix Salviae Miltiorrhizae    丹参

Semen Persicae    桃仁

## 46. Prescription No.2 for Extrauterine Pregnancy    宫外孕
### Ⅱ号方                                        163,166,409

Ingredients:

Radix Paeoniae Rubra    赤芍

Radix Salviae Miltiorrhizae    丹参

Semen Persicae    桃仁

Rhizoma Zedoariae    莪术

Rhizoma Sparganii    三棱

## 47. *Qi Gong Wang*    启宫丸                          96,378

Ingredients:

Rhizoma Pinelliae    半夏

Rhizoma Cyperi    香附

Rhizoma Atractylodis    苍术

Pericarpium Citri Reticulatae    陈皮

Massa Fermentata Medicinalis    神曲

Rhizoma Ligustici Chuanxiong    川芎

Poria　茯苓

(From *Jingyan Fang* 《经验方》,"Classical Proved Prescriptions")

## 48. *Qinggan Yinjing Tang*　清肝引经汤　　　131,392

Ingredients:

    Radix Angelicae Sinensis　当归

    Radix Paeoniae Alba　白芍

    Radix Rehmanniae　生地

    Cortex Moutan Radicis　丹皮

    Fructus Gardeniae　栀子

    Radix Scutellariae　黄芩

    Fructus Meliae Toosendan　川楝子

    Radix Rubiae　茜草

    Rhizoma Lmperatae　白茅根

    Radix Achyranthis Bidentatae　牛膝

    Radix Glycyrrhizae　甘草

(From "Traditional Chinese Gynecology", 1979.)

## 49. *Qi Ju Dihuang Tang*　杞菊地黄汤　　　102,380

Ingredients:

    Radix Rehmanniae Praeparata　熟地

    Rhizoma Dioscoreae　山药

    Fructus Corni　山茱萸

    Poria　茯苓

    Rhizoma Alismatis　泽泻

    Cortex Moutan Radicis　丹皮

    Fructus Lycii　枸杞

    Flos Chrysanthemi　菊花

(From *Yi Ji* 《医级》,"Medical Classics")

**50.** *Qingjin Jianghuo Tang*　清金降火汤　　　　200,424

Ingredients:

Radix Scutellariae　黄芩

Semen Armeniacae Amarum　北杏

Bulbus Fritillariae Thunbergii　贝母

Radix Peucedani　前胡

Semen Trichosanthis　瓜蒌仁

Gypsum Fibrosum　石膏

Pericarpium Citri Reticulatae　陈皮

Radix Glycyrrhizae Praeparata　炙甘草

Poria　茯苓

Rhizoma Pinelliae Praeparatae　法半夏

Radix Platycodi　桔梗

Rhizoma Zingiberis Recens　生姜

Fructus Aurantii　枳壳

(From *Gu Jin Yijian*《古今医鉴》, "A Medical Reference of the Past and Present")

**51.** *Qing Jing Tang*　清经汤　　　　110,384

Ingredients:

Cortex Moutan Radicis　丹皮

Cortex Lycii Radicis　地骨皮

Radix Paeoniae Alba　白芍

Radix Rehmanniae Praeparata　熟地

Herba Artemisiae　青蒿

Poria　茯苓

Cortex Phellodendri　黄柏

(From *Fu Qingzhu Nuke*《傅青主女科》, "Fu Qingzhu's Obstetrics

and Gynecology")

## 52. *Qingluo Yin* 清络饮 223,435

Ingredients:

Fresh Folium Netumbinis 鲜荷叶边

Fresh Flos Lonicerae 鲜金银花

Exocarpium Citrulli 西瓜翠衣

Exocarpium Luffae 丝瓜皮

Fresh bud of Herba Lophatheri 鲜竹叶心

Fresh Flos Dolichoris 鲜扁豆花

(From *Wenbing Tiaobian*《温病条辨》, "Treatise on

Differentiation and Treatment of Epidemic Febrile Diseases")

## 53. *Qingre Gujin Tang* 清热固经汤 69,366

Ingredients:

Cortex Lycii Radicis 地骨皮

Radix Rehmanniae 生地

Plastrum Testudinis 龟板

Concha Ostreae 牡蛎

Colla Corii Asini 阿胶

Fructus Gardeniae 栀子

Radix Sanguisorbae 地榆

Radix Scutellariae 黄芩

Nodus Nelumbinis Rhizomatis 藕节

Charcoal of Trachycarpi 棕榈炭

Radix Glycyrrhizae 甘草

(From "The Concise Traditional Chinese Gynecology")

**54.** *Qingshu Yiqi Tang*　清暑益气汤　　　　　**224,435**

Ingredients:

　　Radix Panacis Quinquefolii　西洋参

　　Herba Dendrobii　石斛

　　Radix Ophiopogonis　麦门冬

　　Rhizoma Coptidis　黄连

　　Herba Lophatheri　竹叶

　　Rhizoma Anemarrhenae　知母

　　Radix Glycyrrhizae　甘草

　　Semen Oryzae Sativae　粳米

　　Exocarpium Citrulli　西瓜翠衣

　　Petiolus Nelumbinis　荷梗

　　(From *Wenbing Tiaobian*《温病条辨》, "Treatise on
　　Differentiation and Treatment of Epidemic Febrile Diseases")

**55.** *Qingying Tang*　清营汤　　　　　**217,218,432**

Ingredients:

　　Cornu Rhinocerotis　犀角

　　Radix Rehmanniae　生地

　　Radix Scrophulariae　玄参

　　Herba Lophatheri　竹叶

　　Radix Ophiopogonis　麦冬

　　Radix Salviae Miltiorrhizae　丹参

　　Rhizoma Coptidis　黄连

　　Fructus Forsythiae　连翘

　　Flos Lonicerae　银花

　　(From *Wenbing Tiaobian*《温病条辨》, "Treatise on
　　Differentiation and Treatment of Epidemic Febrile Diseases")

**56.** *Renshen Huangqi Tang*　人参黄芪汤　　145,399

Ingredients:

    Radix Ginseng　人参

    Radix Astragali seu Hedysari　黄芪

    Radix Angelicae Sinensis　当归

    Rhizoma Atractylodis Macrocephalae　白术

    Radix Paeoniae Alba　白芍药

    Folium Artemisiae Argyi　艾叶

    Colla Corii Asini　阿胶

    (From *Ji Yin Gangmu*《济阴纲目》, "Synopsis of Treating Women's Diseases")

**57.** *Renshen Maidong San*　人参麦冬散　　192,420

Ingredients:

    Radix Ginseng　人参

    Radix Ophiopogonis　麦冬

    Poria　茯苓

    Radix Scutellariae　黄芩

    Rhizoma Anemarrhenae　知母

    Radix Rehmanniae　生地

    Radix Glycyrrhizae Praeparata　炙甘草

    Caulis Bambusae in Taeniam　竹茹

    (From *Furen Mike*《妇人秘科》, "Secret Therapies for Women")

**58.** *Renshen Yangrong Tang*　人参养荣汤　　93,126,377,390

Ingredients:

    Radix Paeoniae Alba　白芍

    Radix Angelicae Sinensis　当归

Pericarpium Citri Reticulatae　陈皮

Radix Astragali seu Hedysari　黄芪

Cortex Cinnamomi　桂心

Radix Ginseng　人参

Rhizoma Atractylodis Macrocephalae　白术

Radix Rehmanniae Praeparata　熟地黄

Fructus Schisandrae　五味子

Poria　茯苓

Radix Polygalae　远志

Radix Glycyrrhizae Pareparata　炙甘草

Rhizoma Zingiberis Recens　生姜

Fructus Ziziphi Jujubae　大枣

(From *He Ji Ju Fang*《和剂局方》, "Formularies")

## 59. *Shen Fu Tang*　参附汤                    164,408

Ingredients:

Radix Ginseng　人参

Radix Aconiti Praeparata　附子

(From *Jiaozhu Furen Liang Fang*《校注妇人良方》, "Revised Effective Prescriptions for Women with Notes")

## 60. *Shaofu Zhuyu Tang*　少腹逐瘀汤            85,373

Ingredients:

Fructus Foenicuii　小茴香

Rhizoma Zingiberis　干姜

Rhizoma Corydalis　延胡索

Myrrha　没药

Radix Angelicae Sinensis　当归

Rhizoma Ligustici Chuanxiong　川芎

Cortex Cinnamomi　肉桂

Radix Paeoniae Rubra　赤芍

Pollen Typhae　蒲黄

Faeces Trogopterorum　五灵脂

(From *Yilin Gaicuo*《医林改错》,"Corrections on the Errors of
Medical Works")

## 61. *Shenghua Tang*　生化汤　　147,220,229,236,400,432,437,440

Ingredients:

Radix Angelicae Sinensis　当归

Rhizoma Ligustici Chuanxiong　川芎

Semen Persicae　桃仁

Rhizoma Zingiberis Recens Praeparata　炮姜

Radix Glycyrrhizae Praeparata　炙甘草

(From *Fu Qingzhu Nuke*《傅青主女科》,"Fu Qingzhu's
Obstetrics and Gynecology")

## 62. *Shunjing Tang*　顺经汤　　　　　　132,392

Ingredients:

Rhizoma Angelicae Sinensis　当归

Radix Rehmanniae Praeparata　熟地

Radix Paeoniae Alba　白芍

Cortex Moutan Radicis　丹皮

Poria　茯苓

Radix Adenophorae　南沙参

Schizonepeta Tenuifolia　黑芥穗

(From *Fu Qingzhu Nüke*《傅青主女科》,"Fu Qingzhu's Obstetrics and
Gynecology")

63. *Si Ling San*  四苓散                                    174,412

   Ingredients:

       Poria  茯苓

       Polyporus Umbellatus  猪苓

       Rhizoma Alismatis  泽泻

       Rhizoma Atractylodis Macrocephalae  白术

       (From *Danxi Xin Fa*《丹溪心法》, "Danxi's Experiential Therapy")

64. *Shengmai San*  生脉散           161,164,225,406,408,435

   Ingredients:

       Radix Ginseng  人参

       Radix Ophiopogonis  麦冬

       Fructus Schisandrae  五味子

       (From *Nei Wai Shang Bianhuo Lun*《内外伤辨惑论》,

         "Differentiation of Internal and External Injuries")

65. *Sini San*  四逆散                                      277,458

   Ingredients:

       Radix Bupleuri  柴胡

       Fructus Aurantii Immaturus  枳实

       Radix Paeoniae Alba  白芍药

       Radix Glycyrrhizae  甘草

       (From *Shanghan Lun*《伤寒论》, "Treatise on Febrile Diseases")

66. *Shenqi Wan*  肾气丸                       207,249,425,445

   Ingredients:

       Radix Rehmanniae  干地黄

       Rhizoma Dioscoreae  山药

Fructus Corni　山茱萸

Poria　茯苓

Cortex Moutan Radicis　丹皮

Ramulus Cinnamomi　桂枝

Rhizoma Alismatis　泽泻

Radix Aconiti Praeparata　制附子

(From *Jinkui Yaolue*《金匮要略》, "Synopsis of Prescriptions of
the Golden Chamber")

## 67. *Shou Tai Wan*　寿胎丸　　　　　　　138,141,396,397

Ingredients:

Semen Cuscutae　菟丝子

Radix Dipsaci　续断

Ramulus Loranthi　桑寄生

Colla Corii Asini　阿胶

(From *Yixue Zhongzhong Canxi lu*《医学衷中参西录》, "Records
of Traditional Chinese and Western Medicine in Combination")

## 68. *Shentong Zhuyu Tang*　身痛逐瘀汤　　　　243,442

Ingredients:

Radix Gentianae Macrophyllae　秦艽

Rhizoma Ligustici Chuanxiong　川芎

Semen Persicae　桃仁

Flos Carthami　红花

Radix Glycyrrhizae　甘草

Rhizoma seu Radix Notopterygii　羌活

Myrrha　没药

Radix Angelicae Sinensis　当归

Faeces Trogopterorum　灵脂

Lumbricus    地龙

Rhizoma Cyperi    香附

Radix Achyranthis Bidentatae    牛膝

(From *Yilin Gaicuo*《医林改错》,"Corrections on the Errors of
Medical Works")

69. *Siwu Tang*    四物汤                    72,231,368,438

Ingredients:

Radix Rehmanniae Praeparata    熟地

Radix Angelicae Sinensis    当归

Rhizoma Ligustici Chuanxiong    川芎

Radix Paeoniae Alba    白芍

(From *He Ji Ju Fang*《和剂局方》,"Formularies")

70. *Shixiao San*    失笑散              72,124,145,368,389,399

Ingredients:

Pollen Typhae    蒲黄

Faeces Trogopterorum    五灵脂

(From *He Ji Ju Fang*《和剂局方》,"Formularies")

71. *Suye Huanglian Tang*    苏叶黄连汤                159,405

Ingredients:

Rhizoma Coptidis    黄连

Folium Perillae    苏叶

(From *Wenre Jingwei*《温热经纬》,"Compendium on Epidemic
Febrile Diseases")

72. *Sheng Yu Tang*    圣愈汤                86,141,374,397

Ingredients:

Radix Ginseng 人参

Radix Astragali seu Hedysari 黄芪

Radix Angelicae Sinensis 当归

Rhizoma Ligustici Chuanxiong 川芎

Radix Rehmanniae Praeparata 熟地

Radix Paeoniae Alba 白芍

(From *Lanshi Micang*《兰室秘藏》,"Secret Records of the Chamber of Orchids")

## 73. *Tiao Gan Tang* 调肝汤          88,374

Ingredients:

Rhizoma Dioscoreae 山药

Colla Corii Asini 阿胶

Radix Angelicae Sinensis 当归

Radix Paeoniae Alba 白芍

Fructus Corni 山茱萸

Radix Morindae Officinalis 巴戟天

Radix Glycyrrhizae 甘草

(From *Fu Qingzhu Nüke*《傅青主女科》,"Fu Qingzhu's Obstetrics and Gynecology")

## 74. *Tuo Hua Jian* 脱花煎      143,149,398,401

Ingredients:

Radix Angelicae Sinensis 当归

Cortex Cinnamomi 肉桂

Rhizoma Ligustici Chuanxiong 川芎

Radix Achyranthis Bidentatae 牛膝

Flos Carthami 红花

Herba Plantaginis 车前子

(From *Jingyue Quanshu*《景岳全书》, " Jing Yue's Complete Works")

## 75. *Tao Hong Siwu Tang* 桃红四物汤      128,266,391,453

Ingredients:

Semen Persicae 桃仁

Flos Carthami 红花

Radix Angelicae Sinensis 当归

Rhizoma Ligustici Chuanxiong 川芎

Radix Paeoniae Rubra 赤芍

Radix Rehmanniae Praeparata 熟地

(From *Yi Zong Jin Jian*《医宗金鉴》, "The Golden Mirror of Medicine")

## 76. *Tongru Dan* 通乳丹      242,443

Ingredients:

Radix Ginseng 人参

Radix Astragali seu Hedysari 黄芪

Radix Angelicae Sinensis 当归

Radix Ophiopogonis 麦冬

Caulis Clematidis Armandii 川木通

Radix Platycodi 桔梗

Sus Scrofa domestica 猪蹄跤

(From *Fu Qingzhu Nüke*《傅青主女科》, "Fu Qingzhu's Obstetrics and Gynecology")

## 77. *Taishan Panshi San* 泰山磐石散      154,403

Ingredients:

Radix Ginseng 人参

Radix Astragali seu Hedysari　黄芪

Radix Angelicae Sinensis　当归

Radix Dipsaci　续断

Radix Scutellariae　黄芩

Radix Rehmanniae Praeparata　熟地

Rhizoma Ligustici Chuanxiong　川芎

Radix Paeoniae Albe　白芍

Rhizoma Atractylodis Macrocephalae　白术

Fructus Amomi　砂仁

Semen Oryzae Glutinosae　糯米

Radix Glycyrrhizae Praeparata　炙甘草

(From *Jingyue Quanshu*《景岳全书》,"Jing Yue's Complete Works")

## 78. *Tianxianteng San*　天仙藤散　174,412

Ingredients:

Caulis Aristolochiae　天仙藤

Rhizoma Cyperi　香附子

Pericarpium Citri Reticulatae　陈皮

Radix Linderae　乌药

Rhizoma Zingiberis Recens　生姜

Fructus Chaenomelis　木瓜

Folium Perillae　紫苏叶

Radix Glycyrrhizae　甘草

(From *Jiaozhu Furen Liang Fang*《校注妇人良方》,"Revised Effective Prescriptions for Women with Notes")

## 79. *Ta Yang Tang*　塌痒汤　49,358

Ingredients:

Fructus Carpesii 鹤虱

Radix Sophorae Flavescentis 苦参

Radix Clematidis 威灵仙

The tip of Radix Angelicae Sinensis 归尾

Fructus Cnidii 蛇床子

Radix Euphorbiae Ebracteolatae 狼毒

(From *Yang Yi Daquan*《疡医大全》,"Encyclopedia of Treatment of Diseases")

## 80. *Tai Yuan Yin* 胎元饮        139,396

Ingredients:

Radix Ginseng 人参

Radix Angelicae Sinensis 当归

Cortex Eucommiae 杜仲

Radix Paeoniae Alba 白芍

Radix Rehmanniae Praeparata 熟地

Rhizoma Atractylodis Macrocephalae 白术

Pericarpium Citri Reticulatae 陈皮

Radix Glycyrrhizae Praeparata 炙甘草

(From *Jingyue Quanshu*《景岳全书》,"Jing Yue's Complete Works")

## 81. *Wandai Tang* 完带汤        40,354

Ingredients:

Rhizoma Atractylodis Macrocephalae 白术

Rhizoma Dioscoreae 山药

Radix Ginseng 人参

Radix Paeoniae Alba 白芍

Rhizoma Atractylodis 苍术

Semen Plantaginis　车前子

Pericarpium Citri Reticulatae　陈皮

Radix Bupleuri　柴胡

Spica Schizonepetae　荆芥穗

Radix Glycyrrhizae　甘草

(From *Fu Qingzhu Nüke*《傅青主女科》,"Fu Qingzhu's Obstetrics and Gynecology")

## 82. *Wenjing Tang*　温经汤            113,385

Ingredients:

Ramulus Cinnamomi　桂枝

Fructus Euodiae　吴茱萸

Radix Angelicae Sinensis　当归

Radix Paeoniae　芍药

Rhizoma Ligustici Chuanxiong　川芎

Radix Ginseng　人参

Rhizoma Zingiberis Recens　生姜

Radix Ophiopogonis　麦门冬

Rhizoma Pinelliae　半夏

Cortex Moutan Radicis　牡丹皮

Colla Corii Asini　阿胶

Radix Glycyrrhizae　甘草

(From *Jinkui Yaolüe*《金匮要略》,"Synopsis of Prescriptions of the Golden Chamber")

## 83. Augmented *Wulin San*　加味五淋散         203,425

Ingredients:

Fructus Gardeniae　黑栀子

Poria Rubra　赤茯苓

Radix Angelicae Sinensis　当归

Radix Paeoniae Alba　白芍

Radix Glycyrrhizae　甘草梢

Semen Plantaginis · 车前子

Radix Scutellariae　黄芩

Radix Rehmanniae　生地

Rhizoma Alismatis　泽泻

Talcum　滑石

Caulis Clematidis Armandii　川木通

(From *Yi Zong Jin Jian*《医宗金鉴》, "The Golden Mirror of Medicine")

## 84. *Wuren Wan*　五仁丸　　　　　　　　　　275,457

Ingredients:

Semen Persicae　桃仁

Semen Armeniacae Amarum　杏仁

Semen Pinus · 松子仁

Semen Biotae　柏子仁

Semen Pruni　郁李仁

(From *Shiyi Dexiao Fang*《世医得效方》, "Effective Formulas Handed Down for Generations")

## 85. *Wentu Yulin Tang*　温土毓麟汤　　　　　191,420

Ingredients:

Radix Morindae Officinalis　巴戟天

Fructus Rubi　复盆子

Rhizoma Atractylodis Macrocephalae　白术

Radix Ginseng　人参

Rhizoma Dioscoreae　山药

Massa Fermentata Medicinalis 神曲

(From *Fu Qingzhu Nüke*《傅青主女科》, "Fu Qingzhu's Obstetrics and Gynecology")

**86.** *Wuwei Xiaodu Yin*　五味消毒饮　　44,151,215,356,402,431

　　Ingredients:

　　　　Flos Lonicerae　金银花

　　　　Flos Chrysanthemi Indici　野菊花

　　　　Herba Taraxaci　蒲公英

　　　　Herba Violae　紫花地丁

　　　　Radix Semiaquilegiae　紫背天葵子

　　　　(From *Yi Zong Jin Jian*《医宗金鉴》, "The Golden Mirror of Medicine")

**87. Angmented** *Wuyao Tang*　加味乌药汤　　　117,387

　　Ingredients:

　　　　Radix Linderae　乌药

　　　　Fructus Amomi　砂仁

　　　　Rhizoma Corydalis　延胡

　　　　Rhizoma Cyperi　香附

　　　　Semen Arecae　槟榔

　　　　Radix Aucklandiae　木香

　　　　Rhizoma Zingiberis Recens　生姜

　　　　Radix Glycyrrhizae　甘草

　　　　(From *Yi Zong Jin Jian*《医宗金鉴》, "The Golden Mirror of Medicine")

**88.** *Xiao* **Banxia** *Plus Fuling Tang*　小半夏加茯苓汤　　160,406

　　Ingredients:

Rhizoma Pinelliae　半夏

Rhizoma Zingiberis Recens　生姜

Poria　茯苓

(From *Jinkui Yaolue*《金匮要略》, "Synopsis of Prescriptions of the Golden Chamber")

## 89. *Xiao Chaihu Tang*　小柴胡汤　　　　235,440

Ingredients:

Radix Bupleuri　柴胡

Radix Scutellariae　黄芩

Radix Ginseng　人参

Radix Glycyrrhizae Praeparata　炙甘草

Rhizoma Pinelliae　半夏

Rhizoma Zingiberis Recens　生姜

Fructus Ziziphi Jujubae　大枣

(From *Shanghan Lun*《伤寒论》, "Treatise on Febrile Diseases")

## 90. *Xuefu Zhuyu Tang*　血府逐瘀汤　　　　94,377

Ingredients:

Radix Angelicae Sinensis　当归

Radix Rehmanniae　生地

Semen Persicae　桃仁

Flos Carthami　红花

Fructus Aurantii　枳壳

Radix Paeoniae Rubra　赤芍

Radix Bupleuri　柴胡

Radix Platycodi　桔梗

Rhizoma Ligustici Chuanxiong　川芎

Radix Achyranthis Bidentatae　牛膝

Radix Glycyrrhizae 甘草

(From *Yilin Gaicuo*《医林改错》, " Corrections on the Errors of Medical Works")

## 91. *Xiang Ling Wan* 香棱丸 253,447

Ingredients:

Radix Aucklandiae 木香

Flos Caryophylli 丁香

Rhizoma Sparganii 三棱

Rhizoma Zedoariae 莪术

Fructus Aurantii 枳壳

Pericarpium Citri Reticulatae Viride 青皮

Fructus Meliae Toosendan 川楝子

Fructus Foenicuii 小茴香

(From *Ji Sheng Fang*《济生方》, "Prescriptions for Succouring the Sick")

## 92. *Xiaru Yongquan San* 下乳涌泉散 243,443

Ingredients:

Radix Angelicae Sinensis 当归

Rhizoma Ligustici Chuanxiong 川芎

Radix Trichosanthis 花粉

Radix Paeoniae Alba 白芍

Radix Rehmanniae 生地

Radix Bupleuri 柴胡

Pericarpium Citri Reticulatae Viride 青皮

Radix Rhapontici seu Echinopsis 漏芦

Radix Platycodi 桔梗

Medulla 通草

Radix Angelicae Dahuricae　白芷

Squama Manitis　穿山甲

Semen Vaccariae　王不留行

Radix Glycyrrhizae　甘草

(From "Medical Formulas of Taiyi Hospital of the Qing Dynasty")
《清太乙医院配方》)

## 93. *Xiangsha Liujunzi Tang*　香砂六君子汤　　　158,405

Ingredients:

Radix Ginseng　人参

Rhizoma Atractylodis Macrocephalae　白术

Poria　茯苓

Radix Aucklandiae　木香

Fructus Amomi　砂仁

Pericarpium Citri Reticulatae　陈皮

Rhizoma Pinelliae　半夏

Radix Glycyrrhizae　甘草

Rhizoma Zingiberis Recens　生姜

Fructus Ziziphi Jujubae　大枣

(From *Mingyi Fanglun*《名医方论》, "A Research Manual of Prescriptions of Famous Physicians")

## 94. *Xiaoyao San*　逍遥散　　　119,187,387,418

Ingredients:

Radix Bupleuri　柴胡

Radix Angelicae Sinensis　当归

Radix Paeoniae Alba　白芍

Rhizoma Atractylodis Macrocephalae　白术

Poria　茯苓

Radix Glycyrrhizae  甘草

Rhizoma Zingiberis Recens Praeparata  煨姜

Herba Menthae  薄荷

(From *He Ji Ju Fang* 《和济局方》, "Formularies")

## 95. *Yiguan Jian*  一贯煎                                    176,413

Ingredients:

Radix Adenophorae  南沙参

Radix Ophiopogonis  麦冬

Radix Angelicae Sinensis  当归

Radix Rehmanniae  生地

Fructus Meliae Toosendan  川楝子

Fructus Lycii  枸杞

(From *Liuzhou Yihua* 《柳州医话》, "Medical Notes in Liuzhou")

## 96. *Yougui Wan*  右归丸                              77,106,370,382

Ingredients:

Radix Rehmanniae Praeparata  熟地

Rhizoma Dioscoreae  山药

Fructus Corni  山茱萸

Fructus Lycii  枸杞

Colla Cornus Cervi  鹿角胶

Semen Cuscutae  菟丝子

Cortex Eucommiae  杜仲

Radix Angelicae Sinensis  当归

Corter Cinnamomi  肉桂

Radix Aconiti Praeparata  制附子

(From *Jingyue Quanshu* 《景岳全书》, "Jing Yue's Complete Works")

## 97. *Yinhua Jicai Yin*　银花蕺菜饮　　　　　　　151,402

Ingredients:

　　Flos Lonicerae　金银花

　　Herba Houttuyniae　蕺菜（即鱼腥草）

　　Rhizoma Smilacis Glabrae　土茯苓

　　Herba Menthae　薄荷

　　Radix Glycyrrhizae　生甘草

　　(From "Traditional Chinese Gynecological Therapeutics")

## 98. *Yulin Zhu*　毓麟珠　　　　　　　267,453

Ingredients:

　　Cornu Cervi Degelatinatum　鹿角霜

　　Rhizoma Ligustici Chuanxiong　川芎

　　Radix Paeoniae Alba　白芍

　　Rhizoma Atractylodis Macrocephalae　白术

　　Poria　茯苓

　　Pericarpium Zanthoxyli　川椒

　　Radix Ginseng　人参

　　Radix Angelicae Sinensis　当归

　　Cortex Eucommiae　杜仲

　　Radix Glycyrrhizae　甘草

　　Semen Cuscutae　菟丝子

　　Radix Rehmanniae Praeparata　熟地

　　(From *Jingyue Quanshu*《景岳全书》, "Jing Yue's Complete
　　Works")

## 99. *Yunü Jian*　玉女煎　　　　　　　274,456

Ingredients:

Gypsum Fibrosum  生石膏

Radix Rehmanniae Praeparata  熟地

Radix Ophiopogonis  麦冬

Rhizoma Anemarrhenae  知母

Radix Achyranthis Bidentatae  牛膝

(From *Jingyue Quanshu*《景岳全书》,"Jing Yue's Complete Works")

## 100. *Yiqi Daoniao Tang*　益气导溺汤　　　　　206,426

Ingredients:

Radix Codonopsis Pilosulae  党参

Rhizoma Atractylodis Macrocephala  白术

Semen Dolichoris  扁豆

Ramulus Cinnamomi  桂枝

Poria  茯苓

Rhizoma Cimicifugae Praeparata  炙升麻

Radix Platycodi  桔梗

Tetrapanacis  通草

Radix Linderae  乌药

(From "Traditional Chinese Gynecological Therapeutics")

## 101. *Yinqiao San*　银翘散　　　　　　　　234,439

Ingredients:

Flos Lonicerae  金银花

Fructus Forsythiae  连翘

Radix Platycodi  桔梗

Fructus Arctii  牛蒡子

Spica Schizonepetae  荆芥穗

Herba Menthae  薄荷

Herba Lophatheri　竹叶

Semen Sojae Praeparatum　豆豉

Fresh Rhizoma Phragmitis　鲜苇根

Radix Glycyrrhizae　甘草

(From *Wenbing Tiaobian*《温病条辨》, "Treatise on

Differentiation and Treatment of Epidemic Febrile Diseases")

## 102. Modified *Yi Yin Jian*　加减一阴煎　　　　92,376

Ingredients:

Radix Rehmanniae　生地

Radix Rehmanniae Praeparata　熟地

Radix Paeoniae Alba　白芍

Rhizoma Anemarrhenae　知母

Radix Ophiopogonis　麦冬

Cortex Lycii Radicis　地骨皮

Radix Glycyrrhizae　甘草

(From *Jingyue Quanshu*《景岳全书》, "Jing Yue's Complete
Works")

## 103. *Zhi Bai Dihuang Tang*　知柏地黄汤　　47,65,134,204,357,
364,393,426

Ingredients:

Radix Rehmanniae Praeparata　熟地

Rhizoma Dioscoreae　山药

Fructus Corni　山茱萸

Poria　茯苓

Rhizoma Alismatis　泽泻

Cortex Moutan Radicis　丹皮

Cortex Phellodendri　黄柏

Rhizoma Anemarrhenae　知母

(From *Zheng Yin Mai Zhi* 《症因脉治》, "Etiological Analysis by Pulse Conditions")

## 104. *Zhidai Fang* 止带方        41,355

Ingredients:

Poria 茯苓

Polyporus Umbellatus 猪苓

Rhizoma Alismatis 泽泻

Radix Paeoniae Rubra 赤芍

Cortex Moutan Radicis 丹皮

Herba Artemisiae Capillaris 茵陈

Cortex Phellodendri 黄柏

Fructus Gardeniae 栀子

Radix Achyranthis Bidentatae 牛膝

Semen Plantaginis 车前子

(From *Shibu Zhai Bu Xie Fang* 《世补斋·不谢方》, "Shibu Zhai's Everlasting Prescriptions")

## 105. *Zuogui Wan* 左归丸        75,369

Ingredients:

Radix Rehmanniae Praeparata 熟地

Rhizoma Dioscoreae 山药

Fructus Corni 山萸萸

Fructus Lycii 枸杞

Radix Achyranthis Bidentatae 川牛膝

Semen Cuscutae 菟丝子

Colla Cornus Cervi 鹿胶

Plastrum Testudinis 龟板

(From *Jingyue Quanshu* 《景岳全书》, "Jing Yue's Complete

Works")

## 106. *Zuogui Ying* 左归饮       104,381

Ingredients:

     Radix Rehmanniae Praeparata    熟地

     Rhizoma Dioscoreae    山药

     Fructus Corni    山茱萸

     Fructus Lycii    枸杞

     Poria    茯苓

     Radix Glycyrrhizae Praeparata    炙甘草

     (From *Jingyue Quanshu*《景岳全书》, "Jing Yue's Complete
       Works")

## 107. *Zhuli Tang* 竹沥汤       193,421

Ingredients:

     Succus Bambosae    竹沥

     Radix Scutellariae    黄芩

     Radix Ophiopogonis    麦冬

     Poria    茯苓

     Radix Ledebouriellae    防风

     (From *Beiji Qianjin Yaofang*《千金要方》, "Prescriptions Worth a
       Thousand Gold for Emergencies")

## 108. *Zisu Yin* 紫苏饮       196,422

Ingredients:

     Folium Perillae    紫苏

     Pericarpium citri Reticulatae    陈皮

     Pericarpium Arecae    大腹皮

     Radix Angelicae Sinensis    当归

Radix Paeoniae Alba　白芍

Rhizoma Ligustici Chuanxiong　川芎

Radix Ginseng　人参

Radix Glycyrrhizae　甘草

(From *Puji Benshi Fang*《普济本事方》,"Effective Prescriptions
  for Universal Relief")

## 109. *Zhen Wu Tang*　真武汤　　　　　　　　173,412

Ingredients:

Poria　茯苓

Rhizoma Atractylodis Macrocephalae　白术

Radix Paeoniae Alba　白芍

Rhizoma Zingiberis Recens　生姜

Radix Aconiti Praeparata　附子

(From *Shanghan Lun*《伤寒论》,"Treatise on Febrile Diseases")

## 110. *Zi Xue Tang*　滋血汤　　　　　　　　116,386

Ingredients:

Radix Ginseng　人参

Rhizoma Dioscoreae　山药

Radix Astragali seu Hedysari　黄芪

Poria　白茯苓

Rhizoma Ligustici Chuanxiong　川芎

Radix Angelicae Sinensis　当归

Radix Paeoniae Alba　白芍药

Radix Rehmanniae Praeparata　熟地黄

(From *Zhengzhi Zhunsheng*《证治准绳》, "Standards of
  Diagnosis and Treatment")

## 111. *Zengye Tang*　增液汤

Ingredients:

Radix Rehmanniae　生地

Radix Scrophulariae　玄参

Radix Ophiopogonis　麦冬

(From *Wenbing Tiaobian*《温病条辨》, " Treatise on Differentiation and Treatment of Epidemic Febrile Diseases")

# 12

# 妇 科 学

# 序

　　《英汉实用中医药大全》即将问世，吾为之高兴。

　　歧黄之道，历经沧桑，永盛不衰。吾中华民族之强盛，由之。世界医学之丰富和发展，亦由之。然而，世界民族之差异，国别之不同，语言之障碍，使中医中药的传播和交流受到了严重束缚。当前，世界各国人民学习、研究、运用中医药的热潮方兴未艾。为使吾中华民族优秀文化遗产之一的歧黄之道走向世界，光大其业，为世界人民造福，徐象才君集省内外精英于一堂，主持编译了《英汉实用中医药大全》。是书之问世将使海内外同道欢呼雀跃。

　　世界医学发展之日，当是歧黄之道光大之时。

　　吾欣然序之。

中华人民共和国卫生部副部长
　兼国家中医药管理局局长
世界针灸学会联合会主席
中国科学技术协会委员
中华全国中医学会副会长
中国针灸学会会长

一九八九年十二月

# 序

中华民族有同疾病长期作斗争的光辉历程，故而有自己的传统医学——中国医药学。中国医药学有一套完整的从理论到实践的独特科学体系。几千年来，它不但被完好地保存下来，而且得到了发扬光大。它具有疗效显著、副作用小等优点，是人们防病治病，强身健体的有效工具。

任何一个国家在医学进步中所取得的成就，都是人类共同的财富，是没有国界的。医学成果的交流比任何其他科学成果的交流都应进行得更及时，更准确。我从事中医工作30多年来，一直盼望着有朝一日中国医药学能全面走向世界，为全人类解除病痛疾苦作出其应有的贡献。但由于用外语表达中医难度较大，中国医药学对外传播的速度一直不能令人满意。

山东中医学院的徐象才老师发起并主持了大型系列丛书《英汉实用中医药大全》的编译工作。这个工作是一项巨大工程，是一种大型科研活动，是一个大胆的尝试，是一件新事物。对徐象才老师及与其合作的全体编译者夜以继日地长期工作所付出的艰苦劳动，克服重重困难所表现出的坚韧不拔的毅力，以及因此而取得的重大成绩，我甚为敬佩。作为一个中医界的领导者，对他们的工作给予全力支持是我应尽的责任。

我相信《英汉实用中医药大全》无疑会在中国医学史和世界科学技术史上找到它应有的位置。

中华全国中医学会常务理事
山东省卫生厅副厅长
张秀文
1990 年 3 月

# 出 版 前 言

　　中国医药学是我中华民族优秀文化遗产之一，建国以来由于党和国家对待中医药采取了正确的政策，使中医药理论宝库不断得到了发掘整理，取得了巨大的成绩。当前，世界各国人民对中国医药学的学习和研究热潮日益高涨。为促进这一热潮更加蓬勃的发展，为使中国医药学能更好地为全人类解除病痛服务，就必须促进中医中药在世界范围内的传播和交流，而要使这一传播和交流进行得更及时、更准确，就必须首先排除语言障碍。因此，编译一套英汉对照的中医药基本知识的书籍，供国内外学习、研究中医药时使用，已成为国内外医药学界和医药学教育界许多人士的迫切需要。

　　多年来，在卫生部门的号召下，在"中医英语表达研究"方面，已经作出了一些可喜的成绩。本书《英汉实用中医药大全》的编辑出版就是在调查上述研究工作的历史和现状的基础上，继续对中医药英语表达作较系统、较全面的研究，以适应中国医药学对外传播交流的需要。

　　这部"大全"的版本为英汉对照，共有 21 个分册，一个分册介绍论述中国医药学的一个分科。在编著上注意了中医药汉文稿的编写特色，在内容上注意了科学性、实用性、全面性和简明易读。汉文稿的执笔撰写者主要是有 20 年以上实践经验的教授、副教授、主任医师和副主任医师。各分册汉文稿撰写成后，均经各学科专家逐一审订。各分册英文主译、主审主要是国内既懂中医又懂英语的权威人士，还有许多中医院校的英语教师及医药卫生部门的专业翻译人员。英译稿脱稿后，经过了复审、终审，有些译稿还召开全国 22 所院校和单位人员参加的英译稿统稿定稿研讨会，对英译稿进行细致的研讨和推敲，对如何较全面、较系统、较准确地用英语表达中国医药学进行了探讨，从而推动整个译文达到较高水平，因此，这部"大全"可供中医院校高年级学生作为泛读教材使用。

这部"大全"的编纂得到了国家教育委员会、国家中医药管理局、山东省教育委员会、山东省卫生厅等各部门有关领导的支持。在国家教委高等教育司的指导下，成立了《英汉实用中医药大全》编译领导委员会。还得到了全国许多中医院校和中药生产厂家领导的支持。

希望这部"大全"的出版，对中医院校加强中医英语教学，对国内卫生界培养外向型中医药人才，以及在推动世界各国人民对中医药的学习和研究方面，都将产生良好的影响。

高等教育出版社

1990 年 3 月

# 前　言

　　《英汉实用中医药大全》是一部以中医基本理论为基础，以中医临床为重点，较为全面系统、简明扼要、易读实用的中级英汉学术性著作。它的主要读者是：中医药院校高年级学生和中青年教师，中医院的中青年医生和中医药科研单位的科研人员，从事中医对外函授工作的人员和出国讲学或行医的中医人员，西学中人员，来华学习中医的外国留学生和各类进修人员。

　　由于中国医药学为我中华民族之独有，因此，英译便成了本《大全》编译工作的重点。为确保译文能准确表达中医的确切含义，我们邀集熟悉中医的英语人员、医学专业翻译人员、懂英语的中医药人员乃至医古文人员于一堂，共同翻译、共同对译文进行研讨推敲的集体翻译法，这样，就把众人之长融进了译文质量之中。然而，即使这样，也难确保译文都能尽如人意。汉文稿虽反映了中国医药学的精髓和概貌，但也难能十全十美。我衷心地盼望读者能提出批评和建议，以便《大全》再版时修改。

　　参加本《大全》编、译、审工作的人员达 200 余名，他们来自全国 28 个单位，其中有山东、北京、上海、天津、南京、浙江、安徽、河南、湖北、广西、贵阳、甘肃、成都、山西、长春等 15 所中医学院，还有中国中医研究院，山东省中医药研究所等中医药科研单位。

　　山东省教育委员会把本《大全》的编译列入了科研计划并拨发了科研经费，山东省卫生厅和一些中药生产厂家也给了很大支持，济南中药厂的资助为编译工作的开端提供了条件。

　　本《大全》的编译成功是全体编译审者集体劳动的结晶，是各有关单位主管领导支持的结果。在《大全》各分册即将陆续出版之际，我诚挚地感谢全体编译审者的真诚合作，感谢许多专家、教授、各级领导和生产厂家的热情支持。

愿本《大全》的出版能在培养通晓英语的中医人才和使中医早日全面走向世界方面起到我所期望的作用。

主编　　徐象才

于山东中医学院
一九九〇年三月

# 目　录

# 说　明

　　《妇科学》是《英汉实用中医药大全》的第12分册。

　　本分册共有六章，其内容为：概论，女性生殖系统炎症，月经失调，妊娠病理，异常分娩与异常产褥和其他妇科疾病。

　　为给世界范围内的读者在阅读时提供方便，本分册仍采用妇科疾病的现代医学分类法，但就内容的编写乃是根据中医治疗妇科疾病的基本理论和方法。

　　本分册的汉文稿曾经山东中医杂志的王文玉女士校阅，最后由中国已故的中医妇科权威哈荔田教授审定。其英文稿经过了懂中医的英语教授和懂英语的中医教授的集体研讨推敲，力求准确。

编　者

1990年3月

# 1 概 论

## 1.1 中医妇科概况

中医妇科学是根据中医学的理论，认识妇女的解剖生理、病理特点、诊断规律和研究妇女特有疾病的一门临床医学学科。

中医妇科学研究的范围为调经、嗣育、胎前、临产、产后、崩漏、带下、杂病等项。概括为经、带、胎、产、杂五个方面。

中医妇科学是祖国医学的重要组成部分，有着悠久的历史，丰富的经验。几千年来为我国妇女保健事业起着重大的作用，对我们民族的繁衍和昌盛做出了贡献。

中医妇科的起源，根据现有文献证明，早在3千年前的殷商时代，甲骨文中就有"疾育"的记载。周初《诗经》中就有 茹（茜草）、蓷（益母草）、茉苢（车前草）等妇科常用药物的采集。先秦战国时代的《山海经》记载了"䳡"食之"宜子"，而"蓍蓉"食之使人"无子"。《曲礼》指出"取妻不取同姓"，"男女同姓，其生不蕃"。认识到近亲婚配的危害性。

公元前221年成书的《黄帝内经》中，已有妇女解剖、生理、诊断妇科病的描述，指出女子14岁月经可以来潮，21岁发育成熟，49岁左右月经即不来潮。详细地论述了月经产生的机理及女性一生生长发育和衰老的过程。并记载了妇科第一个方剂"四乌鲗骨——藘茹丸"。战国时代就有了妇科医生，《史记·扁鹊仓公列传》记载了名医扁鹊，过邯郸闻贵妇人，即为带下医。带下医指治疗裙带以下疾病而言，即妇科医生。

现存医籍中最早有妇科专篇论述的是汉代张仲景的《金匮要略》对妇女妊娠病、产后病、杂病脉证并治的三篇论述，至今对妇科临床影响很大。书中记载了阴道冲洗和阴道栓剂的外治法。同时代的神医华佗，凭脉证对一生一死的双胎进行了正确的诊断，并用针药合治方法下死胎。

公元3世纪，晋代名医王叔和著有《脉经》，记载了妇人妊娠、产后、带下、月经病及妇女杂病的脉法和辨证。并观察到临产的"离经之脉"及月经的异常现象：三月一潮的"居经"及一年一潮的"避年"。

南齐褚澄著《褚氏遗书》，他在求嗣一门中提倡：男"必三十而娶"，女"必二十而嫁"，只有这样后代才"坚壮强寿"。并提出"合男子多则沥枯虚人，产乳众则血枯杀人"这种对晚婚、节欲、节育的认识，对保证妇女的健康及民族的昌盛起了重大作用。

北齐徐之才著《十月养胎方》（即逐月养胎方），记述了胎儿逐月发育的情况、孕妇各月饮食起居应注意的问题及针灸禁忌等，并附养胎方以防流产。

公元610年隋代以太医博士巢元方为首集体编写的《诸病源候论》，论述了妇产科疾病283种，明确了妊娠为10个阴历月，并提出母病"既不能养胎，兼害妊妇，故去之"，主张人工去胎，以保母亲的安全。

公元652年，唐代孙思邈著《备急千金要方》，将妇人方列为卷首，明确提出妇科应设专科研究，并指出不孕与男女双方都有关系。认为"凡人无子，当为夫妻俱有五劳七伤，虚羸百疾所致"。强调产房要清洁安静，"凡欲产时，特忌多人瞻视"。提倡"凡产后满百日，乃可会合，不尔，至死虚羸，百病滋长，慎之"。极其重视产褥期的卫生。

《产宝》是现存最早的产科专著，即现传本《经效产宝》。公元852年由唐代昝殷所撰写，分上、中、下3卷及续编1卷，全部内容均围绕着妊娠、分娩、产后病加以论述，并有治法。

公元14世纪，宋代有了管理医事的太医局，产科为所设九科之一，并设产科教授。这是世界医事制度上妇科最早的独立分科，明确了分科，促进了妇产科的发展。宋代产科专著颇多，最著名的有杨子建的《十产论》，陈自明的《妇人良方大全》。

公元 13～14 世纪的金元时代，是我国医学的百家争鸣时代，刘（完素）、李（东垣）、朱（丹溪）、张（子和）四大家，他们对妇科各有独到见解。刘氏提出妇女在少年时代着重于肾经，中年重肝经，老年重脾经的理论和治法，对后世影响很大。李氏主张补脾升阳，益气补血之法，为妇科广泛应用。朱氏以他"阳常有余，阴常不足"理论，提出"产前当清热养血"，认为"产前安胎黄芩、白术为妙药"，并延用至今。张氏的"养生当论食补，治病当论药攻"理论，用吐、下法驱逐痰水以治月经病。

明代妇科专著很多，有王肯堂的《证治准绳·女科》，薛立斋的《女科撮要》，万全（密斋）的《广嗣纪要》，张景岳的《妇人规》等。万氏提出"种子者，男则清心寡欲以养其精，女则平心定气以养其血"。指出女子先天性生理缺陷而造成的不孕症有五：螺、纹、鼓、角、脉，称之为五不女。张景岳对"天癸"的论述十分详细，认为天癸是来自先天经过后天逐渐滋养而产生的一种阴液，对人体生长、发育、月经来潮与终止有直接作用。明代伟大医药学家李时珍在《本草纲目》中，论述女性月经如月之盈亏，潮之朝夕一样有规律，指出"女人之经，一月一行，其常也"。

清代将妇科统称之为女科，著作很多。对后世影响较大的有《傅青主女科》、《医宗金鉴·妇科心法要诀》、《达生编》、《女科辑要》等。亟斋居士的《达生编》提出临产时要"睡、忍痛、慢临盆"的六字真言，对产妇起到精神保护性作用。

清末民国初年，由于西方医学的输入，"中西医汇通"的代表作有唐容川的《血证论》、张锡纯的《医学衷中参西录》、张山雷的《沈氏女科辑要笺正》等。

中华人民共和国成立以来，妇科学取得了巨大成就，如中西医结合非手术治疗宫外孕、中药引产、针灸纠正胎位等等。自

1956 年成立中医学院以来，至今已编写出版了五版中医妇科学统一教材，出版了《中国医学百科全书·中医妇科学》培养了大批中医妇科人才，为妇女的保健事业做出了巨大贡献。

## 1.2　女性的解剖生理特点

### 1.2.1　女性内、外生殖器官

胞宫，即子宫，又称女子胞、胞脏、子脏、子处，简称脏或胞等。因其对月经、妊娠有不同的定期藏泻作用，既藏又泻，而且无与其他脏腑表里相配，故称之为奇恒之府。

胞脉、胞络是联系胞宫的脉络，附属于胞宫，与脏腑有着密切的联系，它们与胞宫共同完成主月经，孕育胎儿的功能。

子门，指子宫颈口。

产道，即阴道。

子肠，概指子宫及阴道壁。"子肠不收"系子宫脱垂或阴道壁膨出。

阴户，指妇女外阴。

阴门，亦称产门，即阴道口。

阴器，外生殖器官。

毛际，外阴阴毛丛生之处。

交骨，即耻骨联合处。

### 1.2.2　冲、任、督、带脉

冲脉，起于胞中，循会阴上行到头，下行至足，前行腹部，后行脊里，是十二经脉汇聚之所，具有调节月经的功能。

任脉，任脉主胞胎，起于胞中，下出会阴，沿腹正中线上行至唇及眼眶下。凡精、血、津、液均属任脉所司，只有任脉之气通，才能促使月经来潮和孕育的正常。

督脉，有总督之意，起于胞中，与任脉同出会阴，沿脊柱上行至头部。督脉贯脊属肾，肾为先天之本，元气之根，所以督脉又维系一身之元气。任脉、督脉相交会于龈交穴，循环往复，维持着阴阳脉气的平衡，调节月经的正常来潮。

带脉，始于季胁，绕身一周，状如束带，故称之为带脉。其功能约束诸经，使经脉、气血循行保持常度。

冲、任、督三脉皆起于胞中，由带脉约束，外连十二经脉，使之与脏腑相通，调节着月经的产生和维持着正常生理功能。

## 1.2.3　月经及其产生机理

月经是指有规律的、周期性的子宫出血。每月一次，如月之盈亏，潮之朝夕，经常不变，故有月汛、月信、月水之称。

早在两千年前《内经》就记载有："女子七岁肾气盛，齿更发长；二七而天癸至，任脉通，太冲脉盛，月事以时下，故有子…。七七任脉虚，太冲脉衰少，天癸竭，地道不通，故形坏而无子也。"详细地论述了女性生殖功能的发育、成熟和衰退的过程。健康女子，一般在14岁左右月经来潮，称为初潮，是青春发育期的标志。初潮年龄可因地区、气候、民族、营养等不同而有差异，早者11岁，迟者18岁。除妊娠、哺乳以外，直至49岁左右月经才终止。

月经一般28天一个周期，提前、错后不应超过7天，持续3～7天，量约50～80毫升，色暗红，开始和最后色淡红，第2、3天量较多，质不稀不稠，血不凝固，无特殊臭气。定期2月一次者，称"并月"；3个月一潮者，称"居经"或"季经"；一年一行，称"避年"；终生不来潮而能受孕者，称"暗经"；受孕后，初期仍按月有少量流血，而无损胎儿者，称"激经"、又称"垢胎"或"盛胎"。

月经的产生是天癸、脏腑、气血、经络协调作用于子宫的生理现象。天癸，男女皆有，是影响人体生长、发育和生殖的一种阴精，它来源于先天肾气，靠后天水谷精气的滋养，逐渐成熟。

天癸禀受于父母，但必须在肾气盛，并到一定年龄时才蓄极而生，它使任脉所司精血津液充沛，并与冲脉相资。冲脉得肾精充实，聚脏腑之血，依时由满而溢于子宫，使月经来潮。月经的主要成分是血，血由脏腑所化生；肾藏精，精化血，心主血，肝藏血，脾统血，肺主气，气帅血，故月经的产生与肾、肝、脾（胃）的关系最密切。血是月经的物质基础，气是运行血脉的动力，只有气血和调，才能经候如常。经络是内属脏腑，外络肢节，沟通内外，贯串上下信息的径路，把人体各部分联成一个有机的整体，运行气血，营养全身。冲任督带脉与妇女的生理、病理特点联系最为密切，调节十二经气血的运行，在月经的产生中起了很大的作用。

肾是产生月经的根本，气血是月经的物质基础，冲任是化月经之所，子宫乃是行月经之处。故只有在肾气盛，天癸至，任脉通，太冲脉盛的情况下，月经方可以时而下。

# 1.3  治法概要

妇科疾病的治疗方法是从人的整体观出发，遵循中医的四诊八纲、辨证论治的原则，根据女性的生理特点，结合妇科经、带、胎、产、杂特有疾病的病因病机，本着"治病必求其本"，以"急则治其标，缓则治其本"，"虚者补之"、"实者泻之"、"寒者热之"、"热者寒之"的原则，对不同的疾病，采用不同的具体治疗方法。若全身病变，应以内服药为主。属局部病变，可兼用外治法。常用治疗方法如下。

## 1.3.1  内治法

### 1.补肾法

补肾法是针对肾虚而立的治疗大法，肾为女子之先天，肾在女性生理上的重要作用，决定了补肾法的重要性。若肾气虚，精血耗损，冲任失调，则经、带、胎、产、杂诸疾丛生。通过补肾，使肾之阴阳平衡协调，以维持正常生理功能。

（1）补肾阳

若肾阳不足，胞宫失于温煦，则出现阴部寒冷，性欲低下，宫寒不孕、胎萎不长、堕胎、小产等病。

常用药物：肉桂、附子、破故纸、仙灵脾、仙茅、菟丝子、巴戟、锁阳、复盆子等。

代表方剂：肾气丸、右归丸、右归饮等。

（2）滋肾阴

肾阴不足，冲任失养，致使月经量少，闭经，阴中干涩，崩漏，月经提前或延后，不孕，胎萎不长等病发生。

常用药物：地黄、黄精、阿胶、山茱萸、女贞子、何首乌、龟板胶、枸杞、冬虫夏草等。

代表方剂：六味地黄丸，左归丸等。

应用补肾药时，根据临床辩证，无论是补肾阳，或是滋肾阴，或阴阳双补，都必须遵循在滋阴时不忘补阳，补阳中不忘滋阴，即在补阴方中少佐温阳药物，补阳方中少佐益阴之品，使阴阳互相依存，以利疾病的恢复。

**2. 调肝法**

调肝法指调节肝的功能，使其恢复正常。肝藏血，主疏泄。其功能正常，月经才能按时来潮。肝病在妇科主要表现于肝气郁结和肝阴不足两方面。治以疏肝和养肝为主。

（1）疏肝

①疏肝解郁

妇人因经、带、胎、产屡伤于血，故常血分不足，气分偏盛，情志致病较多。若抑郁愤怒，则肝失条达，肝郁气滞，血行不畅，脉络受阻。出现痛经、闭经、经前乳房胀痛、产后缺乳等疾病。若疏泄无度则月经先后不定期。必治以疏肝解郁。

常用药物：柴胡、香附、郁金、川楝子、乌药、青皮、橘叶、薄荷等。

代表方剂：逍遥散、柴胡疏肝散等。

②清肝泻热

肝郁化火，肝气上逆，迫血妄行，引起月经先期、月经量多、经期延长、崩漏、经行吐衄、经行头痛等病证。治疗时必须在疏肝的基础上加入清肝泻热药物。如丹皮、栀子、菊花、夏枯草等。

代表方剂：丹栀逍遥散。

③清热利湿

肝经湿热下注，引起带下、阴痒、阴疮等病。治宜清利肝经湿热。

常用药物：龙胆草、茵陈、车前子、黄柏。

代表方剂：龙胆泻肝汤。

(2) 养肝

①养血柔肝

肝阴不足，则出现月经后期、月经量少、闭经、崩漏、月经前后诸证、绝经前后诸证等病。

常用药物：枸杞、白芍、女贞子、旱莲草、桑椹、五味子、当归、地黄等。

代表方剂：二至丸、一贯煎、杞菊地黄丸等。

②平肝潜阳，镇肝熄风

肝阴不足，肝阳上亢，致使经行头痛、先兆子痫及肝风内动所致妊娠痫证等。宜在滋补肝阴的基础上，加入平肝潜阳、镇肝熄风的药物。如代赭石、白芍、龙骨、牡蛎、珍珠母、龟板、刺蒺藜、地龙、钩藤、羚羊角、牛黄等。

代表方剂：三甲复脉汤、羚羊钩藤汤、羚羊角汤等。

**3. 健脾法**

健脾法是针对脾虚而设的治疗大法。脾统血，主运化，是气血生化之源，水液代谢之枢纽。脾虚引起许多妇科疾患，必须用健脾法治之。

(1) 健脾益气

脾气虚弱，化源不足，常出现月经后期、月经量少、闭经、缺乳、恶阻等病。

常用药物：人参、党参、黄芪、山药、大枣、甘草等。

代表方剂：四君子汤、参苓白术散。

(2) 健脾利湿

脾虚不运，水湿停滞常致带下、妊娠水肿、经行泄泻、经行水肿，或湿聚成痰引起痰湿闭经、不孕等病。

常用药物：苍术、茯苓、猪苓、半夏、白术、车前子、大腹皮、薏苡仁、赤小豆、藿香、厚朴等。

代表方剂：完带汤、全生白术散、启宫丸等。

(3) 健脾升陷

脾虚中气下陷，统摄无权，所致崩漏、月经量多、堕胎、滑胎、恶露不绝、子宫脱垂等，宜用健脾升举中气治之。

常用药物：党参、黄芪、白术、柴胡、升麻等。

代表方剂：补中益气汤、举元煎、固本止崩汤等。

(4) 健脾和胃

脾胃互为表里。若脾胃不和，胃失和降则上逆，引起恶阻等疾。治宜健脾和胃以降逆。若肝郁气结，肝气上逆犯胃者，加入抑肝之品。

常用药物：陈皮、半夏、砂仁、苏叶、黄连、代赭石、竹茹、吴茱萸、生姜等。

代表方剂：香砂六君子汤、苏叶黄连汤。

**4. 调理气血**

气血是维持人体生命活动的基本物质和动力。气血调和，人体生理功能正常，气血失调，影响冲任为病，导致经、带、胎、产诸疾丛生。调理气血是治疗妇科病的重要方法之一。

调理气血，首先分辨病在气还是在血，然后确定治法。气病有气虚、气滞、气陷、气逆之不同。虚者补之，郁者散之，陷者举之升之，逆者降之。气虚、气陷、气逆均在健脾法中论述，不再赘述。

(1) 理气行滞

气郁运行不畅，冲任受阻，可致闭经、痛经、月经先后不定期、症瘕、不孕、妊娠腹痛等病。治宜理气通滞，行气散结。

常用药物：香附、枳壳、厚朴、木香、乌药、青皮、川楝子、橘核、荔枝核、佛手等。

代表方剂：加味乌药散等。

(2) 补血养血

血虚冲任虚损所致月经量少、月经后期、闭经、妊娠腹痛、产后身痛等病。

常用药物：当归、熟地、白芍、首乌、阿胶、桂圆肉、鸡血藤、枸杞子、桑椹子、大枣等。

代表方剂：四物汤、当归补血汤、人参滋血汤等。

(3) 清热凉血

血分蕴热，热扰冲任，迫血妄行，常致月经量多，月经先期，经期延长、崩漏、胎漏、产后恶露不绝。治宜清热凉血以止血。

常用药物：生地、玄参、丹皮、紫草、白薇、栀子、地榆、侧柏叶、白芍、麦冬等。

代表方剂：清经汤、两地汤等。

(4) 温经和血

寒主收引凝涩。寒邪客于胞宫，血行不畅，冲任受阻所致月经量少、月经后期、闭经、痛经、妊娠腹痛、恶露不下等。

常用药物：肉桂、附子、桂枝、艾叶、小茴香、吴茱萸、炮姜、乌药等。

代表方剂：温经汤、艾附暖宫丸等。

(5) 活血化瘀

气滞、寒凝、血热灼津均可造成血瘀。血瘀则冲任阻滞，引起痛经、闭经、崩漏、症瘕、产后发热、产后恶露不绝等。

常用药物：当归、川芎、益母草、蒲黄、五灵脂、红花、桃仁、丹参、泽兰、牛膝、三七、乳香、没药、王不留行等。

代表方剂：桃红四物汤、少腹逐瘀汤、生化汤等。

**5. 清热解毒**

感受热邪，蕴结成毒，可致带下、阴痒、阴疮、产后发热、产后发痉等病。

常用药物：金银花、蒲公英、紫花地丁、败酱草、鱼腥草、红藤、土茯苓、苦参、野菊花、黄柏、板蓝根、大青叶、贯众等。

代表方剂：五味消毒饮、银翘红酱解毒汤。

若热邪伤阴，常在清热解毒方中，配伍滋阴药，如生地、玄参、沙参、麦冬、芦根等。热毒蕴结，常致血瘀，故在清热解毒方中加入赤芍、丹皮、鳖甲、海藻、昆布、刘寄奴、牡蛎、乳香、没药等活血化瘀，软坚散结药物，可收到更好的疗效。

## 1.3.2 外治法

早在公元 219 年成书的《金匮要略》一书中，张仲景就用外治法治疗妇女杂病。以蛇床子散坐药，治疗寒湿带下；狼牙汤淋洗阴部，治疗下焦湿热、阴中生疮；矾石纳入阴中治内有干血，阴中时下白带；膏发煎导肠治胃气下泄，阴吹正喧。后世对妇科病的外治法有了很大发展，主要有以下几法。

**1. 熏洗法**

作用：清热解毒、活血化瘀、软坚散结、祛风杀虫止痒。

用法：将配好的中药放入盆内，倒入 2000～2500 毫升的水，浸泡半小时，然后加热，煮沸 15～20 分钟，去掉药渣，先熏蒸局部，待水温适宜时，坐入盆中 15～20 分钟，日一次。

适应证：外阴瘙痒、外阴炎、巴氏腺囊肿、巴氏腺脓肿、外阴疖肿、慢性外阴营养不良症、滴虫性阴道炎、霉菌性阴道炎、老年性阴道炎等。

**2. 外敷法**

作用：活血化瘀、软坚散结、清热解毒。

用法：中药捣碎装袋蒸煮后放在局部热敷，或将药物制成膏剂外贴患处或某些穴位上。

适应证：痛经、盆腔炎块、输卵管积水、月经失调等。

**3. 纳入法**

作用：清热解毒、去腐生肌、杀虫止痒。

用法：睡觉前洗净外阴阴道，将药栓或药片、药粉纳入阴道深处，臀部垫一布垫，以防用药后液体流出污染床铺，每晚一次。若腐蚀性药物，必须由医生放置，用棉球保护好周围的好组织后，将蘸上药粉的带线棉球敷在患处，定期取出。

适应证：阴道炎、宫颈炎、宫颈癌等。

**4. 导肠法**

作用：清热解毒，活血化瘀祛湿，润肠通腑。

用法：将栓剂放入肛内或将汤剂注入肠内，用药前最好排便或清洁灌肠，以利于药物吸收。汤剂温度在 37 度左右，量不可过多，一般在 100～200 毫升即可。每日一次，保留时间越长越好。

适应证：产后感染发热、盆腔炎、阴吹等证。

**注意事项**：

阴道内用药宜在月经干净后 3～7 天，经期、新产禁用。

妊娠期不用导肠法或外敷少腹法。

用药期间禁性生活，阴道内用药期间不坐浴。

一切药品、工具必须严格消毒。

(李竹兰)

# 2 女性生殖系统炎症

## 2.1 外阴炎及前庭大腺炎

### 2.1.1 外阴炎

外阴部的皮肤粘膜发炎称为外阴炎。可分为急、慢性两种。由于阴道分泌物的增多、经血、月经垫的刺激、糖尿病人的糖尿、粪瘘及尿瘘患者的粪便、尿液的刺激和浸渍，以及由此所造成的混合感染所引起。临床主要以外阴瘙痒、疼痛、烧灼、局部肿胀、溃烂为特点。属中医的"阴痒""阴疮"（亦称"阴蚀"、"䘌"）的范畴。

中医认为足厥阴肝经绕阴器而行，阴部为肝经之分野，外阴疾患乃肝经湿热，或肝郁脾虚化火生湿，湿热之邪随经下注，蕴结于阴部所引起。

**临床表现** 外阴皮肤瘙痒、疼痛、焮红灼热。活动、排尿、性交时加重。或少腹急痛，或两胁胀痛，口苦、咽干、心烦易怒、时有寒热。舌红苔黄腻，脉滑数。妇科检查：外阴局部充血、肿胀、有抓痕，有时可见溃疡。严重时腹股沟淋巴结肿大、压痛。慢性外阴炎皮肤粘膜增厚、粗糙、苔藓化。

治法：清热利湿，解毒止痒。

方药：龙胆泻肝汤（38）。

龙胆草 6 克，山栀子 9 克，黄芩 12 克，车前子 12 克（包），木通 6 克，泽泻 9 克，生地 15 克，当归 12 克，柴胡 9 克，甘草 6 克。水煎 200～300 毫升，早晚分服。

加减：发热，化验白细胞增高时，加金银花 30 克、土茯苓 15 克、丹皮 15 克。

小便涩痛、量少、色黄者，加滑石 15 克，淡竹叶 12 克。

大便秘结者，加大黄 6 克（后入）、芦荟 9 克。

外治法：清热燥湿，解毒止痒。

方药：I 号外阴洗剂。

野菊花 30 克，苦参 30 克，蛇床子 30 克，金银花 30 克，黄柏 15 克，土茯苓 15 克，川椒 12 克，丹皮 12 克，冰片 3 克（冲入）。

以上各药（冰片除外）用水 2000～2500 毫升，浸泡半小时～1 小时后加热，煮开 15～20 分钟，将水倾入浴盆内，倒掉药渣，放冰片于盆内化开，先熏后洗外阴部，待水温适度时，坐浴 15～20 分钟，每日一次。

加减：皮肤粘膜被抓破或有溃疡者，去川椒，加紫草 15 克，白芨 12 克。

痒甚，皮肤粘膜呈苔藓样变者加赤芍 15 克，当归 15 克，荆芥、防风各 9 克。

## 2.1.2  前庭大腺炎

前庭大腺炎多发生于生育期年龄，婴幼儿及绝经后很少发生。多属葡萄球菌、大肠杆菌、链球菌及肠球菌等混合感染所致。临床主要以一侧大阴唇肿胀、疼痛为特点。属中医"阴肿"范畴。亦称"阴户肿胀"、"子户肿胀"。

由于肝经湿热循经下流，乘于阴户，与血气相搏，腠理壅闭，不得泄越而肿胀。

**临床表现**  外阴一侧疼痛、肿胀、活动受限，严重时发热、口苦。苔黄腻，脉弦数。妇科检查：一侧大阴唇下方皮肤红肿、发热、压痛明显，肿块直径可达 5～6 厘米，有波动感。

治法：清热解毒，消肿排脓。

方药：柴芩芷桔汤。

柴胡 9 克，黄芩 12 克，土茯苓 15 克，薏苡仁 30 克，连翘 15 克，当归 15 克，白芷 12 克，桔梗 9 克，木通 6 克，生甘草 6 克。水煎 200～300 毫升，早晚分服。

外治法：清热解毒，活血化瘀消肿。

方药：Ⅱ号外阴洗剂。

野菊花 30 克，蒲公英 30 克，连翘 15 克，当归 15 克，丹皮 15 克，赤芍 15 克，苏木 15 克，白芷 12 克，黄柏 12 克，穿山甲 9 克，皂刺 9 克，冰片 3 克（冲入）。水煎熏洗、坐浴，每日一次，方法同前。

**单方验方**

川椒 15 克，艾叶 15 克，野菊花 30 克。水煎熏洗，每日 1～2 次，方法同前。用于止痒。

青黛 30 克，蛤粉 30 克，黄柏 15 克。共研细粉，用植物油调匀后，涂于患处，治疗外阴溃疡。

艾叶 30 克，防风 15 克，大戟 12 克。水煎熏洗。陈皮 30 克，枳实 30 克，研末炒热装袋后外敷患处。用以消肿止痛。

**预防**　不过食辛辣刺激性食物。

勤洗外阴，换洗内裤，养成良好的卫生习惯。月经垫、纸应消毒后使用，保持外阴清洁干燥。

积极治疗阴道炎、宫颈炎、糖尿病、尿瘘、粪瘘等病，防止过多分泌物的刺激。

## 2.2　阴道炎症

女性青春期后，阴道的酸碱度（pH）在 4.2～5 之间，本身有自净作用。当这种防御功能遭到破坏时，病原菌即可侵入，导致阴道炎。临床以阴道烧灼、疼痛、阴痒、白带增多为特点。属中医的"带下病"、"阴痒"范畴。

"带下"有广义和狭义之分，广义带下指妇女的经、带、胎、产诸疾而言，狭义带下指妇女阴道内少量白色或无色、质粘、无臭气的阴液。这是肾气充盛、脾气健运、任脉通畅、带脉健固的表现，是女性进入青春期的标志，属正常生理现象。

若带下绵绵不断，量多，色、质、臭气异常，并伴有全身或局部症状者，称"带下病"。湿邪为患是其主要病因，脾虚失运，痰湿内停肝经湿热下注，或肾虚不固以及经行产后胞脉空虚，摄生不洁，手术损伤后，湿邪乘虚而入，蕴而化热，损伤任、带二脉，以致带脉失约，任脉不固，导致带下病。古代有青、白、黄、赤、黑五种带下及五色兼杂的"五色带"之分，但临床以白带、黄带为多。若有赤白带下或五色杂下时，应仔细检查，排除恶变。

## 辨证论治

### 1. 脾虚型

**临床表现** 带下色白或淡黄，质粘稠，无臭气，绵绵不断，面色萎黄，四肢不温，精神疲倦，纳少便溏，两足跗肿，舌淡苔白腻，脉缓弱。妇科检查往往无异常。

治法：健脾益气，升阳除湿。

方药：完带汤 (81)。

白术 15 克，山药 12 克，人参 9 克 (先煎)，白芍 12 克，苍术 9 克，陈皮 12 克，甘草 6 克，车前子 12 克 (包)，柴胡 9 克，黑芥穗 6 克。水煎 200～300 毫升，早晚分服。

加减：若带下色黄者，加薏苡仁 30 克，黄柏 9 克。

兼有腰痛者，加芡实 30 克，菟丝子 15 克，杜仲 15 克。

带下日久，滑脱不止者，加乌贼骨 30 克，金樱子 15 克，白果 9 克。

中成药：白带丸，每次一丸，日三次，水冲服。

### 2. 湿热型

(1) 湿热下注

**临床表现** 带下量多，色黄或黄白，质粘腻有臭气。胸闷口腻，小腹作痛，或带下色白质粘如豆腐渣、凝乳状、阴痒，小便量少，涩痛，舌苔黄厚或腻，脉濡数或弦滑。若妇科检查见小阴唇、阴道粘膜上有白色膜状物，擦去后局部红肿，或有溃疡者，并在分泌物中找到白色念珠菌时，为霉菌性阴道炎。

治法：清利湿热。

方药：止带方 (104)。

猪苓12克，茯苓18克，车前子12克 (包)，泽泻9克，茵陈12克，赤芍15克，丹皮12克，黄柏9克，栀子9克，牛膝12克。水煎200～300毫升，早晚分服。

加减：小便量少色黄、涩痛者，加滑石15克，淡竹叶9克。

胸闷口腻，苔黄腻者，加薏苡仁30克，萆薢12克，苍术9克。

外治法：清热利湿，杀虫止痒。

方药：Ⅰ号阴道洗剂。

地肤子30克，木槿皮30克，苦参30克，土茯苓30克，蛇床子15克，川椒12克，野菊花30克，艾叶9克，冰片3克 (冲入)。每日一剂，水煎熏洗、坐浴，方法同外阴炎。

(2) 肝胆湿热

**临床表现** 带下量多，色黄或黄绿，质粘或呈泡沫状，有臭气。阴部痒痛、灼热感。精神抑郁，口苦咽干，心烦少寐，便秘，尿赤，胁痛。舌质红，苔薄黄，脉弦细数。月经前后、妊娠期及产后加重。妇科检查：阴道及宫颈粘膜红肿，常有散在出血点，或草莓状突起，后穹窿有多量泡沫样或脓性分泌物，白带化验找到滴虫者，为滴虫性阴道炎。

治法：清肝泻热，杀虫止痒。

方药：龙胆泻肝汤 (38) (方见外阴炎) 加百部15克，土茯苓15克。

外治法：清热解毒，杀虫止痒。

方药：Ⅱ号阴道洗剂。

白头翁 30 克，苦参 30 克，百部 30 克，石榴皮 15 克，蛇床子 15 克，黄柏 12 克，白矾 15 克，艾叶 9 克，冰片 3 克（后入），野菊花 30 克。每日一剂，水煎熏洗、坐浴，方法同外阴炎。

中成药：龙胆泻肝丸，每次 9 克，每日 2 次，温水冲服。

（3）热毒型

**临床表现**　带下量多，或赤白相兼，或五色杂下，质粘腻。或如脓样，有臭气，或腐臭难闻。小腹作痛，烘热口干，头昏晕，大便干结或秽臭，小便黄少。舌红苔黄干，脉数。妇科检查可见宫颈水肿、充血，或有结节状、菜花、空洞样变。多为急性炎症或宫颈癌。

治法：清热解毒。

方药：五味消毒饮（86）加味。

蒲公英 15 克，金银花 15 克，野菊花 30 克，紫花地丁 30 克，天葵子 15 克，白花蛇舌草 30 克，薏苡仁 5 克，蚤休 15 克，樗根白皮 30 克，土茯苓 15 克，香附 12 克，半枝莲 30 克。水煎 200～300 毫升，早晚分服。

加减：大便干结、数日不下者，加大黄 6 克（后入），芒硝 3 克（冲）。

口干舌燥、小便涩痛量少者，加生地 15 克，淡竹叶 12 克，黄连 6 克，生甘草 9 克。

带下脓样，腹痛甚者，加鱼腥草 30 克，元胡 12 克，车前草 15 克。

**3. 肾虚型**

（1）肾阳虚

**临床表现**　白带清冷、量多、质稀薄，终日淋漓不断，腰酸如折，小腹冷感，小便频数清长，夜间尤甚，大便溏薄。舌质淡，苔薄白，脉沉迟。妇科检查常无异常发现。

治法：温肾固涩止带。

方药：内补丸（43）。

鹿茸9克，菟丝子24克，沙苑蒺藜15克，黄芪15克，肉桂6克，桑螵蛸30克，肉苁蓉15克，制附子6克，白蒺藜15克，紫菀茸9克。水煎200～300毫升，早晚分服。

加减：夜尿多，便溏者，加益智仁30克，补骨脂15克，白术18克。

胸闷纳少、乏力者，加茯苓15克，陈皮12克，厚朴9克，砂仁6克。

（2）肾阴虚

**临床表现**　外阴干涩灼热感，痒或痛。带下少，色黄或赤白，质粘无味。头晕目眩，烘热汗出，腰酸耳鸣，五心烦热，口干便燥，尿黄，舌红少苔，脉弦细数。妇科检查：外阴萎缩状，阴道分泌物多，呈黄水状、血性或脓性。阴道皱襞消失，粘膜充血，有点状出血或溃疡。

治法：益肾滋阴，清热止带。

方药：知柏地黄汤（103）。

生地18克，丹皮12克，茯苓15克，泽泻9克，山茱萸12克，山药15克，知母6克，黄柏9克。水煎200～300毫升，早晚分服。

加减：带下量多淋漓不断者，加芡实30克，金樱子15克，莲须12克。

头晕目眩，心烦失眠者，加菊花9克，麦冬12克，五味子12克，生龙骨30克。

带下血性者，加旱莲草18克，地榆15克。

外治法：清热解毒，益肾凉血止带。

方药：Ⅲ号阴道洗剂。

野菊花30克，金银花30克，仙灵脾30克，紫草15克，黄柏 15 克，当归 15 克，蛇床子 30 克，赤芍 15 克，丹皮 12 克，乌梅 15 克，艾叶 9 克，冰片 3 克（后入）。每日一剂，水煎熏洗，坐浴。方法同外阴炎。

**中成药及单验方**

冰硼散一管，甘油调匀后，棉棒蘸药涂抹阴道及外阴，每日 1～2 次。治疗霉菌性阴道炎。

地肤子 45 克，野菊花 30 克。水煎熏洗、坐浴，每日一次，治疗霉菌性阴道炎。

百部 30 克，白头翁 30 克，苦参 30 克。水煎熏洗，每日一次。治疗滴虫性阴道炎。

塌痒汤（79）：鹤虱 30 克，苦参 30 克，威灵仙 15 克，当归尾 30 克，狼牙 9 克，蛇床子 15 克，猪胆汁二个。水煎熏洗，每日一次，治疗外阴阴道搔痒。

仙灵脾 30 克，紫草 15 克，黄柏 15 克，野菊花 30 克，水煎熏洗，每日一次，治疗老年性阴道炎。

**预防** 内裤、月经垫常洗换、日晒，存放清洁干燥处。

要有专用的浴盆、浴巾，不到公共浴池洗盆浴，不用公共浴巾，防止传染病。

医者妇科检查严格无菌操作，以防交叉感染。

# 2.3 子宫颈炎

子宫颈炎是生育年龄妇女的常见病，有急、慢性两种。急性宫颈炎常与产褥感染、感染性流产或急性阴道炎同时发生。临床以白带增多，子宫颈肥大、充血、糜烂、囊肿为特点。属中医"带下病"范畴。故辨证施治参考阴道炎部分，内服中药治疗。本节侧重于宫颈炎的局部治疗。

**临床表现** 白带增多呈脓性，腰骶酸痛，小腹坠痛，月经期、排便或性交后加重。或有尿涩量少色黄，或有不孕史。妇科检查：急性宫颈炎可见宫颈充血、水肿，慢性炎症可见宫颈呈单纯型、滤泡型或乳突状不同程度的糜烂，宫颈肥大，外翻、息肉或腺体囊肿，颈管内有脓性白带。

治法：清热解毒，活血去腐生肌。

方药：宫颈炎Ⅰ号粉。

作用：清热解毒，燥湿止带。

黄柏 30 克，黄连 30 克，黄芩 30 克，大黄 15 克，冰片 3 克。将前四味药焙干后研细粉，加入研好的冰片，充分混合后，装入喷粉器内备用。用阴道窥器暴露好宫颈，用干棉球拭净阴道分泌物，用喷粉器均匀地把药粉喷撒在宫颈上，或用带线棉球蘸上药粉，敷在宫颈表面，24 小时后取出。每日 1 次，7 天 1 个疗程。

本方用于糜烂表浅，充血明显的单纯型糜烂，或经宫颈Ⅱ号粉去腐后充血明显者。

方药：宫颈炎Ⅱ号粉

作用：活血化瘀，祛腐生新。

明矾 30 克，硇砂 6 克，乳香 9 克，没药 9 克，儿茶 15 克，雄黄 15 克，硼砂 1.5 克，冰片 3 克，共研细粉备用。暴露宫颈，拭净阴道分泌物，用棉球保护好穹窿及阴道，用带线棉球蘸上少许药粉，敷于宫颈糜烂面上，勿使药物撒在周围皮肤粘膜上，24 小时后由医生取出。每日 1 次，连用 2~3 次。

适应于宫颈呈颗粒状、乳突状糜烂者。

方药：宫颈炎Ⅲ号粉

作用：收敛生肌。

蛤粉 30 克，白芨 12 克，五倍子 9 克，黄柏 30 克，乌贼骨 30 克，象皮 15 克，冰片 3 克，共研细粉备用。

用法：同宫颈炎Ⅰ号粉。以上三种宫颈炎粉,使用时根据宫颈糜烂情况可交替使用。炎症明显时使用Ⅰ号粉，结节乳突明显时用Ⅱ号粉，去腐后可用Ⅰ号粉或Ⅲ号粉。在宫颈消除了充血、水肿后可用Ⅲ号粉。

**中成药及单验方**

苦参栓每晚一粒，塞入阴道深处。有清热利湿、祛风杀虫止痒作用。

白带丸每日 2 次，每次 1 丸，白开水冲服。

**预防** 分娩或人工引产、流产及其他宫内手术操作时，严格遵守操作规章及无菌，以防宫颈损伤、感染。

讲究个人卫生，勤洗外阴，勤换内裤，保持外阴清洁干燥，防止感染。

## 2.4 盆腔炎

女性内生殖器及其周围的结缔组织、盆腔腹膜发炎时，称为盆腔炎。炎症可限于一个部位，或几个部位同时发病。根据发病过程、临床表现，可分为急性盆腔炎、慢性盆腔炎和结核性盆腔炎三类。多因分娩、流产及其他宫内手术操作消毒不严，或经期、产后不注意卫生所引起。临床表现以下腹疼痛、发热、腰骶酸痛、白带多、月经失调、不孕为特点。盆腔炎概括于中医的"热入血室"、"带下病"、"经水不调"、"症积"、"不孕"等病之中。

经期、产后胞脉空虚，邪毒乘虚内侵，湿浊热毒蓄积下焦，容于胞中，与气血相搏，因而发病。正邪交争，营卫不和，邪毒壅盛，致使恶寒发热，腹痛，瘀毒内结，形成积块。

### 辨证论治

#### 1. 湿热型

**临床表现** 高热、寒战，下腹疼痛拒按。带下量多，色黄或脓样，质稠味臭。口干苦，尿涩少，肛门下坠，排便困难。舌质红，苔薄黄或黄腻，脉滑数或弦细数。妇科检查：外阴正常，阴道充血，大量脓性分泌物，穹窿触痛明显，宫颈充血，水肿，举痛明显。子宫略大或正常、压痛，活动受限。子宫两旁压痛，有时可触及包块，或片状增厚。或后穹窿触及囊性包块。血化验白细胞在 $10\sim20\times10^9$ / L。

治法：清热解毒利湿，佐以活血化瘀。

方药：急盆汤。

柴胡 12 克，黄芩 15 克，金银花 30 克，败酱草 30 克，连翘 24 克，丹皮 15 克，黄柏 9 克，丹参 15 克，元胡 12 克，制乳香 9 克，制没药 9 克，赤芍 15 克，川楝子 9 克。每日 2 剂，早晚各 1 剂，水煎 200～300 毫升，1 次服。热退后可以每日 1 剂。

加减：大便干结者，加大黄 6 克（后入）元明粉 3 克（冲服）。

尿痛、尿急者，加淡竹叶 12 克，生甘草梢 9 克，滑石 12 克。

脓性白带多者，加冬瓜仁 30 克，鱼腥草 24 克，薏苡仁 15 克。

包块者，加山楂 15 克，鸡内金 9 克，三棱 12 克，莪术 12 克。

心烦口渴、舌绛发斑者，加犀角粉 3 克（冲），生地 18 克，栀子 12 克，白茅根 30 克，黄连 6 克。去柴胡，制乳香，制没药，川楝子。

**2. 气滞血瘀型**

**临床表现**　下腹坠痛或胀痛，拒按，腰酸。劳累、性交、月经前后加重，月经量多，有块，块下痛减。胸胁、乳房胀痛。白带多，色白或黄。脉弦涩，舌质黯，有瘀点或瘀斑，舌苔薄白。妇科检查：子宫多后位，活动受限，或粘连固定，压痛。可触及附件增厚，索条或包块，或囊性肿块。B 型超声往往可以协助诊断。

治法：活血化瘀，理气止痛。

方药：慢盆汤 I 号。

生蒲黄 12 克，炒灵脂 12 克，当归 15 克，桃仁 12 克，红花 12 克，乳香 9 克，没药 9 克，赤芍 15 克，丹参 30 克，香附 12 克，金银花藤 30 克，土茯苓 15 克。每日 1 剂，水煎 200～300 毫升，分 2 次服。

加减：乳房、胸胁胀痛重者，加橘叶 12 克，川楝子 12 克。

白带量多色黄者，加车前子 12 克（包），泽泻 9 克。

腰痛者，加牛膝 15 克，川断 15 克。

### 3. 寒凝血滞型

**临床表现** 下腹冷痛，得热则痛减，按之痛甚。月经延后，量少，色黯有块，脉沉弦或沉紧，舌苔白薄。妇科检查同气滞血瘀型。

治法：温经散寒，活血化瘀。

方药：慢盆汤 II 号。

小茴香 9 克，桂枝 9 克，茯苓 15 克，当归 15 克，川芎 9 克，丹皮 9 克，乌药 12 克，桃仁 12 克，鸡血藤 15 克。水煎 200～300 毫升，早晚分服。

加减：腹冷甚者，加炮姜 6 克，吴茱萸 9 克。

经期延后，量少块多，腹痛甚者，加牛膝 15 克，改鸡血藤为 30 克，肉桂 9 克。

### 4. 阴虚血热型

**临床表现** 月经量渐渐减少或闭经，下腹坠痛，经后加剧。午后潮热，乏力，盗汗，手足心热，纳呆。舌质红无苔或黄薄苔，脉细数，多有原发性不孕及结核病史。妇科检查：子宫一般发育差，活动受限，或固定粘连。附件区可触及大小不等、不规则的包块，质硬，表面结节感。血化验血沉可快或正常，刮宫病理切片可找到典型的结核结节，碘油造影可见盆腔钙化点，宫腔狭窄或畸形，边缘呈锯齿状，输卵管呈串珠状或僵直、狭窄。

治法：养阴清热，活血化瘀。

方药：慢盆汤 III 号。

生地 15 克，鳖甲 30 克，生龟板 30 克，野菊花 30 克，百部 15 克，地榆 15 克，夏枯草 12 克，鸡血藤 15 克，地骨皮 12 克，青蒿 9 克，丹皮 9 克，元（玄）参 15 克。水煎 200～300 毫升，早晚分服。

加减：输卵管积水者，加赤小豆 30 克，防已 12 克，车前子 12 克（包），泽泻 9 克，肉桂 6 克。

包块者，加生牡蛎 30 克，浙贝母 12 克，连翘 24 克，鸡内金 9 克，山楂 15 克。

输卵管通水显示不通畅者，可用丹参 30 克，连翘 24 克，丹皮 15 克，当归 15 克，川芎 9 克，苏木 15 克，车前子 12 克（包），王不留行 12 克，穿山甲 12 克，肉桂 9 克，牛膝 15 克，鸡血藤 30 克，川楝子 12 克。自月经干净后，每日 1 剂，水煎 200～300 毫升，早晚分服。每月 18～24 剂，连服 2～3 个月。

**其他治疗　中药保留灌肠法**

①丹参 30 克，败酱草 30 克，连翘 30 克，紫花地丁 30 克，赤芍 15 克，制乳香 15 克，制没药 15 克，川楝子 15 克。水煎 100～200 毫升，温度在 37 度左右。病人睡前取左侧卧位，用肛管插入肛门，用 100 毫升针管吸取中药液，缓缓推入肠管内，每日一次，10 次为一疗程。灌药前最好清洁灌肠或服少量缓泻剂，以排空粪便，利于药液吸收。灌药后，保留时间越长效果越好。

②中药外敷法：芒硝半斤，鲜大蒜 6～7 头，大黄末 250 克，醋 200 克。将去皮大蒜与芒硝放入蒜窝内，捣烂如泥。把纱布放在炎性包块的部位上，将捣烂的药物平摊在纱布上，约 5～10 分钟，炎症包块处的皮肤即出现 Ⅰ 度烫伤（发红、皮肤烧灼感）后，取下药物，把大黄与醋调成稀糊状，敷于包块处，约半小时以上。用于炎性包块或脓肿。

③丹参注射液：丹参注射液 2 毫升，肌肉注射，日 2 次，10

天为 1 疗程。或丹参注射液 10 毫升，加入 10%的葡萄糖溶液 500 毫升中，静脉点滴，10 天为 1 疗程。一般 2～3 个疗程。

金鸡冲剂（金樱子，千斤拔，鸡血藤）：每日 2 次，每次 1 包冲服。10 天一个疗程，一般 2～3 个疗程。或金鸡片剂，每日 3 次，每次 6 片。

康妇消炎栓：睡前取左侧卧位，将栓剂推入肛门，每晚 1 次，10 日 1 疗程。

**预防**　经期，产褥期注意卫生，不坐浴，禁性生活，月经垫及纸要消毒，保持干燥。

严格宫腔内无菌操作。

# 附：慢性外阴营养不良

慢性外阴营养不良，指一组女阴皮肤、粘膜营养障碍而致的组织变性及色素改变的疾病。属中医的"阴痒"范畴，肝经循阴器，肾主二阴。肝肾不足，精血亏少，阴虚化燥，血虚生风，发为阴痒。

## 辨证论治

### 1. 肝肾阴亏型

**临床表现**　阴部干涩烧灼感，痒甚，带下量少，色黄或血性带下，五心烦热，头晕目眩，烘热汗出，腰酸耳鸣，舌红少苔，脉细数无力。妇科检查：外阴皮肤和粘膜变白，变薄、干裂，失去弹性，阴蒂或小阴唇萎缩状，阴道口狭窄。

**治法**　益肾降火，养血祛风。

**方药**　知柏地黄汤（103）加味。

知母 6 克，黄柏 9 克，生地 15 克，山药 12 克，丹皮 9 克，山茱萸 12 克，泽泻 9 克，茯苓 15 克，制首乌 30 克，白藓皮 15 克，当归 15 克。水煎 200～300 毫升，早晚分服。

外治法：益肾养血，解毒止痒。

方　药：Ⅳ号外阴洗剂

仙灵脾 15 克，当归 15 克，紫草 15 克，黄柏 12 克，丹皮 12 克，白花蛇舌草 30 克，蚤休 30 克，鸡血藤 15 克，艾叶 15 克，冰片 3 克（冲）。每日一剂，水煎熏洗、坐浴，方法同外阴炎。

**2. 血虚生风**

**临床表现**　外阴瘙痒，精神疲倦，夜寐不安，饮食少思，形体消瘦，舌淡苔白薄，脉细弱。病久则皮肤粘膜变厚而粗糙，检查时可见大阴唇、阴唇沟、阴蒂、后联合处皮肤增厚，呈粉红或暗红色，有界限清晰的白斑。

治法：养血活血，祛风止痒。

方药：当归饮子（17）。

当归 15 克，川芎 9 克，白芍 15 克，生地 15 克，防风 9 克，荆芥 9 克，黄芪 30 克，甘草 6 克，白蒺藜 30 克，制首乌 30 克。水煎 200～300 毫升，早晚分服。

外治法：活血祛风止痒。

方　药：Ⅴ号外阴洗剂。

荆芥 9 克，防风 9 克，透骨草 15 克，丹参 30 克，鸡血藤 30 克，苏木 15 克，赤芍 15 克，丹皮 12 克，川椒 12 克，艾叶 12 克，冰片 3 克（冲），当归 15 克。每日 1 剂，水煎熏洗、坐浴，方法同前。

**单方验方**

仙灵脾 30 克，鹿含草 30 克。水煎熏洗，每日 1 次。

竹红菌软膏涂于患处，竹红菌光疗灯泡照射，每日 1 次，每次 30～40 分钟，30 天为 1 疗程。可止痒，恢复色泽和软度。

（李竹兰）

# 3 月 经 失 调

## 3.1 功能失调性子宫出血

凡月经不正常，经检查无妊娠、肿瘤、炎症、外伤或全身出血疾病等，而系内分泌失调所引起的子宫内膜异常出血，称为功能失调性子宫出血，简称"功血"。"功血"临床分无排卵型与有排卵型两种，前者多发于青春期、更年期妇女，后者多发于生育期妇女。功血属中医崩漏病的范畴。崩漏指妇女不在行经期间阴道大量流血，或持续下血，淋漓不断。发病急，来势猛，流血量多的为崩，亦称崩中。发病慢，来势缓，流血量少的为漏，亦称漏下。崩与漏可以互相转化，久漏可崩，崩后又可漏。其病因是由于血热、血瘀、脾虚、肾虚，导致冲任损伤不能制约经血而引起。

### 辨证论治

崩漏的治疗以"急则治其标，缓则治其本"为原则，灵活掌握"塞流"、"澄源"、"复旧"三法。"塞流"即止血，"澄源"即求因治本，"复旧"即固本，善后调理。三者可侧重一方，而不可断然分开。

#### 1. 血热型

(1) 实热型

**临床表现** 阴道大量流血或淋漓不断，血色深红、质稠，口渴喜饮，身热面赤，大便干结，小便色黄，烦躁不寐。舌质红，苔黄或黄腻，脉洪数。平时月经先期而至或月经量多。

治法：清热凉血，止血调经。

方药：清热固经汤（53）。

黄芩 12 克，焦栀子 12 克，生地 30 克，地骨皮 12 克，地榆 30 克，阿胶 12 克（烊化），生藕节 9 克，陈棕炭 12 克，炙龟板 30 克，牡蛎粉 30 克，生甘草 6 克。水煎 200～300 毫升，早晚分服。若流血量多可日服 2 剂，早晚各 1 剂。

加减：壮热口渴，面红目赤者，加石膏 30 克，知母 6 克，白茅根 30 克。

大便干结，数日不下者，加大黄 6 克（后入），芒硝 3 克（冲）。

胸胁胀满，口苦、心烦易怒者，加柴胡 9 克，白芍 15 克。

脘腹胀闷，经血质稠臭秽、苔黄腻者，加鱼腥草 15 克，薏苡仁 5 克，黄柏 9 克。

(2) 虚热型

**临床表现** 经血非时而下，量少，色鲜红，质粘稠，心烦潮热，手足心热，小便色黄，大便干结，舌质红，苔薄黄，脉细数。

治法：滋阴清热，止血调经。

方药：保阴煎（5）加味。

生地 30 克，熟地 15 克，白芍 18 克，山药 15 克，续断 15 克，黄芩 12 克，黄柏 9 克，甘草 6 克，地骨皮 12 克，玄参 15 克，丹皮 9 克。水煎，200～300 毫升，早晚分服。若流血多可以日服 2 剂，早晚各服 1 剂。

加减：心烦少寐者，加生龙骨 30 克，生牡蛎 30 克，五味子 12 克。

流血量多者，加地榆 30 克，仙鹤草 15 克，乌贼骨 30 克。

出血日久，气短倦怠、头晕心悸者，加黄芪 30 克，太子参 12 克。

**2. 血瘀型**

临床表现　流血时下时止，或淋漓不断，或闭经数月后又突然大量流血，血色紫黑，夹有血块，小腹疼痛拒按，血块下后痛减。舌质紫黯有瘀斑或瘀点，脉沉涩。

治法：活血化瘀，止血调经。

方药：四物汤（69）合失笑散（70）加味。

熟地15克，当归15克，川芎12克，赤芍15克，蒲黄12克，五灵脂12克，益母草30克，茜草12克，红花12克，元胡9克。水煎200～300毫升，早晚分服。流血多时可以每日2剂，早晚各1剂。

加减：胸胁、乳房及少腹胀痛者，加川楝子9克，香附12克。

小腹痛剧、血块多者，加牛膝15克，刘寄奴15克。

口干苦，面色红而量多者，加夏枯草12克，丹参15克，地榆30克。

腹冷痛，经色黯而稠者，加艾叶12克，乌药12克。

中成药：保坤丹，每次服30片，每日1次。忌生冷食物及辛辣、荞麦面。

三七片，每次服5～10片，最多不超过30片，每日1次。若血不止时，可隔6小时加服一次。

益母草膏，每次1汤匙（约10毫升）每日3次。

云南白药，每次0.2～0.3克，最大量0.5克，每隔4小时服1次。

### 3. 脾虚型

临床表现　突然流血量多或淋漓不止，血色淡而质薄，面色苍白或浮肿，神疲肢倦，手足不温，纳少便溏，心悸。舌胖质淡，苔白薄，脉缓弱。

治法：补气摄血，止血调经。

方药：固本止崩汤（24）加减。

人参15克（先煎），黄芪30克，白术18克，熟地炭15

克，黑姜9克，莲子肉12克，生龙牡各30克，炙升麻6克。水煎200～300毫升，早晚分服，流血多时每日2剂，早晚各1剂。

加减：胁胀脘闷，纳少便溏者，去熟地，加柴胡9克，白芍15克，砂仁6克。

出血日久，淋漓不止者加乌贼骨30克，乌梅炭12克。

心慌气短者，加五味子12克，麦门冬12克。

**中成药及单方** 归脾丸，每次1丸，日三次。

补中益气丸，每次1丸，日3次。

人参归脾丸，每次1丸，日3次。

人参30克，先水浸泡后水煎，吃参喝汤。

### 4. 肾虚型

(1) 肾阴虚型

**临床表现** 经乱无期，出血淋漓不止或量多，色鲜红，质粘稠。头晕耳鸣，腰膝酸软，五心烦热，舌质红，少苔或无苔，脉细数。

治法：滋水益阴，止血调经。

方药：左归丸（105）合二至丸（22）加减。

生熟地各15克，山药15克，枸杞18克，山茱萸12克，菟丝子24克，龟板胶15克（烊化），女贞子15克，旱莲草30克，鹿角胶12克，玄参12克，丹皮12克，地榆15克。水煎200～300毫升，早晚分服。流血量多者日2剂，早晚各1剂。

加减：咽干，目眩耳鸣者加生牡蛎30克，夏枯草12克。

胁痛乳胀，心烦易怒者，加川楝子12克，白芍15克，柴胡9克。

尿黄，大便干结，舌苔黄者加黄柏6克，沙参15克。

中成药：六味地黄丸，每次1丸，日2次。若小蜜丸，每次服 9 克，日 2 次。

(2) 肾阳虚型

**临床表现** 经来无期，血量多或淋漓不断，色淡质清。畏寒肢冷，面色晦暗，腰膝酸软，小便清长，夜尿多。舌质淡，苔薄白，脉沉细。

治法：温肾固冲，止血调经。

方药：右归丸（96）加减。

制附子 6 克，肉桂 6 克，熟地 15 克，山药 15 克，山茱萸 12 克，枸杞 15 克，菟丝子 24 克，鹿角胶 12 克，杜仲 30 克，赤石脂 30 克，复盆子 30 克，水煎 200～300 毫升，早晚分服。流血量多可每日 2 剂，早晚各 1 剂。

加减：血量多时去肉桂，加黄芪 30 克，乌贼骨 30 克。

小腹冷痛，血多色暗有块者，加乳香 9 克，没药 9 克，炒小茴香 6 克。

浮肿纳差，四肢不温者，加茯苓 15 克，炮姜 6 克，砂仁 6 克。

中成药：金匮肾气丸，每次 1 丸，日 2 次，淡盐水冲服。

艾附暖宫丸，每次 1 丸，日 2 次。

**关于中药人工周期的应用**

当"功血"血止后，应重视月经周期的调节。大量临床实践和实验证明：以益肾为主，根据临床症状，佐以调肝、健脾、活血法，可促使卵泡发育，按时排卵，维持黄体功能，使子宫内膜剥脱完整。

(1) 经后期（月经周期的第 6～10 天）

治法：益肾养血，调补冲任。

方药：促卵泡汤。

熟地 15 克，山药 15 克，续断 30 克，菟丝子 24 克，首乌 30 克，枸杞子 15 克，黄芪 30 克，当归 15 克，香附 12 克。水煎 200～300 毫升，早晚分服。连服 5～6 剂。

加减：月经后期、量少，兼见肾阳虚者，加仙灵脾 15 克，仙茅 12 克，紫河车 12 克，肉桂 6 克。

月经先期、量多，兼有肾阴虚者，改熟地为生地，加女贞子 15 克，旱莲草 15 克，龟板 30 克，鳖甲 30 克。

乏力，纳呆气虚者，加党参 30 克，白术 18 克，砂仁 9 克，去熟地。

(2) 排卵前期或排卵期（月经周期的第 11～16 天）

治法：益肾养血，佐以活血化瘀。

方药：促排卵汤。

山药 15 克，续断 30 克，菟丝子 24 克，枸杞子 15 克，肉苁蓉 30 克，仙灵脾 15 克，丹参 15 克，赤芍 12 克，红花 12 克，刘寄奴 12 克，川芎 9 克，香附 12 克。水煎 200～300 毫升，早晚分服，连服 6 剂。

(3) 排卵后期（月经周期的第 17～25 天）

治法：补益肝肾，健脾固冲任。

方药：助黄体汤。

黄芪 30 克，山药 15 克，白芍 15 克，续断 30 克，旱莲草 15 克，女贞子 15 克，生龙牡各 30 克，首乌 15 克，菟丝子 24 克，复盆子 30 克，丹参 12 克。水煎 200～300 毫升，早晚分服，连服 6～8 剂。

(4) 经前期（月经周期的第 25～28 天）

治法：活血通经。

方药：通经汤。

当归 15 克，川芎 12 克，赤芍 15 克，红花 12 克，丹参 30 克，泽兰 15 克，牛膝 15 克，鸡血藤 30 克，生蒲黄 12 克，茺蔚子 12 克，香附 12 克，肉桂 6 克。水煎 200～300 毫升，早晚分服，连服 3～5 剂。

## 3.2  痛经

凡在经期前后或经期中，发生腹部疼痛或其他不适，以致影响了工作和日常生活者，称为痛经。临床分原发性痛经和继发性痛经两种。生殖器官无器质性病变者，称原发性痛经或功能性痛经；继发性痛经指生殖器官有明显的器质性病变者，引起继发性痛经的多为子宫内膜异位症、急慢性盆腔器官炎症，或子宫颈狭窄阻塞等。

中医认为"不通则痛"。由于情志抑郁、起居不慎，或六淫为害，导致了冲任瘀阻或寒凝经脉，均可引起气血运行不畅，胞宫经血流通受阻，引起痛经。另外，气血虚弱，肝肾亏损，使胞脉失于濡养，亦可引起痛经。

### 辨证论治

临床根据疼痛发生的时间、性质、部位以及痛的程度，结合月经的期、量、色、质及兼证，舌苔、脉象，而辨其寒热虚实。一般疼痛发生在经前、经期，疼痛剧烈拒按者属实；痛在经后，隐隐作痛、喜按喜揉者属虚；绞痛、冷痛、得热痛减属寒；灼痛、得热痛剧者属热；胀甚于痛者是气滞；痛甚于胀者，刺痛、跳痛、血块排出后痛减者是血瘀；痛在两侧少腹，病在肝；痛连及腰，病在肾。

**1. 气滞血瘀型**

**临床表现**  经前 1~2 日或经期小腹胀痛、拒按，月经量少，经色紫黯挟有血块，血块排出后痛减。胸胁、乳房胀痛，舌质紫黯边有瘀斑或斑点，脉弦涩。

治法：疏肝理气，化瘀止痛。

方药：膈下逐瘀汤（25）加味。

当归 15 克，川芎 12 克，赤芍 15 克，桃仁 12 克，红花 12

克，枳壳 9 克，延胡索 12 克，五灵脂 12 克，丹皮 9 克，乌药 12 克，香附 12 克，甘草 6 克，刘寄奴 15 克，牛膝 15 克，丹参 30 克。于经前 7～10 天开始服，每日 1 剂，水煎 200～300 毫升，早晚分服，服至月经来潮。

加减：伴有恶心呕吐者，加吴茱萸 12 克，姜竹茹 9 克，黄连 6 克。

口苦，苔黄，脉数者，加栀子 9 克，夏枯草 12 克。

胸闷，食少者，加焦山楂 15 克，鸡内金 6 克，白术 12 克。

中成药：元胡止痛片，每次 4 片，日 3 次。

益母草膏，10 毫升冲服，每日 3 次。

## 2. 寒湿凝滞型

**临床表现** 经前、经期小腹冷痛，按之痛甚，得热痛减。月经量少，色黯有块，畏寒便溏，舌苔白腻，脉沉紧。

治法：温经散寒除湿，化瘀止痛。

方药：少腹逐瘀汤（60）加苍术、茯苓。

小茴香 6 克，干姜 6 克，延胡索 9 克，没药 12 克，当归 15 克，川芎 9 克，肉桂 6 克，赤芍 12 克，蒲黄 12 克，五灵脂 12 克，苍术 9 克，茯苓 12 克，乌药 12 克，吴茱萸 12 克。经前 7～10 天开始服药，每日 1 剂，水煎 200～300 毫升，早晚分服，服至月经来潮。

加减：痛甚而厥，手足不温，冷汗淋漓者，加附子 9 克，艾叶 12 克。

经量少、腰痛者，加牛膝 15 克，杜仲 15 克，鸡血藤 30 克。

中成药：艾附暖宫丸，每次 1 丸，日 2 次，温水冲服。

## 3. 气血虚弱型

**临床表现** 经后 1～2 日或经期小腹隐隐作痛，或小腹、外阴下坠，小腹喜按喜揉，月经量少，色淡质稀。神疲乏力，面色少华，食少便溏，舌质淡，脉沉弱。

治法：益气补血止痛。

方药：圣愈汤（72）加减。

人参 15 克（先煎），黄芪 30 克，当归 15 克，川芎 9 克，熟地 15 克，白芍 18 克，香附 9 克，延胡索 9 克，炙甘草 9 克，鸡血藤 15 克，红花 12 克。每日 1 剂，水煎 200～300 毫升，每日 2 次温服。

加减：头晕心悸，失眠者，加柏子仁 15 克，炒枣仁 30 克。

纳呆便溏者，加白术 18 克，焦山楂 15 克，茯苓 15 克。

经量明显少而淡者，改鸡血藤 30 克，加何首乌 30 克，阿胶 12 克（烊化）。

中成药：八珍益母丸，每次 1 丸，日 2 次。

鸡血藤片，每次 5 片，日三次。

### 4. 肝肾亏损型

**临床表现** 经后 1～2 日小腹疠痛，腰骶疼痛酸胀，经色黯淡而量少，质稀薄。头晕耳鸣，或潮热，脉细弱，舌苔薄白或薄黄。

治法：益肾养肝止痛。

方药：调肝汤（73）加味。

当归 12 克，白芍 15 克，山茱萸 12 克，巴戟天 15 克，阿胶 12 克（烊化），山药 12 克，甘草 6 克，枸杞子 30 克，熟地 15 克，丹皮 9 克，香附 12 克。每日 1 剂，水煎 200～300 毫升，分 2 次温服。

加减：胁胀，少腹胀痛者，加川楝子 12 克，延胡索 9 克，橘核 9 克。

颧红潮热，口干者，加青蒿 9 克，鳖甲 30 克，地骨皮 12 克，去巴戟天。

痛及腰骶，夜尿频而清长者，加益智仁 15 克，桑螵蛸 30 克。

**注意事项**：经期不可冒雨、涉水、游泳或经行之时过食生冷食物。注意经期卫生，勤换纸垫，冲洗外阴，保持外阴清洁。经期禁性生活。

## 3.3 闭经

闭经系指妇女应有月经而超过一定时限仍未来潮者。而青春期前、妊娠期、哺乳期以及绝经期后等生理情况应除外。病理性闭经有原发性闭经和继发性闭经两种：前者为女子年过 18 岁仍未行经者；后者指曾有过正常月经，现闭经 3 个月以上者。精神因素、环境改变、全身慢性消耗性疾病，以及内分泌紊乱，或子宫发育异常、内膜严重损伤等均可引起闭经。

闭经即中医的"女子不月"、"月事不来"、"月水不通"、"经闭"。根据临床症状，可分为血枯经闭和血滞经闭虚实两种。虚者多因肝肾不足，气血虚弱，阴虚血燥而使精血不足，无血可下。而实者多因气滞血瘀、痰湿阻滞、邪气阻隔，脉气不通，使经血不得下行所致。

### 辨证论治

#### 1. 肝肾不足型

**临床表现**　年过 18 岁而月经尚未来潮，或月经后期、量少，逐渐经闭不行。腰酸腿软，头晕耳鸣，面色黯或两颧潮红，舌质淡红，苔少，脉沉弱。妇科检查：子宫发育不良或幼稚子宫。阴道细胞学检查雌激素轻度影响或轻度低落。

**治法**：滋补肝肾，养血调经。

**方药**：归肾丸（26）加味。

熟地 15 克，山药 15 克，山茱萸 12 克，茯苓 15 克，当归 15 克，枸杞 30 克，杜仲 30 克，菟丝子 24 克，川续断 30 克，仙灵脾15克。每日1剂，水煎200～300毫升，分2次服。

加减：形寒肢冷、小便清长，大便溏泻者，加巴戟天12克，附子9克。

腹胀，食少便溏者，去熟地，加扁豆30克，焦山楂15克，砂仁9克。

口干、咽燥，脉细数者，改熟地为生地，加旱莲草15克，女贞子15克，麦冬12克。

中成药：六味地黄丸，每日3次，每次1丸。

乌鸡白凤丸，每日2次，每次1丸。

**2. 阴虚血燥型**

**临床表现** 月经延后，量少渐渐闭止，手足心热，两颧潮红，盗汗，或咳嗽唾血，口干咽燥，舌红无苔或苔少，脉弦细数。多可询问到结核病史。妇科检查：可能无异常发现或可触及盆腔包块，质硬，与周围粘连而触痛不明显，子宫往往发育不全。

治法：养阴清热调经。

方药：加减一阴煎（102）加减。

生地15克，白芍15克，麦门冬12克，知母9克，地骨皮12克，炙甘草6克，百部15克，地榆15克，元参12克，鳖甲30克，龟板30克，每日1剂，水煎200～300毫升，分2次温服。

加减：干咳咯血者，加沙参30克，川贝母12克，百合30克，白芨12克，五味子12克。

心悸、少寐者，加夜交藤15克，柏子仁15克。

触到包块者，加鸡内金9克，连翘30克，夏枯草15克，生牡蛎30克。

**3. 气血虚弱型**

**临床表现** 月经延后量少，色淡质稀薄，继则月经不来，头昏眼花，心悸气短，神疲肢倦，面黄羸瘦，纳呆，毛发不泽易脱落，舌淡苔薄白，脉缓弱。妇科检查：子宫发育不良或萎缩。

治法：补气养血调经。

方药：人参养荣汤（58）加味。

人参 15 克（先煎），黄芪 30 克，煨白术 30 克，茯苓 15 克，远志 9 克，陈皮 12 克，五味子 12 克，当归 15 克，白芍 15 克，熟地 15 克，桂心 9 克，炙甘草 6 克，何首乌 30 克，柏子仁 15 克，鸡血藤 30 克，桂圆肉 12 克。每日 1 剂，水煎 200～300 毫升，分 2 次温服。

加减：失眠、多梦者，加枣仁 30 克。

口干，舌红或口舌生疮者，加黄芩 9 克，黄连 9 克。

产后大出血引起的闭经，兼见畏寒肢冷，性欲低下，生殖器官萎缩者，加仙灵脾 30 克，紫河车 15 克，鹿角霜 12 克，菟丝子 30 克。

中成药：当归丸，每日 3 次，每次 1 丸。

首乌片，每日 3 次，每次 3～5 片。

### 4. 气滞血瘀型

**临床表现**　月经数月不行，精神抑郁，烦躁易怒，胸胁胀满，少腹胀痛拒按，舌紫黯有瘀斑或瘀点，脉沉涩。

治法：理气活血，祛瘀通经。

方药：血府逐瘀汤（90）加味。

桃仁 12 克，红花 12 克，当归 15 克，生地 15 克，川芎 9 克，赤芍 15 克，牛膝 15 克，桔梗 12 克，柴胡 9 克，枳壳 9 克，甘草 6 克，丹参 30 克，苏木 15 克，泽兰 18 克。每日 1 剂，水煎 200～300 毫升，分 2 次温服。

加减：胸胁、少腹胀甚者，加青皮 12 克，川楝子 12 克。

腹痛甚拒按者，加益母草 30 克，三棱 12 克，刘寄奴 15 克。

小腹冷痛、四肢不温、舌苔白、脉沉紧者，加肉桂 6 克，炒小茴香 9 克，去丹参、生地。

小腹痛而灼热、黄带多、苔黄、脉数者，加败酱草30克，丹皮12克，黄柏9克。

中成药：保坤丹，每次30片，每日1次。

丹参膏，每次一汤匙，冲服，日3次。

**5. 痰湿阻滞型**

**临床表现**　月经停闭，形体肥胖，胸胁满闷，呕恶痰多，神疲肢倦，面浮足肿，带下量多，舌苔腻，脉滑。妇科检查：子宫发育不良或可触到卵巢胀大、质韧，子宫正常大，内分泌化验往往不正常。

治法：祛痰除湿，调气活血通经。

方药：启宫丸（47）（经验方）加味。

茯苓18克，半夏12克，陈皮12克，苍术15克，香附12克，神曲12克，川芎9克，仙灵脾30克，鸡血藤30克，川断30克，牛膝15克，桃仁12克，车前子12克（包），肉桂6克，王不留行12克。每日1剂，水煎200～300毫升，分2次温服。

加减：白带少，子宫发育不良者，加菟丝子24克，肉苁蓉30克。

检查双侧卵巢胀大者，加丹参15克，生牡蛎30克，苏木15克，三棱12克。

带下量多色黄、苔黄腻者，加泽泻9克，黄柏6克。


# 3.4　经前期紧张综合征

经前期紧张综合征系指周期性出现的一系列症状，如精神紧张，情绪不稳定，注意力不集中，烦躁易怒，或抑郁焦虑，失眠，头晕头痛，胸胁乳房胀痛，浮肿泄泻等，一般经前7至14天开始出现，经前2至3天加重，行经后消失。可能与体内孕激素减少，雌激素相对过多，引起的水、盐潴留；精神紧张致使血中的催乳素过多；个体对经前期醛固酮升高的敏感性不同等因素所引起。

经前期紧张综合征包括在中医的"月经前后诸证"之中，古代医籍中，对经前、经后、经期出现的不同症状，分别称"经行乳房胀痛"、"经行浮肿"、"经行泄泻"、"经行头痛"、"经行身痛"、"经行发热"。由于肝郁气滞，脾肾阳虚，血虚肝旺所引起。

## 辨证论治

### 1. 肝郁气滞型

**临床表现**　经前乳头、乳房胀大疼痛，甚则不能触衣，胸闷胁胀，小腹胀满，烦躁易怒或精神抑郁。舌淡苔薄白，脉弦。检查乳房胀硬，有结节、触痛。

治法：疏肝理气，活血调经。

方药：柴胡疏肝散（9）加味。

柴胡 9 克，白芍 15 克，川芎 9 克，香附 12 克，陈皮 12 克，枳壳 9 克，炙甘草 6 克，橘叶 12 克，川楝子 12 克，郁金 9 克，丹参 15 克。症状出现前开始服药，每日 1 剂，水煎 200～300 毫升，分 2 次服。服至月经来潮，下次月经来前，重复服药。

加减：排经不畅、腹痛者，加牛膝 15 克，桃仁 12 克，苏木 15 克。

口干苦，头痛发热，尿黄便艰、舌苔黄薄者，去川芎，加丹皮 9 克，栀子 9 克，石决明 15 克。

乳房胀硬有块者，加王不留行 12 克，橘核 12 克，荔枝核 12 克，路路通 12 克。

精神抑郁，长叹息，不寐者，加合欢花 15 克。

中成药：逍遥丸，每次 6～9 克，每日 2 次，经前 7～10 天服。

七制香附丸，每次 1 丸，每日 3 次，经前 7～10 天服。

## 2. 脾肾阳虚型

**临床表现** 经前经期面目四肢浮肿，经行泄泻，纳少腹胀，倦怠乏力，或腰膝酸软，月经量多色淡，苔白腻，脉沉缓。

治法：温肾健脾。

方药：健固汤 (32) 加味。

党参30克，白术15克，茯苓15克，薏苡仁15克，巴戟天15克，肉桂6克，补骨脂15克，扁豆30克，山药12克，莲子肉12克，桔梗9克，砂仁9克，车前子12克（包），甘草6克。症状出现前开始服药，每日1剂，水煎200～300毫升，分2次服，至直月经来潮。下个周期重复服药。

加减：畏寒肢冷者，加桂枝9克。

下肢肿甚者，加防已15克，赤小豆30克。

腹痛即泻，两胁胀痛者，加白芍15克，防风9克。或者用痛泻要方：白术18克，白芍15克，陈皮12克，防风9克。

泄泻日久或五更泻者，加五味子12克，肉豆蔻15克。

## 3. 血虚肝旺型

**临床表现** 经前后或经期烦躁失眠，头晕头痛，身体疼痛，舌淡苔薄，脉弦细数。

治法：养血柔肝。

方药：杞菊地黄汤 (49) 加味。

熟地15克，山茱萸15克，山药12克，泽泻9克，牡丹皮9克，茯苓12克，枸杞15克，菊花9克，白芍15克，生龙牡各30克，石决明15克，薄荷6克。症状出现前开始服药，每日1剂，水煎200～300毫升，分2次服。直至月经来潮，下个周期重复服药。

加减：口苦咽干，舌红苔黄者，加夏枯草12克，栀子9克。

经行肢体疼痛麻木者，加鸡血藤 30 克，黄芪 30 克，当归 15 克。

烦躁，心悸少寐者，加桂圆肉 12 克，何首乌 15 克，枣仁 30 克。

中成药：杞菊地黄丸，每次 1 丸，每日 3 次，治经行头晕。

鸡血藤浸膏片，每次 5 片，每日 3 次。治经行身痛。

逍遥丸，每次 1 袋，每日 2 次，治经前乳房胀痛。

# 3.5 更年期综合征

更年期为妇女卵巢功能逐渐消退直至完全消失的一个过渡时期。在更年期过程中，月经停止来潮，称"绝经"。绝经一般发生在 45～55 岁之间。部分妇女在绝经这个生理过程的前后，常出现月经紊乱，心烦失眠，心悸出汗，手足心烦热，便溏、浮肿，腰膝酸痛等症状。这些症状往往三三两两的出现，症状多少，轻重程度，因人而异。更年期综合征即中医"绝经前后诸证"。由于肾气渐衰，任脉虚，太冲脉衰少，天癸将竭，体内阴阳失于平衡，脏腑气血失调所致。治疗以益肾为主，佐以疏肝、健脾。

## 辨证论治

### 1. 肾阴虚型

**临床表现** 头晕目眩，耳鸣，头部及面颊阵阵烘热汗出，目干涩，视物不清，五心烦热，腰膝酸痛，月经先期或先后不定期，经量或多或少，色鲜红。大便干结，尿少色黄，舌红少苔，脉细数。

治法：滋养肾阴。

方药：左归饮（106）加味。

熟地 15 克，山药 15 克，枸杞 18 克，山茱萸 12 克，茯苓 12 克，甘草 6 克，生龙骨 30 克，生牡蛎 30 克，白芍药 15 克。

每日 1 剂，水煎 200～300 毫升，分 2 次服。

加减：月经量多而色红者，加旱莲草 18 克，女贞子 15 克，地榆 30 克。

月经淋漓不断、色紫黑有块者，加益母草 30 克，茜草 12 克。

口干苦，目胀赤、头痛者，改熟地为生地，加菊花 9 克，珍珠母 30 克，夏枯草 12 克。

喜怒无常，情志不能自制者，加浮小麦 30 克，炙甘草 12 克，大枣 7 枚，合欢皮 15 克，去甘草。

烘热汗出过多者，加黄芪 30 克，浮小麦 15 克。

**2. 肾阳虚型**

**临床表现** 面色晦黯，精神萎靡，形寒肢冷，纳呆腹胀，面浮肢肿，大便溏薄，尿频失禁，夜尿多，月经量多或崩中漏下，色黯淡，带下清稀。舌淡而胖嫩，边有齿痕，舌苔薄白，脉沉细无力。

治法：温肾扶阳。

方药：右归丸 (96) (见功能失调性子宫出血)，每日 1 剂，水煎 200～300 毫升，分 2 次服。

加减：尿频失禁，夜尿甚多者，加益智仁 30 克，海螵蛸 15 克，复盆子 15 克。

面目及四肢浮肿甚者，加车前子 12 克 (包)，泽泻 9 克。

性欲低下者，加仙灵脾 30 克，仙茅 15 克。

大便溏薄、泄泻日久者，加炮姜 6 克，肉豆蔻 15 克，莲子肉 12 克，赤石脂 15 克。

**中成药及单方验方**

更年康，每日 2 次，每次 4 片。

益肾宁，每日 2 次，每次 2 片。

浮小麦 30 克，大枣七枚，甘草 12 克。水煎 200 毫升，早晚分服。用于情志不畅，哭笑无常者。

# 3.6  其他月经病证

## 3.6.1  月经先期

月经周期提前 7 天以上，甚至 10 余天一行者，称为"月经先期"，亦称"经水先期"、"经期超前"、"经早"等。多由气虚、血热所致。因饮食失节，劳倦思虑过度，损伤脾气，致使中气统摄无权，冲任不固，或素体阳盛，过食辛辣，或阴血亏损。水亏火旺以致热扰冲任，迫血妄行，均可导致月经提前来潮。

### 辨证论治

**1. 气虚型**

**临床表现**  月经提前，量多、色淡，质稀。倦怠嗜睡，神疲乏力，小腹空坠，纳少便溏，舌质淡，脉细弱。

治法：补气摄血，固冲任。

方药：补中益气汤 (7) 加减。

人参 15 克（先煎），黄芪 30 克，白术 15 克，炙甘草 9 克，生龙骨 30 克，生牡蛎 30 克，血余炭 12 克，陈皮 12 克，柴胡 6 克，升麻 6 克。每日 1 剂，水煎 200～300 毫升，分 2 次服。

加减：心悸失眠多梦者，去升麻、柴胡，加桂圆肉 12 克，枣仁 30 克，远志 9 克。

腰痛、腹冷、尿多便溏者，去升麻、柴胡，加益智仁 15 克，补骨脂 15 克，炮姜 6 克。

中成药：人参归脾丸，每次 1 丸，每日三次。

**2. 血热型**

(1) 实热

**临床表现**  月经提前，量多，色鲜红或紫红，质粘稠，面红口干，喜冷饮，心烦，大便燥结，小便少黄。舌质红，苔薄黄，脉滑数有力。

治法：清热凉血调经。

方药：清经汤（51）加减。

牡丹皮12克，地骨皮12克，白芍药15克，生地15克，青蒿9克，黄柏9克，小蓟15克，黄芩9克，地榆30克。每日1剂，水煎200～300毫升，分2次服。

加减：壮热面红，口渴，便燥尿赤者，加石膏15克，大黄6克（后入）。

(2) 肝郁血热

临床表现：月经提前，量或多或少，色紫红有块，质粘稠。心烦易怒，少腹胀痛，胸闷胁胀，乳房胀痛，口苦咽干，舌质红，苔黄薄，脉弦数。

治法：清肝解郁调经。

方药：丹栀逍遥散（21）加减。

牡丹皮12克，栀子9克，白芍药15克，当归12克，白术12克，柴胡9克，茯苓12克，炙甘草6克，薄荷9克，生地15克，川楝子12克，香附12克。每日1剂，水煎200～300毫升，分2次服。

加减：乳房胀痛有块者，加王不留行12克，丝瓜络9克，荔枝核12克，橘核9克。

经行不畅、血块多者，加丹参15克，泽兰18克，川芎9克。

口干目眩，失眠者，加菊花9克，石决明15克，生牡蛎30克。

(3) 阴虚血热型

临床表现：月经提前，量少，色红，质稠。两颧潮红，手足心热，咽干口燥，心烦不眠，舌质红，少苔或剥苔，脉细数。

治法：养阴清热调经。

方药：两地汤（37）加味。

生地 15 克，地骨皮 12 克，玄参 15 克，麦冬 12 克，阿胶 12 克（溶化），白芍药 15 克，沙参 15 克，丹皮 9 克，旱莲草 15 克，女贞子 15 克，黄芩 9 克。每日 1 剂，水煎 200～300 毫升，分 2 次服。

加减：月经很少，潮热、不寐者，加丹参 15 克，青蒿 9 克，龟板 30 克，柏子仁 15 克。

## 3.6.2　月经后期

月经周期延后 7 天以上，甚至四、五十天一至者，称"月经后期"、"经水过期"、"经期错后"、"经迟"等。病因有虚实之分，虚者多因营、血亏损，阳气虚衰，以致化源不足，血海不能按时满盈；而实者多因气郁血滞，寒凝血瘀，冲任受阻，以致经期延后。

### 辨证论治

#### 1. 血寒型

**临床表现**　经期延后，量少，色黯有块，小腹冷痛，得热则减，畏寒肢冷，苔白，脉沉紧。

治法：温经散寒，活血行滞。

方药：温经汤（82）加味。

人参 15 克（先煎），当归 12 克，川芎 9 克，白芍 15 克，桂心 6 克，牛膝 15 克，牡丹皮 12 克，莪术 12 克，甘草 6 克，鸡血藤 30 克，乌药 12 克。每日 1 剂，水煎 200～300 毫升，分 2 次服。

加减：腹痛拒按、块多者，加蒲黄 12 克，益母草 30 克，苏木 15 克，香附 12 克。

月经量多者，去牛膝、莪术，加艾叶 12 克，炮姜 6 克。

中成药：乌鸡白凤丸，每次 1 丸，每日 2 次。

女金丹，每日 2 次，每次 1 丸。

**2. 虚寒型**

**临床表现** 经期延后，量少，色淡红、质清稀，无血块，小腹隐痛，喜按喜暖，腰酸无力，舌淡苔白，脉沉迟。

治法：扶阳散寒，养血调经。

方药：艾附暖宫丸（1）。

艾叶 9 克，香附 12 克，当归 12 克，续断 15 克，吴茱萸 12 克，川芎 9 克，白芍药 15 克，黄芪 15 克，熟地 12 克，肉桂 6 克。每日 1 剂，水煎 200～300 毫升，分 2 次服。

加减：小便清长，大便溏薄者，加补骨脂 15 克，白术 15 克。

宫寒多年不孕者，加紫石英 30 克。

**3. 血虚型**

**临床表现** 经期延后，量少，色淡，无块。小腹空坠、隐痛，面色无华，头晕眼花，心悸少寐，舌淡苔薄白，脉细弱。

治法：补气养血。

方药：滋血汤（110）加味。

人参 15 克（先煎），山药 12 克，黄芪 30 克，茯苓 12 克，川芎 9 克，当归 15 克，白芍药 18 克，熟地 30 克，首乌 30 克，鸡血藤 30 克，生枣仁 15 克，阿胶 12 克（烊化）。每日 1 剂，水煎 200～300 毫升，分 2 次服。

加减：心烦口干，手足心热者，去熟地、人参，加生地 15 克，太子参 15 克，旱莲草 15 克，女贞子 12 克。

心悸少寐者，加柏子仁 15 克，五味子 12 克。

食少便溏者，去熟地，加白术 15 克，扁豆 30 克，莲子肉 12 克。

中成药：首乌片，每次 5 片，每日 3 次。

八珍益母丸，每次 1 丸，每日 3 次。

**4. 气滞型**

**临床表现** 月经延后，量少、色黯红、有血块，小腹胀痛，胸胁、乳房胀痛，精神抑郁，舌质正常，脉弦或涩。

治法：理气调经。

方药：加味乌药汤（87）加减。

乌药 12 克，砂仁 9 克，延胡索 12 克，香附 12 克，甘草 6 克，槟榔 9 克，木香 9 克，牛膝 15 克，肉桂 6 克。每日 1 剂，水煎 200～300 毫升，分 2 次服。

加减：血块多，腹痛甚者，加当归 15 克，川芎 9 克，鸡血藤 15 克。

胸胁胀闷、精神抑郁者，加柴胡 9 克，郁金 9 克。

中成药：七制香附丸，每次 1 丸，每日 3 次。

元胡止痛片，每次 5 片，每日 3 次。

### 3.6.3　月经先后无定期

月经周期提前或错后 7 天以上者，称为"月经先后无定期"，或称"经水先后无定期"、"经乱"。本病与肝、肾关系密切，肝主疏泄、司血海，肾主封藏，为月经之本。肝郁疏泄无度，肾虚封藏失职，以致气血失调，血海蓄溢失常，引起月经先后无定期。

**辨证论治**

**1. 肝郁型**

**临床表现** 月经周期不定或前或后，量或多或少，色紫红有块，经行不畅，胸胁、乳房、少腹胀痛，胸闷不舒，善叹息，嗳气食少，苔薄白或黄，脉弦。

治法：疏肝理气调经。

方药：逍遥散（94）加减。

柴胡 9 克，白术 15 克，茯苓 12 克，当归 12 克，白芍 15 克，薄荷 9 克，牛膝 15 克，苏木 15 克，香附 12 克，郁金 9 克。每日 1 剂，水煎 200～300 毫升，分 2 次服。

加减：胸闷纳呆者，加厚朴 9 克，砂仁 6 克，陈皮 12 克。

量多者，去牛膝、苏木。

中成药：保坤丸，每次30片，每日1次。

**2. 肾虚型**

**临床表现**　经来先后不定，量少，色黯，质清，头晕耳鸣，腰骶酸痛，舌淡苔少，脉沉细。

治法：补肾调经。

方药：固阴煎（27）加味。

人参15克（先煎），熟地15克，山药12克，山茱萸15克，菟丝子24克，远志9克，五味子12克，炙甘草6克，肉苁蓉15克，川断30克，仙灵脾15克。每日1剂，水煎200～300毫升，分2次服。

加减：量少、色鲜红，舌红少苔、脉沉细数者，加牡丹皮，旱莲草15克，改熟地为生地15克。

小便清长、大便溏薄，腰膝冷痛者，去肉苁蓉，熟地，加肉桂6克，巴戟天12克，补骨脂15克。

中成药：桂附地黄丸，每次1丸，日2次，淡盐水送下。

### 3.6.4　月经量多

月经量明显增多而月经周期正常者，称为"月经量多"或"经水过多"。多因气虚统摄无权，或血热扰动血海，以致冲任不固，或瘀血内阻，血不归经所致。

**辨证论治**

**1. 气虚型**

**临床表现**　月经量多，色淡红，质清稀。面色㿠白，气短懒言，肢软无力，小腹空坠，心悸怔忡，舌淡，脉细弱。

治法：补气摄血固冲。

方药：举元煎（35）加味。

人参15克（先煎），黄芪30克，白术18克，升麻6克，炙甘草9克，生龙牡各30克，五味子15克，炒白芍15克。每日

1剂，水煎 200～300 毫升，分 2 次服。

加减：量过多者，加乌贼骨 30 克，炒艾叶 9 克，炮姜 6 克。

心悸失眠者，加柏子仁 15 克，炒枣仁 30 克。

中成药：补中益气丸，每次 1 丸，每日 3 次。

**2. 血热型**

**临床表现** 月经量多，色深红或鲜红，质稠粘，或有血块。心烦口渴，尿黄，便结，舌红苔黄，脉滑数。

治法：清热凉血止血。

方药：保阴煎（5）加减。

生地 18 克，黄芩 12 克，黄柏 9 克；白芍药 15 克，山药 12 克，炒续断 15 克，地榆 30 克，生牡蛎 30 克，白茅根 30 克，小蓟 30 克。每日 1 剂，水煎 200～300 毫升，每 2 次服。

加减：心烦，便结尿黄者，加淡竹叶 12 克，栀子 9 克，大黄 6 克（后入）。

潮热汗出，口干咽燥者，加沙参 15 克，地骨皮 9 克，麦冬 12 克。

气短懒言，倦怠乏力者，加黄芪 30 克，白术 15 克。

**3. 血瘀型**

**临床表现** 经来量多，色紫黑，有血块，小腹疼痛拒按，舌质紫有瘀点或瘀斑。脉细涩。

治法：活血化瘀止血。

方药：失笑散（70）加味。

五灵脂 12 克，蒲黄 12 克，益母草 30 克，茜草 12 克，丹参 15 克，牡丹皮 9 克，桃仁 12 克，黄芪 15 克。每日 1 剂，水煎 200～300 毫升，分 2 次服。

加减：小腹冷痛者，去丹参，加艾叶 9 克，乌药 12 克。

胸胁、少腹胀满者，加青皮 12 克，川楝子 12 克。

中成药：三七片，每次 5～10 片，最多不超过 30 片，日一次，血太多，可隔 6 小时加服 1 次。

### 3.6.5 月经量少

月经周期正常，月经量明显减少，甚或点滴即净，或经期缩短不足两天，经量亦少者，称为"月经过少"，亦称"经水涩少"。病因有虚实之分，虚者为化源不足，精血衰少，以致血海亏虚。实者多由瘀血内停，痰湿阻滞，以致经脉壅阻，血行不畅所致。

**辨证论治**

**1. 血虚型**

**临床表现** 月经量少，或点滴即净，色淡无块，伴头晕眼花，心悸怔忡，面色萎黄，唇、舌、爪甲苍白无华，小腹空坠，皮肤不泽，舌质淡红、苔白薄，脉细。

治法：养血调经。

方药：人参养荣汤（58）加味。

白芍药 18 克，当归 15 克，陈皮 12 克，黄芪 30 克，桂心 6 克，人参 15 克（先煎），白术 15 克，炙甘草 9 克，熟地 15 克，五味子 12 克，茯苓 15 克，远志 9 克，首乌 30 克，丹参 30 克，鸡血藤 30 克，生姜 6 克，大枣 7 枚。每日 1 剂，水煎 200～300 毫升，分 2 次服。

加减：心悸失眠者，加柏子仁 15 克，麦门冬 12 克。

中成药，人参健脾丸，每次 1 丸，每日 3 次。

**2. 肾虚型**

**临床表现** 初潮过迟，潮后月经量即少，常伴月经周期延后、经量少、色黯淡、质薄。腰膝酸软，足跟痛，头晕耳鸣，或小腹冷，夜尿多，舌淡，脉沉迟或沉弱。

治法：益肾养血调经。

方药：归肾丸（26）加味。

熟地 15 克，山药 15 克，山茱萸 12 克，茯苓 15 克，当归 15 克，菟丝子 24 克，杜仲 30 克，枸杞子 30 克，仙灵脾 30

克，肉桂9克，每日1剂，水煎200~300毫升，分2次服。

加减：经色红，手足心热，咽干口燥，舌红苔少者，去熟地、杜仲、肉桂、仙灵脾，加生地15克，玄参15克，女贞子12克，旱莲草15克。

腹冷尿多者，加巴戟天15克，益智仁30克。

中成药：六味地黄丸，每次1丸，日2次，适用于肾阴虚型。

桂附地黄丸，每次1丸，日2次，适用于肾阳虚型。

### 3. 血瘀型

**临床表现**　月经量少，色紫黑，有血块，小腹胀痛拒按，血块下而痛减，舌质紫黯，有瘀点或瘀斑，脉涩。

治法：活血化瘀调经。

方药：桃红四物汤（75）加减。

桃仁12克，红花12克，当归15克，川芎9克，白芍药15克，泽兰15克，益母草30克，牛膝15克，三棱12克，每日1剂，水煎200~300毫升，分2次服。

加减：胸胁胀满、腹胀痛者，加香附12克，乌药12克，枳壳9克。

腹冷痛者，加桂枝9克，艾叶12克，吴茱萸12克。

### 4. 痰湿型

**临床表现**　月经量少，色淡红，质粘腻，形体肥胖，胸闷呕恶，带下量多，舌淡苔白腻，脉滑。

治法：祛痰渗湿，活血通络。

方药：苍附导痰丸（10）加味。

茯苓18克，姜半夏12克，陈皮12克，苍术12克，香附12克，胆南星12克，枳壳12克，神曲12克，甘草6克，生姜6克，鸡血藤15克，牛膝12克，川芎9克，车前子12克（包），肉桂6克。每日1剂，水煎200~300毫升，分2次服。

加减：腰酸痛者，加川断 30 克，菟丝子 24 克。

　　　　面目四肢肿胀者，加白术 15 克，防己 12 克，赤小豆 30 克。

### 3.6.6　经行吐衄

　　经行前 2 至 3 日或经期出现吐血或衄血，而经后数日即可自行消失者，称"经行吐衄"，亦称"逆经"、"倒经"。经前、经期冲气旺盛，冲脉丽于阳明胃而附于肝，别络出于颃颡穴（即鼻后孔），肺开窍于鼻。若情志不遂，肝郁化火，或素体阴虚，虚火上炎，冲气挟肝气上逆，热灼络脉而致吐血衄血。

**辨证论治**

**1. 肝郁化火型**

**临床表现**　经前或经期口鼻出血，量多，色红，有块，心烦易怒，口苦咽干，头昏目眩，乳胀胁痛，月经提前量少，舌红苔黄，脉弦数。

治法：疏肝清热，引血下行。

方药：清肝引经汤（48）加减。

白芍药 15 克，生地 15 克，牡丹皮 12 克，栀子 12 克，黄芩 9 克，川楝子 9 克，茜草 12 克，牛膝 15 克，白茅根 30 克，甘草 6 克，小蓟 30 克，藕节 12 克，仙鹤草 15 克。每日 1 剂，水煎 200～300 毫升，分 2 次服，平日隔日 1 剂。

　　加减：经量少而腹痛者，加益母草 30 克，红花 12 克，丹参 15 克。

**2. 肺肾阴虚型**

**临床表现**　经前、经期吐衄，量少色黯红，头晕耳鸣，手足心热，两颧潮红，咽干口燥，潮热咳嗽痰少或无痰，形体消瘦，月经先期量少，舌红或绛，苔剥或无苔，脉细数。

治法：滋肾润肺，清热降逆止血。

方药：顺经汤（62）加味。

当归 12 克，生地 15 克，沙参 18 克，白芍 15 克，茯苓 12 克，黑荆芥 9 克，牡丹皮 12 克，牛膝 15 克，紫草 15 克，白薇 12 克，旱莲草 30 克，地骨皮 12 克，黄芩 9 克，经前 7 日，每日 1 剂，水煎 200～300 毫升，分 2 次服，平时隔日 1 剂。

加减：干咳无痰、潮热者，加麦门冬 12 克，桑叶 12 克，百合 15 克。

咽干口渴，出血量多者，加白茅根 30 克，侧柏叶 12 克。

### 3.6.7  经行口糜

每当月经将至或经行之时，口舌糜烂生疮，如期反复发作者，称"经行口糜"。口，胃之门户，舌，心之苗，多为胃热熏蒸，心火上炎所致。

**辨证论治**

**1. 阴虚火旺型**

**临床表现**  经前或经期口舌糜烂疼痛，口燥咽干，五心烦热，卧不安神，尿少色黄，舌红苔少，脉细数。

治法：滋阴降火。

方药：知柏地黄汤（103）加味。

生地 15 克，牡丹皮 12 克，茯苓 12 克，泽泻 9 克，山茱萸 12 克，山药 12 克，知母 6 克，黄柏 9 克，花粉 12 克，麦冬 12 克，竹叶 9 克，生甘草梢 6 克。每日 1 剂，水煎 200～300 毫升，分 2 次服。

**2. 胃热熏蒸型**

**临床表现**  经行口舌生疮，口臭，口干喜饮，尿黄便结，舌苔黄厚，脉滑数。

治法：清热泻火，荡涤胃热。

方药：凉膈散（39）。

大黄 6 克（后入），芒硝 6 克，生甘草 9 克，栀子 12 克，薄荷9克，黄芩12克，连翘15克，竹叶12克。每日1剂，水煎200～300毫升，分2次服。

中成药：冰硼散，少量吹敷于溃烂处，每日2～3次。

（李竹兰）

# 4 妊娠病理

## 4.1 流产

妊娠于 28 周前终止，胎儿体重不足 1000 克者称为流产。流产发生在 12 周以前者称为早期流产，发生在 12 周至 28 周之间者称晚期流产。人工流产是指用药物或机械性干预等人工方法，而使妊娠终止者。自然流产指胚胎或胎儿因某种原因自动脱离母体而排出。根据自然流产的不同情况，临床上又分为先兆流产、难免流产、不全流产、完全流产、稽留流产、感染性流产、习惯性流产。根据症状先兆流产属中医的"胎漏"、"胎动不安"范畴，早期流产、晚期流产，早产属"堕胎"、"小产"范畴，而习惯性流产即"滑胎"。

### 4.1.1 先兆流产

先兆流产常发生在妊娠早期，以阴道少量流血或伴有轻微下腹痛、腰酸及下坠感为特点。早孕反应存在，检查子宫颈口未开，子宫大小与停经月份相符，妊娠试验阳性。属于中医胎漏、胎动不安范畴。胎漏指阴道少量出血，时下时止而无腰酸腹痛者，胎动不安指仅有腰酸腹痛或下腹坠胀，或伴有阴道少量出血者。由于母体肾气不足、房事不节或气血虚弱、邪热动胎，导致冲任气血不调，以及夫妇精气不足，胎元缺陷，胎元不固所引起。

## 辨证论治

### 1. 肾虚型

**临床表现** 妊娠期间，腰部酸痛，小腹下坠，阴道少量流血，色黯淡。或伴头晕耳鸣，小便频数，夜尿多甚至失禁。舌淡红，苔薄白，脉沉滑尺弱。

治法：固肾安胎，佐以益气。

方药：寿胎丸 (67) 加味。

菟丝子 18 克，桑寄生 15 克，续断 15 克，阿胶 12 克（烊化），杜仲 12 克，党参 15 克，白术 9 克。每日 1 剂，水煎 200～300 毫升，分 2 次服。

加减：下血多者，加艾叶炭 9 克。

小便频数或失禁者，加益智仁 9 克。

腰酸腹痛而有坠感者，加炙升麻 6 克，黄芪 15 克。

### 2. 气血虚弱型

**临床表现** 妊娠期，胎动下坠，阴道少量流血，色淡。伴神疲肢倦，面色㿠白，心悸气短，或腰酸腹痛。舌淡苔薄白，脉细滑或沉弱。

治法：补气养血，固肾安胎。

方药：胎元饮 (80) 加减。

党参 15 克，杜仲 12 克，白术 9 克，白芍 9 克，熟地 12 克，陈皮 9 克，炙黄芪 15 克，阿胶 12 克（烊化），炙甘草 6 克。每日 1 剂，水煎 200～300 毫升，分 2 次服。

加减：腹痛甚者，改白芍 15 克。

阴道下血量多者，加艾叶炭 9 克，仙鹤草 15 克。

食少便溏，苔白而腻者，加砂仁 6 克，山药 12 克。

中成药：保胎丸，每次 1 丸，每日 3 次。

八珍益母丸，每次 1 丸，每日 3 次。

**3.血热型**

**临床表现** 妊娠期阴道流血，色鲜红，或腰酸坠痛，伴口干咽燥，渴喜冷饮，心烦不安，或小便黄，大便干。舌质红，苔黄而干，脉滑数。

治法：滋阴清热，养血安胎。

方药：保阴煎 (5) 加味。

生、熟地各 12 克，白芍 9 克，续断 15 克，炒山药 12 克，黄芩 9 克，黄柏 6 克，苎麻根 12 克，生甘草 6 克。每日 1 剂，水煎 200～300 毫升，分 2 次服。

加减：出血多者，加旱莲草 15 克，莲房炭 12 克。

偏阴虚者，加麦冬 9 克，石斛 9 克。

腰酸痛者，加菟丝子 15 克，杜仲 12 克。

**4.外伤型**

**临床表现** 妊娠期间，跌仆闪挫、外伤之后，小腹坠痛，腰骶酸痛，阴道流血量少色红，脉滑无力。

治法：补气和血，固肾安胎。

方药：圣愈汤 (72) 合寿胎丸 (67)。

炒当归身 9 克，川芎 3 克，熟地 12 克，生地 12 克，党参 18 克，炙黄芪 18 克，菟丝子 15 克，川续断 15 克，桑寄生 15 克，阿胶 12 克 (烊化)。每日 1 剂，水煎 200～300 毫升，分 2 次服。

加减：下血较多者，去炒当归身、川芎，加艾叶炭 9 克，苎麻根 12 克。

小腹刺痛、舌质黯红者，加炒蒲黄 9 克，五灵脂 9 克，三七粉 3 克 (分 2 次冲)。中病即止，不可久服。

**注意事项** 孕妇应注重调饮食，心情舒畅，劳逸适当。

妊娠早期慎戒性生活。

保胎期间卧床休息。

## 4.1.2 难免流产

难免流产是由先兆流产发展而来，以流血量多，腹痛、宫口开大，但胚胎组织尚未排出为特点。多由气血虚弱，胎失所养，肾虚胎失所系，或血热伤胎，跌仆闪挫，伤动胎元引起。因妊娠不能继续下去，以去胎保母为治疗原则。

### 辨证论治

**临床表现** 妊娠期间，阴道流血量多，超过正常月经量，有血块，或伴有液体流出，小腹疼痛拒按。妇科检查：子宫颈口已开大。脉滑或涩或细数，舌黯或有瘀点、瘀斑。

治法：祛瘀下胎。

方药：脱花煎（74）加味。

当归15克，川牛膝15克，川芎9克，红花12克，车前子9克（布包），肉桂6克，益母草30克。每日1剂，水煎200～300毫升，分2次服。

加减：伴面色苍白、神疲乏力者，加党参30克，炙黄芪30克。

小腹冷痛、面色青白，肢冷畏寒者，加干姜6克，小茴香9克。

胸腹胀满较甚者，加香附12克，枳壳9克。

## 4.1.3 不全流产

不全流产由难免流产发展而来，以阴道流血持续不止，腹痛，宫口开大，胚胎组织堵塞于宫口为特点。属中医的"堕胎"、"小产"范畴。一般怀孕3个月以内，胎儿尚未成形而堕者，称为"堕胎"，而怀孕3个月以后，胎儿已成形而坠者，则称"小产"，亦称"半产"。本病多因素体气虚，或产育频繁，耗伤正气，气虚则推动无力，以致瘀血内阻胞宫;亦有流产时感受风寒，或情志郁结，以致气机不畅，瘀血阻于胞宫所致。

## 辨证论治

### 1.气虚血瘀型

**临床表现** 胎儿、胎盘部分排出后，阴道流血不止，并夹有血块及伴有较多的液体，小腹坠痛，面色苍白，神倦乏力，头晕心悸。舌质淡黯，边有齿印，或有瘀点，苔薄白，脉弦涩无力。妇科检查：子宫颈口开大，宫缩欠佳，或有胚胎组织阻塞宫口。

治法：益气逐瘀。

方药：人参黄芪汤（56）合失笑散（70）加味。

人参 6～9 克，黄芪 30 克，白术 9 克，当归 12 克，白芍 9 克，艾叶 4.5 克，阿胶 12 克（烊化），蒲黄 12 克，五灵脂 12 克，川牛膝 15 克，益母草 30 克。每日 1 剂，水煎 200～300 毫升，分 2 次服。

加减：胁腹胀痛者，加枳壳 9 克，香附 12 克。

### 2.气滞血瘀型

**临床表现** 胎儿、胎盘部分排出后，阴道流血时多时少，色紫黯或有块，小腹胀痛拒按，块下痛减，舌质黯或有瘀点，苔薄白，脉弦涩。妇科检查：子宫颈口开大，或有胚胎组织阻塞宫口。

治法：行气祛瘀。

方药：当归汤（16）加味。

当归 15 克，木通 6 克，滑石 15 克，冬葵子 12 克，瞿麦 12 克，川牛膝 12 克，枳壳 9 克。每日 1 剂，水煎 200～300 毫升，分 2 次服。

加减：小腹冷痛者，加肉桂 6 克。

阴道下血量多者，加三七粉 3 克（分 2 次冲服），炒蒲黄 9 克，益母草 30 克。

兼有气短神疲等气虚之象者，加党参 30 克，炙黄芪

30 克。

### 4.1.4　完全流产

完全流产是指通过先兆流产及难免流产过程，以胚胎组织完全排出，阴道出血逐渐停止，腹痛渐渐消失为特点。属中医"堕胎"、"小产"范畴。

#### 辨证论治

完全流产一般不需作特殊处理，倘若仍有腹痛及阴道有少量瘀血流出者，则须调治，以促使子宫的恢复。

**临床表现**　经过剧烈腹痛后阴道流血量多，有块，可见胚胎组织排出，块下痛减，腹痛逐渐消失，或腹痛隐隐，阴道流血减少或停止。妇科检查：子宫颈口已关闭，子宫正常大小。

治法：活血化瘀，佐以益气。

方药：生化汤（61）加味。

当归 12 克，川芎 9 克，桃仁 9 克，炮姜炭 3 克，炙甘草 3 克，益母草 15 克，党参 15 克。每日 1 剂，水煎 200～300 毫升，兑黄酒 30 克，童便一盅，分 2 次服。

中成药：益母草膏，每次 10 毫升，口服，日 2 次。

生化汤丸，每次 1 丸，每日 3 次。

### 4.1.5　稽留流产

本病指胚胎死亡 2 个月以上尚未自然排出者。中医称为"胎死不下"或"死胎"。因素体肾气不足，气血虚弱，或房事不节，或跌仆损伤胎气，胎失所养，停止发育，而气虚无力排胎，或瘀血内阻，阻碍胚胎排出所致。

## 辨证论治

**临床表现** 妊娠后阴道流血，量时多时少，色黯，有块，不再恶心呕吐，原有胎动消失，小腹冷，口臭，面色黯，舌质紫黯，或有瘀斑，脉沉涩。妇科检查：子宫小于妊娠月份，B超或听诊探听不到胎心音。

治法：行气活血，祛瘀下胎。

方药：救母丹（34）合脱花煎（74）加减。

人参9~15克（先煎），当归12~18克，川芎15克，益母草30克，赤石脂6克，炒芥穗9克，牛膝15克，肉桂6克，厚朴9克。

加减：肢肿、胸闷，苔厚腻者，加苍术12克，陈皮12克，车前子12克（包）。

胸胁少腹胀满者，加元胡9克，枳壳9克。

每日早、晚各一剂，每剂水煎150毫升1次服。

**其他治疗方法**

天花粉针剂肌注

用法： 天花粉蛋白针剂1.2~2.4毫克，结晶天花粉蛋白用盐水2毫升稀释后，臀部肌肉注射。

注意： 用前先作皮试，观察20分钟。

试探剂量观察2小时。

治疗剂量1.2~2.4毫克。

用药后48小时卧床休息，严密观察体温、心率、血压等。可服强的松10毫克，日3次，用2天，以预防过敏反应。

副反应治疗常用非那根、安乃近，皮质激素，高渗糖、维生素C等。

禁忌：天花粉皮试的试探剂量阳性者。

过敏体质，对多种药物及食物过敏者。

活动性肝、肾疾病伴功能不全者。

出血性疾病，严重贫血慎用。

急性炎症暂缓使用。

## 4.1.6　感染性流产

在流产过程中，或流产后的短时间内感染病邪热毒者，称为感染性流产，以发热恶寒、腹痛、带下秽臭为特点。各型流产均可并发感染，最多发生在不全流产。它包括在中医的"产后发热"、"热入血室"、"湿热带下"之中。因流产、产后血室大开，邪毒乘虚入侵，热毒积于胞宫，或因瘀血滞于胞宫，蕴久化热所致。

### 辨证论治

**临床表现**　发热恶寒，小腹疼痛拒按，恶露淋漓不净，色黯、有块，或赤白带下有臭味。舌质黯或有瘀点，苔黄腻或黄燥，脉弦数。妇科检查：子宫或附件有明显压痛。血液化验：白细胞总数及中性粒细胞均增高。

治法：清热解毒，活血化瘀。

方药：五味消毒饮（86）合银花蕺菜饮（97）加味。

金银花15克，蒲公英15克，紫花地丁15克，蕺菜（鱼腥草）15克，土茯苓30克，野菊花12克，天葵子9克，丹皮15克，赤芍15克，荆芥6克，生甘草6克。每日1剂，水煎200～300毫升，分2次服。

加减：神疲肢倦、乏力、纳差者，加党参18克。

恶露量多有块者，加茜草15克，乌贼骨30克。

## 4.1.7　习惯性流产

自然流产连续发生三次以上者，称为习惯性流产，即中医的滑胎。因素体脾肾亏虚和阴血不足所致。肾虚胎失所养，脾气虚胎失系载血亏胎失荫养，阴虚生内热，热伤胞络，冲任失固以致屡孕屡堕。

## 辨证论治

本病以孕前服药调治为主，孕后服药保胎，直至超过易堕胎的妊娠月份为止。

### 1.脾肾两虚型

**临床表现** 头晕耳鸣，腰膝酸软，神疲肢倦，气短懒言，纳少便溏，夜尿频多，眼眶黯黑或面有黯斑，月经或前或后，经量或多或少，或滑胎后又不易受孕，舌质淡嫩或苔薄，脉沉弱。

治法：补肾健脾固冲。

方药：补肾固冲丸 (4)。

菟丝子 240 克，续断 90 克，巴戟天 90 克，杜仲 90 克，当归 90 克，熟地 150 克，鹿角霜 90 克，枸杞 90 克，阿胶 120 克，党参 120 克，白术 90 克，大枣 50 枚（去核），砂仁 15 克。制成蜜丸，孕前服，每次 6 克，每日 2 次，经期停服，2 个月为1 疗程。

加减：素体虚弱者，加紫河车粉 90 克。

　　　肢冷畏寒、小腹冷痛者，加仙灵脾 120 克。

中成药：胎产金丹，每次 1 丸，每日 2 次。

### 2. 气血虚弱型

**临床表现** 面色㿠白或萎黄，心悸气短，头晕肢软，神疲乏力，舌质淡苔薄白，脉细弱无力。

治法：益气养血，佐以补肾安胎。

方药：泰山磐石散 (77)。

党参 15 克，黄芪 15 克，续断 18 克，熟地 12 克，当归 9克，川芎 9 克，白术 9 克，白芍 9 克，黄芩 9 克，砂仁 6 克，炙甘草 6 克，糯米 1 撮。每日 1 剂，水煎 200～300 毫升，分 2 次服。

加减：小腹空坠不适者，党参改为30克，黄芪改为30克，加炙升麻6克。

血虚有热者，加生地12克。

心悸失眠者，加炒枣仁30克。

中成药：补中益气丸，每次1丸，每日3次，孕前开始服，至孕后易流产月份止。

保胎丸，每次1丸，日3次。

**3.阴虚血热型**

**临床表现** 两颧潮红，口干咽燥，手足心热，烦躁不宁，形体消瘦，舌红少苔，脉细数。

治法：养阴清热凉血。

方药：保阴煎（5）加味。

生熟地各12克，白芍9克，续断15克，炒山药12克，黄芩9克，黄柏6克，生甘草6克，苎麻根12克，旱莲草15克。

**预防**

对滑胎患者，男女双方均应进行多方面的检查，如：血型、染色体、宫颈机能等，以便给予正确地治疗。

受孕间隔时间不宜太近，最好相隔1年或1年以上。

有习惯性流产史者，首先应解除精神紧张，平时要节制性生活，妊娠期特别是早期妊娠前3个月及最后3个月，应避免房事，以防流产及早产。

艾叶煮鸡蛋平时常服可预防因宫寒所致习惯性流产。

凤凰衣（雏鸡孵化出壳后的卵壳内膜）适量，瓦上文火焙黄，按前次流产月份提前连服5日，每日2次，每次10克，米汤冲服。


## 4.2 妊娠呕吐

妊娠早期恶心、嗜酸、择食，或晨间偶有呕吐等现象，为

"妊娠反应"，不属病态。若呕吐逐渐加重，不仅出现在清晨或进食后，每天反复多次，为妊娠呕吐，甚者呕吐剧烈，饮食不进，造成电解质紊乱及代谢失常，尿酮体阳性，称为妊娠剧吐。中医称为"恶阻"，亦称"阻病"、"食病"等。多由脾胃素虚，孕后经闭而血海不泻，冲任气血旺盛；血聚于下以养胎，血分不足，冲气相对旺盛。冲脉隶属于阳明，冲气上逆犯胃所致，或肝胃不和，胃失和降引起。

## 辨证论治

### 1.脾胃虚弱型

**临床表现**  妊娠早期，恶心呕吐清水，口淡，纳呆，神疲思睡，舌淡苔白润，脉缓滑无力。

治法：健脾和胃，降逆止呕。

方药：香砂六君子汤 (93)。

党参 12 克，白术 9 克，茯苓 9 克，姜半夏 9 克，陈皮 9克，木香 6 克，砂仁 6 克，甘草 3 克，生姜 3 片，大枣 3 枚。每日 1 剂，水煎 100～200 毫升，缓缓频服。

加减：胃寒者，加伏龙肝 18 克 (包煎)。

吐甚伤阴者，去砂仁、茯苓、木香、生姜，加麦门冬 9 克，芦根 9 克，玉竹 9 克。

### 2.肝胃不和型

**临床表现**  呕吐酸水或苦水，胸满胁痛，头胀而晕，烦渴口苦，舌红苔薄黄，脉弦滑。

治法：平肝和胃，降逆止呕。

方药：苏叶黄连汤 (71) 加味。

苏叶 9 克，黄连 6 克，姜半夏 9 克，竹茹 9 克，芦根 15克，煅石决明 12 克，陈皮 9 克。每日 1 剂，水煎 100～200 毫升，缓缓频服。

加减：舌红口干伤津者，去半夏、陈皮、加沙参 12 克，麦冬9克。

　　头晕甚者，加菊花9克，钩藤12克（后入）。

**3. 痰滞型**

**临床表现** 呕吐痰涎，胸脘满闷，不思饮食，口中淡腻，舌淡胖苔白腻，脉弦滑。

治法：健脾化痰，降逆止呕。

方药：小半夏加茯苓汤（88）加味。

姜半夏12克，茯苓12克，生姜15克，白术9克，陈皮6克，砂仁6克。每日1剂，水煎100～200毫升，缓缓频服。

加减：伴乏力神疲等脾胃虚弱者加党参15克。

　　便燥溲黄、苔黄腻者，加黄连6克，黄芩9克。

　　心悸气短者，加苏子9克，炒杏仁9克。

**4.气阴两亏型**

**临床表现** 呕吐剧烈，食入即吐，或呕吐带血样物，发热口渴，尿少便秘，形体消瘦，乏力，唇舌干燥，舌质红，苔薄黄而干或光剥，脉细滑数而无力。

治法：益气养阴，和胃止呕。

方药：生脉散（64）合增液汤（111）加味。

人参6克（先煎），麦冬12克，五味子9克，生地12克，玄参12克，姜竹茹9克，天花粉9克，陈皮6克，乌梅9克。每日1剂，水煎100～200毫升，缓缓频服。

加减：呕吐带血样物者，加藕节9克。

　　伴腰酸腹痛或阴道不时下血者，加炒杜仲12克，川续断15克，苎麻根12克。

**其他治疗方法**

负压壶治疗：对食入即吐，不能进食者，可用负压壶治疗。

负压壶制备方法：用胎头吸引器或小号茶壶一只，使用时将茶壶或胎头吸引器放置中脘穴，壶嘴或胎头吸引器之通气孔处接橡皮管之一端，另一端接上50毫升注射器，一面吸负压，一面鼓励病人进流质和易消化食物。必须注意放置时间不能超过 15 至 20 分钟，防止局部皮肤起泡。

在食前用鲜生姜擦舌头或用姜汁滴舌。

**预防**　孕妇应饮食有节，勿为生冷、油腻所伤。

孕妇应保持心情舒畅。

# 4.3　异位妊娠

受精卵在子宫腔以外的部位着床称"异位妊娠"，亦称"子宫外孕"。临床以停经后（一般在 6 周左右），腹痛，拒按，阴道不规则流血，晕厥或休克，检查时一侧附件肿大，妊娠试验阳性为主要特点。包括在中医"妊娠腹痛"、"胎动不安"、"症瘕"等病中，为"少腹血瘀"之实证。由于七情内伤，肝气郁结，气不能运血，或经期产后，血室正开，湿毒之邪乘虚而入，阻遏经脉而致气滞血瘀，或先天肾气不足，冲脉不盛，任脉不通，以致胎孕位置异常。最常见的是输卵管妊娠。依据输卵管妊娠是否破裂，临床大体分为两类。

**1.未破损型**

**临床表现**　患者可有不同程度的早孕反应，或下腹一侧有隐痛和坠胀不适的感觉。妇科检查可发现一侧输卵管略有膨大或有软性包块，有压痛，尿妊娠试验可为阳性。脉弦滑。

治法：活血化瘀，消症杀胚。

方药：宫外孕Ⅱ号方（46）加味。

赤芍 15 克，丹参 15 克，桃仁 9 克，三棱 6 克，莪术 6 克，牛膝 15 克，蜈蚣 3~6 条。每日 1 剂，水煎 200~300 毫升，分 2 次服。

可同时用天花粉针剂，以提高杀胚效果。天花粉针剂用法见稽留流产篇。

**2.已破损型**

(1) 休克型

**临床表现** 有停经史，或无停经史，或有妊娠反应，突发下腹一侧绞痛，或撕裂样痛，疼痛可呈持续性或反复发作，拒按。伴有面色苍白，四肢厥逆，冷汗淋漓，恶心呕吐，血压下降或不稳定，有时烦躁不安，甚至昏厥。脉微欲绝或细数无力。妇科检查:后穹窿饱满，宫颈摇举痛明显，子宫略大变软，内出血多时，子宫有漂浮感。子宫一侧可触及包块，有压痛，尿妊娠试验可为阳性。后穹窿穿刺可抽出不凝的褐色血液。

治法: 回阳救脱，活血化瘀。

方药: 参附汤 (59) 合生脉散 (64)。

大力参 30 克，熟附子 12 克，麦冬 12 克，五味子 12 克。急煎成浓汁，一次顿服。

如发病急，休克严重者，应立即采取输液、输血，给氧等急救措施。

当宫外孕破损后，血压收缩压维持在 80～90 毫米汞柱，血容量充足的情况下，尽早使用宫外孕 I 号方，促使血块早日吸收，恢复的快。

宫外孕 I 号方 (45)。

丹参 15 克，赤芍 15 克，桃仁 9 克，每日 1 剂，水煎 200～300 毫升，分 2 次服。

(2) 不稳定型

**临床表现** 腹痛拒按，但逐渐减轻。可触及界线不清之包块，或有少量阴道出血，血压稳定，脉细缓。

治法: 活血化瘀，佐以益气。

方药: 宫外孕 I 号方 (45) 加味。

丹参 15 克，赤芍 15 克，桃仁 9 克，党参 18 克，黄芪 15 克。

(3) 包块型

**临床表现** 宫外孕流产或破裂后形成血肿包块，深按及双合诊检查可以触及，有按压痛。有时下腹有坠胀及便意感，腹痛逐渐消失，阴道流血也逐渐停止。脉细涩。

治法：破瘀消癥。

方药：宫外孕Ⅱ号方（46）（方见未破损型）。

加减：身体虚弱者，可加党参18克，黄芪15克。

包块硬者，加炙鳖甲12克，穿山甲9克。

伴低热者，加生地12克，丹皮9克，旱莲草15克。

有感染者，加金银花12克，连翘15克，红藤30克，败酱草30克。

**3.兼证**

在非手术治疗宫外孕的过程中，必须重视对兼证的处理。最常见的兼证是腑实证，主要表现为腹胀便秘，胃脘不适，甚则疼痛拒按，肠鸣音减弱或消失。

（1）热结：腹部硬痛拒按，潮热盗汗，口渴烦躁，大便不通。舌苔黄厚或干黄，脉沉实滑数有力。治宜活血化瘀，清热泻下。可于主方内加生大黄9克（后入），芒硝6克（冲化）。

（2）寒结：脘腹胀满，剧烈疼痛，肢冷畏寒，喜热敷，大便秘结，舌苔白腻，脉沉而弦紧。治宜温经散寒，通便止痛。用大黄附子细辛汤：生大黄9克（后入），熟附子9克，细辛3克。每日1剂，水煎200～300毫升，分2次服。

待寒除结散便通之后仍当活血化瘀，佐以温经法。可于主方中加炮姜1.5克，肉桂1.5克。

（3）胃脘部胀痛甚者，可在疏通胃肠的同时，加枳实9克，厚朴9克。

**其它治疗方法**

①消癥散外敷：艾叶500克，透骨草250克，桑寄生120克，当归尾120克，五加皮120克，续断120克，白芷120克，赤芍药120克，追地风60克，千年健60克，川椒60克，羌活60克，独活60克，血竭60克，乳香60克，没药60克。共研

粗末，250克为1份，装入纱布袋中，封口。同时蒸15分钟，趁热外敷，每日1～2次，10天为1疗程。适用于包块型。

②桃仁15克，丹参15克，赤芍药15克，延胡索15克，三棱15克，莪术15克，地鳖虫15克，制乳香15克，制没药15克。上药浓煎成150～200毫升，保留灌肠。每日1次，7天为一疗程。适用于包块型。

③桃仁15克，赤芍15克，丹参15克，连翘15克，蒲公英15克，红藤30克，败酱草30克。上药浓煎成150～200毫升，再加1%普鲁卡因10毫升，保留灌肠。每日1次，7天为1疗程。或用离子透入法。适用于有炎症者。

④丹参注射液10毫升，加入10%葡萄糖500毫升中静滴，每日1次，7天为一疗程。适用于包块型。

**注意事项**

服药治疗期间应卧床休息，勿过早活动。

严格控制饮食，忌食生冷及少食肥甘食物。

尽量减少增加腹压的因素。

禁止灌肠（陈旧性宫外孕除外）和不必要的盆腔检查。

# 4.4 妊娠高血压综合征

本病的特征是妊娠20周以后，出现高血压、水肿、蛋白尿症候群。由全身小动脉痉挛，导致各脏器的血流不畅和血供不足，造成组织缺血而引起。包括在中医的"子肿"、"子晕"、"子痫"等病之中。多因素体肝肾阴虚，孕后血聚养胎，精血愈亏，肝失所养，肝阳上亢，肝风内动；或因阴虚热盛，炼液成痰，及脾虚失运，水湿内停，聚液成痰，痰火上扰所致。

## 4.4.1　妊娠水肿

妊娠后肢体、面目水肿者，称为妊娠水肿。妊娠水肿属中医的"妊娠肿胀"，根据浮肿的程度和部位不同，又有"子气"、"子肿"、"脆脚"、"皱脚"之分。子气即自膝至足浮肿，小便清长者，属湿气为病。子肿乃头面、全身浮肿，小便短少者，属水气为病。脆脚是两脚肿而皮肤薄者，属水。皱脚为两脚肿而皮肤厚者，属湿。

病在有形之水，其症为皮薄，色白而亮，按之凹陷不起;病在无形之气，其症必皮厚，色不变，随按随起。

因素体脾肾阳虚，脾虚运化失职，肾虚不能温煦脾阳，温化膀胱，以致水道不利，泛溢肌肤，引起水肿。另外，胎儿增大，胎气壅塞，气机阻滞，水湿不化，亦可引起肿胀。临床常用"+"表示水肿的程度。(+) 表示足部及小腿明显凹陷性水肿，经休息而不消退者。(++) 表示水肿延及大腿、皮肤如橘皮样;(+++) 表示水肿涉及外阴及腹部，皮肤薄而发亮;(++++) 指全身水肿，有时伴有腹水。

### 辨证论治

#### 1.脾虚型

**临床表现**　妊娠数月，面目、四肢浮肿，或遍及全身，肤色浅黄，皮薄而光亮，纳呆便溏，精神疲乏，少气懒言。舌淡苔白腻，脉缓滑无力。

治法: 健脾行水。

方药: 白术散 (6) 加味。

生白术 15 克，大腹皮 12 克，茯苓皮 30 克，生姜皮 9 克，陈皮 9 克，砂仁 6 克。日 1 剂，水煎 200～300 毫升，分 2 次服。

加减: 肿甚者, 加黄芪 18 克, 汉防己 9 克。

便溏者, 加淮山药 12 克, 炒扁豆 18 克。

腹胀者, 加苏梗 9 克, 厚朴 9 克。

兼见头晕者, 加钩藤 15 克, 菊花 9 克。

**2.肾虚型**

**临床表现** 孕后数月面浮肢肿, 腰酸乏力, 下肢逆冷, 心悸气短, 头晕耳鸣。舌淡苔白润, 脉沉迟无力。

治法: 温肾行水。

方药: 真武汤 (109)。

熟附子 6~9 克, 生姜 9 克, 茯苓 18 克, 白术 12 克, 白芍药 9 克。日 1 剂, 水煎 200~300 毫升, 分 2 次服。

加减: 浮肿重者, 加车前子 9 克 (包)。

腰痛重者, 加川断 15 克, 杜仲 12 克。

头晕目眩者, 加钩藤 15 克 (后入), 生石决明 30 克。

中成药: 金匮肾气丸, 每次 1 丸, 每日 2 次。

**3.气滞型**

**临床表现** 妊娠中、后期, 下肢浮肿, 甚则全身皆肿, 肤色不变, 随按随起, 胸闷胁胀, 厌食纳少, 头晕胀痛, 苔薄腻, 脉弦滑。

治法: 理气行滞, 健脾化湿。

方药: 天仙藤散 (78) 合四苓散 (63)。

天仙藤 15 克, 香附 12 克, 木瓜 12 克, 生白术 12 克, 紫苏叶 9 克, 陈皮 9 克, 乌药 9 克, 生姜 9 克, 猪苓 9 克, 泽泻 9 克, 茯苓 18 克, 甘草 6 克, 每日 1 剂, 水煎 200~300 毫升, 分 2 次服。

### 4.4.2 妊娠高血压

以往无高血压史，妊娠 20 周后血压升高至 130／90mmHg 以上，或在原水平上，收缩压升高 30mmHg，舒张压升高 15mmHg 以上者，称妊娠高血压。属中医的"子晕"、"子眩"范畴。临床当高血压、蛋白尿、水肿同时存在，又出现头晕、眼花、恶心、胃脘疼痛或呕吐时，为"先兆子痫"，必须提高警惕，积极治疗，防止"子痫"发生。本病多由肝肾阴亏、肝阳上亢所引起。

#### 辨证论治

**1.肝肾阴亏型**

**临床表现**　头晕，口苦心烦，夜寐不安，大便干燥。舌红苔少，脉弦滑而数。测血压在 130／90 mmHg 以上。

治法: 滋肾柔肝。

方药: 一贯煎 (95) 加味。

沙参 12 克，麦冬 12 克，枸杞子 12 克，当归 9 克，生地 15 克，川楝子 6 克，生石决明 30 克，钩藤 18 克 (后入)，黄芩 9 克。日 1 剂，水煎 200～300 毫升，分 2 次服。

中成药: 杞菊地黄丸，每次 1 丸，每日 3 次。

**2.阴虚阳亢型**

**临床表现**　妊娠头晕目眩，面红，心悸失眠，胸闷烦热，口干咽燥，便结尿黄，舌红或绛，脉弦细滑数。测血压往往明显升高，化验尿中可有蛋白，或有轻度水肿。

治法: 滋肾柔肝，育阴潜阳。

方药: 羚角钩藤汤 (40)。

羚羊角粉 5 克 (冲)，生地 30 克，钩藤 15 克 (后入)，白芍药 9 克，竹茹 9 克，茯苓 9 克，菊花 9 克，川贝母 6 克，桑叶 6 克，甘草 6 克。日 1 剂，水煎 200～300 毫升，分 2 次服。

加减：头痛剧烈者，加生石决明 30 克，夏枯草 15 克。

浮肿明显者，加大腹皮 9 克，猪苓 9 克。

便秘者加生大黄 9 克（后入）。

**3.脾虚肝旺型**

**临床表现** 妊娠中、后期，面浮肢肿，头晕头重目眩，胸胁胀满，纳差便溏。苔厚腻，脉弦滑。化验尿中有蛋白，测血压往往升高。

治法：健脾利湿，平肝潜阳。

方药：白术散（6）（方见妊娠水肿）加钩藤 18 克，生石决明 30 克。日 1 剂，水煎 200～300 毫升，分 2 次服。

加减：头晕头痛、眼花目眩甚者，加天麻 9 克，菊花 9 克，生牡蛎 30 克。

面浮肢肿甚者，加泽泻 9 克，猪苓 9 克，赤小豆 30 克。

神疲肢软甚者，加党参 30 克，黄芪 30 克。

中成药：人参健脾丸，每次 1 丸，每日 3 次。

## 4.4.3 子痫

先兆子痫进一步发展而出现抽搐昏迷者称为子痫。多发生于晚期妊娠或临产前，少数发生于临产时，极少数可在产后 24 小时内发生。如不及时抢救，孕、产妇及胎儿均有生命危险，必须重视子痫的防治。子痫一旦发作，应积极抢救，用镇痉熄风或涤痰开窍之剂，采取鼻饲给药方式。

### 辨证论治

**1.肝风内动型**

**临床表现** 妊娠后期，颜面潮红，心悸烦躁，突然四肢抽搐，甚则昏不知人。舌红苔薄黄，脉弦滑数。

治法：平肝熄风。

方药：羚角钩藤汤（40）加减。

羚羊角粉 5 克（冲），生地 30 克，钩藤 15 克（后入），白芍药 9 克，茯苓 9 克，生龟板 30 克，生石决明 30 克，菊花 9 克，生龙骨 30 克，生牡蛎 30 克，白蒺藜 12 克，全蝎 6 克。日 1～2 剂，水煎 200～300 毫升，分 2～4 次鼻饲。

加减：面红目赤、小便短赤，烦躁谵妄者，加黄连 9 克，龙胆草 9 克，焦栀子 9 克。

产后抽搐者，加太子参 30 克，枸杞 12 克。

兼见腹部、四肢有缕红丝，唇色青紫，舌见瘀斑者，加丹参 30 克，赤芍药 12 克，桃仁 9 克。

**2.痰火上扰型**

**临床表现** 妊娠晚期或正值分娩时，卒然昏不知人，四肢抽搐，气粗痰鸣，舌红苔黄腻，脉弦滑。

治法：清热、豁痰、开窍。

方药：牛黄清心丸（44）加味。

牛黄、竹沥、黄连、黄芩、山栀、朱砂、郁金。

牛黄清心丸，每日 2 丸，用竹沥 60 克研调，分 2～4 次鼻饲。

近年来许多报道用活血化瘀方法治疗妊娠高血压综合症，并取得良好效果。如以丹参、赤芍药、川芎、当归、桃仁、枳壳为基础方，根据临床辨证加用补脾、平肝、滋阴潜阳药物。另：丹参、赤芍、刘寄奴、乳香、没药、苏木、茜草为基础方治疗者。

**其它治疗方法**

**1.子痫急救法**

①昏迷不醒者，可用醒脑静针剂 2～4 支加 5% 葡萄糖 500 毫升静滴，或醒脑静 1 支，肌肉注射，每日 2～3 次。

②昏迷抽搐者，可选用：①安宫牛黄丸，每日 2 丸，用凉开水调匀，分 2～4 次鼻饲。适用于心肝火旺及痰热较甚者。②紫雪丹，每日 3 次，每次 0.6～3 克，凉开水调匀，分 2～4 次鼻饲。

适用于抽搐发作较频者。③至宝丹，每次 2 丸，凉开水调匀，分 2～4 次鼻饲。适用于窍闭神昏较深者。

**2.妊娠水肿食疗法**

妊娠后常服淡豆浆或赤小豆粥。

冬瓜皮或西瓜皮煎汤代茶饮。

**预防** 定期做好产前检查，严密观察血压、水肿、尿化验情况。有异常者，应予积极治疗，防止子痫发生。

注意诱发因素，如有原发性高血压、慢性肾炎，糖尿病人，易并发该病。

孕期注意休息和营养.饮食富营养而清淡，补充蛋白，维生素类。因为母体营养不良，低蛋白血症、贫血严重者易发生先兆子痫。

保持心情舒畅。

仔细询问有否家族史，及早提高警惕，防病于未然。

# 4.5  羊水过多

该病以妊娠中、后期，腹部迅速增大，胸胁胀满，胎位不清，胎心遥远为特点。羊水量往往达到或超过 2000 毫升。根据发病速度，临床上有急性和慢性之分。急性羊水过多，多发生在妊娠中期，羊水急剧增加，腹部增大迅速，伴胸闷、气短等。慢性羊水过多，以妊娠后期为多见，发病缓慢，子宫逐渐膨大，常伴胎儿畸形。属中医"子满"、"胎水肿满"范畴。多因素体脾虚，或孕后过食生冷寒凉之物，损伤脾阳，湿聚胞中所致。

若有胎儿畸形者，应及早终止妊娠，无胎儿畸形者，可服中药治疗。

**辨证论治**

**临床表现** 妊娠中、后期，腹部迅速增大，超过妊娠月份，胎位不清，胎心遥远，胸膈满闷，呼吸急促，神疲肢软，腹胀作痛，下肢及外阴部水肿。舌淡胖苔白腻，脉沉滑无力。

治法：健脾行水。

方药：1：鲤鱼汤（42）加味。

鲤鱼一条（250克以上，去鳞、肠），白术15克，生姜、白芍、当归各9克，茯苓30克，陈皮6克。

先取鲤鱼，加水1200毫升，将鲤鱼煮熟，去鱼存汤，用此汤煎药液为200～300毫升，每日1剂，饭前空腹服，并食鱼肉。或先将中药水煎2次，至药液为400～500毫升，滤出药液与鲤鱼同炖，饮汤食鱼，每日1剂，饭前空腹分2次服。适用于体质虚弱者。

加减：畏寒肢冷者，加桂枝6～9克。

气短懒言、神疲乏力者，加党参18克，黄芪15克。

肿甚而小便不利者，加桑白皮9克，大腹皮9克。

方药：2：茯苓导水汤（23）加味。

茯苓30克，白术15克，木瓜12克，陈皮9克，猪苓9克，泽泻9克，苏梗9克，桑白皮9克，大腹皮9克，槟榔9克，葶苈子9克，砂仁6克，木香6克。日1剂，水煎200～300毫升，分2次服。适用于喘满较甚者。

# 4.6 其他妊娠病证

## 4.6.1 妊娠腹痛

妊娠期因胞脉阻滞或失养，气血运行不畅而发生小腹疼痛者，称为"妊娠腹痛"，亦称"胞阻"。由于气郁、血虚、虚寒，以致胞脉受阻或胞脉失养，气血运行不畅所引起。

## 辨证论治

**1.血虚型**

**临床表现** 妊娠后小腹绵绵作痛，按之痛减，面色萎黄，或少寐心悸，舌质淡苔薄白，脉细滑弱。

治法：养血安胎止痛。

方药：当归芍药散（15）加减。

当归9克，白芍药15克，川芎4.5克，茯苓12克，炒白术12克，制首乌15克，桑寄生15克。日1剂，水煎200～300毫升，分2次服。

加减：若小腹冷痛，可加艾叶9克。

神疲肢倦乏力者，加党参15克，黄芪15克。

心烦不寐者，加炒枣仁30克，夜交藤30克。

**2.气郁型**

**临床表现** 小腹胁肋胀痛，或精神抑郁，或烦躁易怒，苔薄腻，脉弦滑。

治法：疏肝解郁，止痛安胎。

方药：逍遥散（94）加减。

当归9克，白芍药12克，柴胡9克，白术9克，茯苓12克，苏梗9克，炙甘草6克。

加减：口苦咽干，舌红苔薄黄，脉滑数者，加栀子9克，黄芩9克。

肢倦神疲、食少便溏者，加党参18克，陈皮9克，淮山药15克。

痛连腰胁者，加续断15克，寄生15克，菟丝子15克，阿胶12克（烊化）。

**3. 虚寒型**

**临床表现** 小腹冷痛，喜温喜按，形寒肢冷，面色㿠白，或纳少便溏，舌淡苔薄白，脉细弱。

治法：暖宫止痛，养血安胎。

方药：胶艾汤（30）加味。

阿胶 12 克（烊化），艾叶 9 克，当归 9 克，川芎 4.5 克，白芍 9 克，熟地 12 克，炙甘草 6 克，巴戟天 9 克，杜仲 12 克，炒白术 9 克。日 1 剂，水煎 200～300 毫升，分 2 次服。

加减：四肢逆冷，小腹冷痛如冰者，加熟附子 6 克。

腰痛者，加菟丝子 15 克，桑寄生 15 克。

## 4.6.2 胎萎不长

妊娠 4～5 个月后，腹形明显小于妊娠月份，胎儿存活而生长迟缓者，称为"胎萎不长"，亦称"妊娠胎萎燥"，即"胎儿宫内发育迟缓"。多因孕妇气血虚弱或素体脾肾不足，以致脏腑气血不足，胎失所养则生长迟缓。该病必须借助妇科检查、听胎心或 B 超，以与"死胎"相鉴别。

### 辨证论治

**1.气血虚弱型**

**临床表现**　身体瘦弱，面色萎黄或㿠白，头晕气短，舌淡嫩少苔，脉细滑无力。

治法：补血益气以养胎。

方药：八珍汤（8）。

党参 12 克，茯苓 12 克，白术 9 克，当归 9 克，白芍药 9 克，熟地 12 克，川芎 4.5 克，炙甘草 6 克。日 1 剂，水煎 200～300 毫升，分 2 次服。

加减：头晕甚者，加枸杞 12 克。

纳差便溏、苔白腻者，加淮山药 12 克，陈皮 9 克。

中成药：八珍益母丸，每次 1 丸，每日 3 次。

人参归脾丸，每次 1 丸，每日 3 次。

**2.脾肾不足型**

临床表现　腰部酸冷，纳少便溏，或形寒怕冷，手足不温，舌淡苔白，脉沉迟。

治法：健脾温肾。

方药：温土毓麟汤（85）加减。

巴戟天 9 克，复盆子 15 克，白术 9 克，人参 6 克（先煎），山药 12 克。日 1 剂，水煎 200～300 毫升，分 2 次服。

加减：腰部冷痛甚者，加杜仲 12 克，川断 18 克，鹿角片 9 克，菟丝子 15 克。

中成药：十全大补丸，每次 1 丸，每日 3 次。

## 4.6.3　子烦

孕妇在妊娠期间出现烦闷不安，郁郁不乐，或烦躁易怒等现象，称为"子烦"，亦称"妊娠心烦"。多由火热乘心，热邪扰心，神明不安所致。但有阴虚、痰火、肝郁之不同。

### 辨证论治

#### 1.阴虚型

临床表现　心中烦闷，坐卧不宁，颧红潮热，咽干口燥，干咳无痰，渴不多饮，小便短黄，舌红苔薄黄而干或无苔，脉细数而滑。

治法：清热养阴，安神除烦。

方药：人参麦冬散（57）加减。

麦冬 9 克，茯苓 9 克，黄芩 9 克，知母 9 克，生地 12 克，竹茹 9 克，炙甘草 6 克，沙参 12 克，莲子心 9 克。日 1 剂，水煎 200～300 毫升，分 2 次服。

加减：心悸胆怯者，加龙齿 15 克，茯神 9 克。

口燥咽干、干咳无痰、潮热盗汗者，加天门冬 9 克，百合 9 克，知母 9 克。

头晕耳鸣，腰膝酸软者，加龟板 9 克，玄参 9 克，女贞子 12 克，旱莲草 15 克。

**2.痰火型**

**临床表现**　心胸烦闷，头晕心悸，胸脘满闷，恶心呕吐，苔黄而腻，脉滑数。

治法：清热涤痰。

方药：竹沥汤（107）加味。

竹沥 30 克（冲兑），麦门冬 9 克，黄芩 9 克，茯苓 12 克，防风 4.5 克，浙贝母 9 克。日 1 剂，水煎 200～300 毫升，分 2 次服。

加减：痰多色黄而稠粘者，加瓜蒌 15 克，黄连 6 克，半夏 9 克。

　　　　呕恶甚者，加枇杷叶 9 克，藿梗 9 克。

**3.　肝郁型**

**临床表现**　心烦不安，郁闷不乐，或烦躁易怒，两胁胀痛。舌质红，苔薄白或黄干，脉弦数。

治法：疏肝解郁，清热除烦。

方药：丹栀逍遥散（21）加减。

当归 9 克，白芍药 9 克，柴胡 9 克，茯苓 12 克，丹皮 9 克，栀子 9 克，薄荷 6 克，白术 9 克，甘草 6 克。日 1 剂，水煎 200～300 毫升，分 2 次服。

加减：头晕目眩者，加钩藤 18 克（后入），菊花 9 克，夏枯草 12 克。

　　　　胸胁胀痛甚者，加炒川楝子 9 克，郁金 9 克。

　　　　心胸烦热甚者，加知母 9 克，竹叶 9 克，莲子心 9 克。

**其他治疗方法**

竹茹汤：青竹茹 30 克，水煎徐徐服之。适用于肝郁胃热之妊娠心烦者。

竹沥 30 克，温开水冲兑，时时服之，适用于痰火内蕴之妊娠心烦者。

## 4.6.4  子悬

妊娠期间,胸腹胀满,甚或喘急,烦躁不安者,称为"子悬"亦名"胎上逼心"、"胎气上逆"。本病的发生主要是素体阴虚,孕后肾阴更虚,肝经失养,肝木乘脾,以致气机升降失常,发为子悬。

### 辨证论治

**临床表现**  妊娠胸腹胀满,痞满不舒,呼吸迫促,坐卧不舒,烦躁不安,苔薄黄,脉弦滑。

治法:疏肝扶脾,理气行滞。

方药:紫苏饮(108)加味。

紫苏叶 6 克,陈皮 9 克,大腹皮 9 克,白芍 9 克,当归 9 克,川芎 4.5 克,党参 12 克,甘草 6 克,黄芩 9 克,香附 12 克。日 1 剂,水煎 200～300 毫升,分 2 次服。

服上方后,若上述症状已解,应滋阴养血以培其本,方用阿胶养血汤:阿胶 12 克(烊化),生地 15 克,沙参 9 克,麦冬 9 克,女贞子 9 克,旱莲草 12 克,桑寄生 12 克。日 1 剂,水煎 200～300 毫升,分 2 次服。

## 4.6.5  子喑

因妊娠而出现声音嘶哑,甚或不能出声者,称为"子喑",亦名"妊娠失音"。本病主要由肾阴不足所致。因声出于肺,根于肾,发于舌本。若肾阴素亏,孕后阴血养胎,肾虚更甚,不能上荣于舌而致失音。多发生在妊娠晚期。

**辨证论治**

**临床表现**　妊娠 8～9 个月声音嘶哑，咽喉干燥，头晕耳鸣，手心灼热，心悸而烦，便结，小便短赤，舌红苔花剥，脉细数。

治法：滋肾养阴。

方药：六味地黄汤（41）加味。

熟地 12 克，生地 12 克，山茱萸 12 克，山药 12 克，泽泻 9克，丹皮 9 克，茯苓 9 克，沙参 12 克，麦冬 12 克。日 1 剂，水煎 200～300 毫升，分 2 次服。

加减：咳吐脓痰、咽干口燥者，去泽泻、山茱萸，加瓜蒌仁15 克，芦根 9 克，桔梗 9 克，川贝母 9 克。

**单方验方**

(1) 豆浆适量，鲜鸡蛋 1 个冲服，每晨 1 次。

(2) 玉蝴蝶 6 克，冰糖 6 克，置入去核梨中，蒸服。

## 4.6.6　子嗽

"子嗽"亦名"妊娠咳嗽"。本病以妊娠期久嗽不已，或伴五心烦热为其特点。由于素体阴虚，孕后血聚养胎，阴血更亏，阴虚火旺，火热上扰，灼肺伤津;或素体阳盛，孕后胎气亦盛，火乘肺金，炼液为痰，壅阻于肺，肺失宣降，引起咳嗽。

**辨证论治**

**1.阴虚肺燥型**

**临床表现**　干咳无痰，甚或痰中带血，口干咽燥，手足心热，舌红少苔，脉细滑数。

治法：养阴润肺，止嗽安胎。

方药：百合固金汤（3）加减。

百合 12 克，生地 12 克，麦冬 9 克，川贝母 9 克，白芍 9

克，玄参9克，桔梗9克，生甘草6克，桑叶9克，炙百部12克，黑芝麻15克。日1剂，水煎200～300毫升，分2次服。

加减：热灼肺络，咯血者，酌加旱莲草15克，白芨9克，阿胶12克（烊化）。

颧红潮热、手足心热甚者，加地骨皮9克，白薇9克，黄精12克。

兼神疲气短，乏力者，加党参15克，黄芪15克。

**2.痰火犯肺型**

**临床表现** 咯痰不爽，痰液黄稠，面红口干，舌红苔黄腻，脉滑数。

治法：清肺化痰，止嗽安胎。

方药：清金降火汤（50）加减。

黄芩9克，炒杏仁9克，川贝母9克，前胡9克，瓜蒌仁15克，陈皮9克，茯苓12克，法半夏9克，桔梗9克，枳壳4.5克，生姜3片，炙甘草6克，桑叶9克，炙杷叶9克。日1剂，水煎200～300毫升，分2次服。

**单方验方**

川贝母粉3克，冰糖6克，置入去核梨中，文火炖烂，喝汤吃梨。

川贝母粉3克，枇杷叶膏酌量开水冲服。

款冬花9克，冰糖适量煎服。

## 4.6.7  子淋

妊娠期间出现尿频、尿急、淋漓涩痛等症状者，称为"子淋"，也称"妊娠小便淋痛"。由于心火偏亢，湿热下注，阴虚火旺，引起膀胱气化失司，水道不利所致。

## 辨证论治

### 1.心火偏亢型

**临床表现**　尿少色深黄，艰涩而痛，面赤心烦，甚至口舌生疮，舌红欠润少苔或无苔，脉细滑数。

治法：泻火通淋。

方药：导赤散（14）加味。

生地 15 克，木通 6 克，甘草梢 9 克，淡竹叶 9 克，玄参 12 克，麦冬 9 克。日 1 剂，水煎 200～300 毫升，分 2 次服。

加减：小便热痛甚者，加山栀仁 9 克，车前草 12 克。

心烦者，加莲子心 9 克，栀子 9 克。

尿中带血者，加白茅根 12 克，藕节 9 克。

### 2.湿热型

**临床表现**　突感小便频数而急，尿黄赤，艰涩不利，灼热刺痛，面色垢黄，口渴而不欲多饮，胸闷食少。舌质红，苔黄腻，脉滑数。

治法：清热利湿通淋。

方药：加味五淋散（83）加减。

黑栀子 9 克，赤茯苓 12 克，当归 9 克，白芍 9 克，黄芩 9 克，甘草梢 6 克，生地 12 克，泽泻 9 克，车前子 9 克（包），木通 6 克。日 1 剂，水煎 200～300 毫升，分 2 次服。

加减：湿热因外感而起者，可加金银花 30 克，蒲公英 30 克。

胸闷腹胀，苔黄厚腻者，加藿香 9 克，佩兰 9 克。

### 3. 阴虚型

**临床表现**　小便频数淋沥，灼热刺痛，量少，色深黄，两颧潮红，手足心热，心烦不寐，大便不畅，舌质红，苔薄黄而干，脉细滑数。

治法：滋阴润燥通淋。

方药：知柏地黄汤（103）加味。

熟地 12 克，山萸肉 12 克，山药 12 克，茯苓 9 克，牡丹皮
9 克，泽泻 9 克，知母 9 克，黄柏 9 克，麦冬 9 克，五味子 9
克，车前草 12 克。日 1 剂，水煎 200～300 毫升，分 2 次服。

加减：潮热盗汗明显者，加玄参 12 克，地骨皮 9 克，白薇
9 克。

尿中带血者，加女贞子 15 克，旱莲草 18 克，白茅根
15 克。

肠燥便结者，加当归 9 克，火麻仁 9 克。

### 4.6.8  妊娠小便不通

妊娠期间，小便不通，甚至小腹胀急疼痛，心烦不得卧，称
为"妊娠小便不通"，亦称"转胞"。由于素体中气不足，或肾气不
足，孕后气虚无力举胎，或肾虚系胎无力，以致胎气下坠，压迫
膀胱，引起膀胱不利，水道不通，尿不得出。

#### 辨证论治

**1.气虚型**

**临床表现**  小便不通或频数量少，小腹胀急疼痛，坐卧不
安，面色㿠白，精神疲倦，头重眩晕，气短懒言，大便不爽，舌
淡苔薄白，脉虚缓滑。

治法：补气、升陷、举胎。

方药：益气导溺汤（100）。

党参 30 克;白术 9 克，白扁豆 15 克，茯苓 12 克，桂枝 6
克，炙升麻 6 克，桔梗 9 克，通草 9 克，乌药 9 克。日 1 剂，水
煎 200～300 毫升，分 2 次服。

加减：面色萎黄者，加阿胶 12 克（烊化）制首乌 15 克。

头晕气短，小腹坠胀者，加黄芪 30 克。

食欲不振、苔白者，加陈皮 9 克，藿梗 9 克，砂仁 6

克。

**2.肾虚型**

**临床表现**　小便频数不畅，继则闭而不通，小腹胀满而痛，坐卧不宁，畏寒肢冷，腰腿酸软。舌质淡，苔薄润，脉沉滑无力。

治法：温肾扶阳，化气行水。

方药：肾气丸（66）加减。

熟地 15 克，山药 12 克，山茱萸 12 克，泽泻 9 克，茯苓 12 克，桂枝 6 克，仙灵脾 9 克。日 1 剂，水煎 200～300 毫升，分 2 次服。

加减：神疲肢倦，气短懒言者，加党参 18 克，黄芪 15 克，炒白术 9 克。

腰酸膝软者，加杜仲 12 克，桑寄生 15 克，菟丝子 12 克。

**其他治疗方法**

针灸：针刺气海、膀胱俞（双）、阴陵泉（双），灸关元穴。

热熨法：①热毛巾敷于耻骨联合上膀胱区。②四季葱（大葱连须），每天用 500 克，洗净用手截断，稍捣烂，放入锅内炒热；分 2 次轮流使用。每次 250 克，用布或毛巾包裹，热熨下腹部（自脐部顺次向耻骨部熨下），冷则换之。每天 1 次，1 次约 30 分钟。

（刘瑞芬）

# 5 异常分娩与异常产褥

## 5.1 产力异常

产力是指将胎儿从子宫逼出的力量。以子宫收缩为主。当产道及胎儿因素正常时，子宫收缩对子宫颈口的扩张及产程的进展，起着决定性作用。如果宫缩失去节律性、对称性和极性，或强度、频率有改变时，称为子宫收缩异常。临床分为子宫收缩乏力和子宫收缩过强两大类，属中医的"难产"范畴。由于孕妇素体虚弱，或产时用力过早，耗气伤力；或临产浆水早破，另外过度紧张，产前过贪安逸，感受寒邪，以致使气血虚弱，或气滞血瘀；气虚不能促胎外出，血瘀阻碍胎体娩出引起难产。

### 辨证论治

#### 1.气血虚弱型

**临床表现** 分娩时阵痛微弱，宫缩时间短，间歇时间长，产程进展缓慢，或下血量多，色淡，面色苍白，神疲肢软，心悸气短，舌淡苔薄白，脉虚大或沉细弱。产科检查：宫缩时子宫肌壁不硬，按压宫底有凹陷感，宫颈口不能如期扩张，胎先露不能如期下降。

治法：大补气血。

方药：蔡松汀难产方（11）。

炙黄芪 30 克，当归 12 克，茯苓 9 克，党参 30 克，龟板 15 克，川芎 9 克，白芍药 12 克，枸杞子 12 克。水煎 200～300 毫升，顿服。

加减：宫缩无力，头汗淋漓，脉微细无力者，改党参为人参3~6克，浓煎后加入以上药液中顿服。2小时可重复煎服1剂。

**2.气滞血瘀型**

**临床表现**　分娩时腰腹疼痛剧烈，宫缩虽强但间歇不匀，产程进展缓慢，或下血色黯红，量少，面色紫黯，精神紧张，胸脘胀闷，时欲呕恶，舌黯红，苔正常或腻，脉弦大而至数不均。产科检查：子宫处于高张状态，甚至子宫有压痛，扪不清胎位，胎心不规律。

治法：理气活血，化瘀催产。

方药：催生饮（12）。

当归12克，川芎9克，大腹皮12克，枳壳12克，白芷12克。水煎200~300毫升，取头煎顿服。4小时后可再服1剂。

加减：产程过长，产妇气虚乏力者，加人参3~6克，浓煎兑服。

　　　　烦躁、腹痛剧者，加茯神12克，炒枣仁15克，钩藤12克，怀牛膝15克，益母草30克。

**其他疗法**：

针刺：在排除产道、胎儿异常后，取合谷、三阴交、太冲穴针刺、强刺久留针。

**预防**　加强产前检查，及时处理异常情况。

临产后不可随意用镇静剂及宫缩剂，以免发生宫缩乏力，过强或不协调。

妊娠到临产，当安神定虑，要安静，莫惊慌，时常步履，不可多睡、饱食，过饮酒醴杂药。

## 5.2 胎位异常

除枕前位为正常胎位外，其余胎位均属异常胎位，可以造成难产。常见的有持续性枕横位、枕后位、面先露、额先露、臀先露、肩先露等。概括在中医"横产"、"碍产"、"偏产"、"坐产"等中。若无产道异常及胎儿异常者，可服用中药以使胎位转正。

**纠正方法：**

妊娠 28 周以后发现胎位异常时，即应及时纠正。

内服中药：

方药：保产无忧散（2）。当归9克，川芎6克，白杭芍9克，黄芪15克，厚朴6克，羌活6克，菟丝子9克，川贝母6克，枳壳9克，芥穗6克，艾叶3克，生姜三片。水煎200～300毫升。待温后分2次服，日1剂。

艾灸法：孕妇仰卧屈膝，松解裤带。取双侧至阴穴（足小趾甲根外一分处），用艾条灸，每次15分钟，每日1～2次，7天为一疗程。转正后停灸。根据临床观察和原理探讨指出：艾灸至阴穴，可以使肾上腺皮质激素分泌增多，子宫活动增强，胎儿活动加剧，有利胎位的转正。

激光照射法：用激光照射双侧至阴穴，每次15分钟，每日1～2次，7天为一疗程。胎位转正后停照。

胸膝卧位：孕妇先自解小便，松解衣带，跪在床上，使胸、膝着床，抬高臀部，每次胸膝卧位10～15分钟，每日2～3次。1周后复查。

**预防**

衣着松软宽舒，勿扎宽、硬腰带，体位舒展，避免过久下蹲及弯腰等姿势。

注意定期产前检查，发现胎位异常应及时纠正。

## 5.3  产褥感染

分娩后由生殖器官感染所引起的疾病称为产褥感染或产褥热。本病有产程长，早破膜以及手术产史，以产后短期内发热，局部疼痛，恶露多，有臭味（溶血性链球菌感染时除外），检查局部红肿，疼痛或子宫压痛，附件增厚压痛为特点。属中医"产后发热"范畴，由分娩时产伤和出血，元气受损；或护理不慎，邪毒乘虚侵入胞宫所引起。

### 辨证论治

#### 1.邪毒壅盛型

**临床表现**　于产后 24 小时至 10 天内出现寒战高热，继而热势不退或起病即高热（体温达 38.5℃以上），小腹疼痛拒按，恶露量多或少，色紫黯如败酱，有臭气，烦躁口干，尿少色黄，大便燥结，舌红苔黄，脉数有力。

治法：清热解毒，凉血化瘀。

方药：五味消毒饮（86）加减。

金银花 12 克，连翘 12 克，公英 12 克，紫花地丁 9 克，败酱草 12 克，红藤 12 克，丹参 30 克，当归 12 克，川芎 9 克，赤芍 15 克，制乳没各 9 克，玄参 12 克，元胡 9 克，生甘草 6 克，水煎 200～300 毫升，分 2 次顿服，日 1 剂。

加减：恶露秽浊或带下脓赤者，加鱼腥草 12 克，生苡仁 30 克，水煎 200～300 毫升，顿服，每日 2 剂。

#### 2.  热毒瘀结胞中型

**临床表现**　小腹剧痛，恶露不畅，有臭气，高热便秘，舌紫黯，脉弦涩而数。

治法：清热泻下逐瘀。

方药：清热逐瘀方。

丹参 30 克，桃仁 9 克，红花 9 克，当归 12 克，丹皮 12 克，赤芍 15 克，枳壳 12 克，生蒲黄 15 克，地榆 12 克，金银花 12 克，公英 9 克，制大黄 9 克。水煎 200～300 毫升，顿服，日 2 剂。

**3. 热入营血型**

**临床表现**　高热汗出，烦躁，斑疹隐隐，舌红绛苔黄燥，脉弦细而数。

治法：清营解毒，凉血养阴。

方药：清营汤（55）。

玄参 12 克，生地 12 克，麦冬 9 克，金银花 12 克，连翘 12 克，竹叶心 9 克，丹参 30 克，川黄连 3 克，犀角 1.5 克（研粉冲服，或羚羊角代替）。浓煎 200 毫升，待冷顿服，每日 2 剂。

**4. 热入心包型**

**临床表现**　高热不退，神昏谵语，甚或昏迷，面色苍白，四肢厥冷，脉数。

治法：清热养阴，芳香开窍。

方药：清营汤（55）（见热入营血），浓煎 200 毫升，立即送服安宫牛黄丸 1 丸（化开）或紫雪丹 3 克，1 次服。

**其它疗法**

红外线照射：用于会阴伤口感染。

切开排脓：用于创口已化脓者，切开后应引流。

祛腐生肌：用于伤口脓液已清除者。以生肌膏涂局部，去腐生新。伤口可迅速愈合。

**预防**

加强孕期保健，增强孕妇的抵抗力。

注意产前卫生，孕末期避免盆浴及性交。

正确处理分娩，严格执行无菌操作。

早破膜者，给予抗生素治疗。

避免或减少损伤，有损伤应及时仔细正确地缝合。

加强产褥护理，保持外阴清洁、干燥。

## 5.4  晚期产后出血

分娩 24 小时后，在产褥期内发生的子宫大量出血，称晚期产后出血。包括在中医"产后血晕"及"产后恶露不绝"之中，应详细检查有无胎盘、胎膜残留，若手术缝合失误，应及时解决。

### 辨证论治

#### 1.  血虚气脱型
**临床表现**  产后失血过多，突然晕眩，面色苍白，心悸，馈闷不适，渐至昏不知人，眼闭口开，甚则四肢厥冷，冷汗淋漓。舌淡无苔，脉微欲绝或浮大而虚。妇科检查：子宫复旧不佳。宫体大而软，宫颈口松，有时可触及残留胎盘、胎膜组织。

治法：益气固脱。

方药：独参汤（20）。

人参 3～6 克，浓煎顿服。

加减：肤冷汗出，可用参附汤以回阳救逆。人参 3 克，制附子 9 克，急煎 100 毫升，待温顿服。

阴道出血不止者，则于参附汤中加用炮姜炭 9 克，艾叶炭 9 克。

#### 2.  血瘀型
**临床表现**  产后出血或多或少，淋漓不净，或突然出血量多，血色紫黯挟块，或挟有组织，伴下腹疼痛、拒按，面、唇、舌质紫黯，脉涩。妇科检查时：宫体大而硬、压痛，有胎盘，胎膜组织残留。

治法：活血祛瘀止血。

方药：生化汤（61）合夺命散（19）。

当归 12 克，川芎 9 克，桃仁 9 克，炮姜 6 克，炙甘草 6

克，没药 9 克，血竭 3 克，水煎服 200 毫升，顿服，每日 1 剂。

加减：兼气虚者，加党参 30 克，黄芪 30 克。

舌红苔黄脉数者，去炮姜，加丹参 30 克，黄芩 9 克，地榆 12 克。

中成药：云南白药，每次服 1 管，日 2 次。用于出血量多者。

三七片，每次口服 6～10 片，日 3 次。用于血量多挟块伴腹痛者。

益母草膏，每次 10 毫升，每日 3 次。

**预防**　胎盘娩出后，必须仔细检查，如有缺残，应即取出。剖腹产作子宫下段横切口时，如切口两侧有明显活跃出血点，以钳挟丝线缝扎为妥。不可大块缝合及缝线过密，以免术后血肿及组织坏死而影响伤口愈合。还应纠正贫血，改善营养状态并预防感染。

# 5.5　产褥中暑

本病是产后产妇体质虚弱，而又受高温、高湿环境的影响，以致中枢性体温调节功能障碍所致的急性热病。本病发生于盛夏季节，以口渴、多汗、恶心、头晕、全身无力、尿频、胸闷开始；不治则体温升高，面色潮红，皮肤干燥，甚者昏迷、谵妄、虚脱为特点。包括在中医"产后发热"中，因产后气血耗伤，体虚未复，暑邪乘虚直中于里，耗气伤津，以阴气卒绝，阳气暴壅，经络不通所致。

## 辨证论治

### 1.　暑热初起型

**临床表现**　口渴、多汗、恶心、头晕、胸闷、心慌、无力，舌红少苔，脉细数。

治法：清热，养阴生津。

方药：清络饮（52）。

西瓜翠衣 50 克，鲜扁豆花 30 克，鲜金银花 30 克，鲜竹叶心 9 克，鲜荷叶边 9 克，丝瓜络 12 克，水煎 200～300 毫升，一次服，每日一剂。

单方：西瓜一只，汤匙挖着吃。

绿豆半斤煮汤频饮。

### 2. 实热型

**临床表现**　壮热面赤，头昏，大汗出，口干渴，烦躁，舌红脉洪大或滑数。

治法：清热祛暑。

方药：祛暑方。

生石膏 30 克（先煎），知母 9 克，黄连 6 克，滑石 9 克（研末），玄参 12 克，藿香 12 克，佩兰 9 克，荷叶 6 克。水煎至 200～300 毫升，分两次服，每日 2 剂。

神昏谵语者：冲服安宫牛黄丸合神犀丹。

### 3. 热邪伤阴型

**临床表现**　身热多汗，心烦口渴，少气无力，溲赤，舌红少津，脉虚大或细数。

治法：清暑益气，养阴生津。

方药：清暑益气汤（54）。

西洋参 3 克（或太子参 15 克），石斛 9 克，麦冬 9 克，黄连 3 克，竹叶 9 克，荷梗 9 克，知母 6 克，粳米 9 克，西瓜翠衣 9 克，生甘草 6 克。水煎至 200～300 毫升，分 2 次服，日 1 剂。

加减：胸满痞闷、头重、舌苔腻浊者，加藿香 9 克，佩兰 9 克，砂仁 6 克。

面色苍白，脉细数者，加生脉散（64）人参、麦冬、五味子以益气生津。

身热抽搐者：清营汤加勾藤 9 克，羚羊角 3 克，地龙

12 克，僵蚕 12 克以镇痉熄风。

**其他疗法**　针刺：轻症针大椎，风池、足三里。重症可采用取十宣速刺放血，配合针刺人中，涌泉。

**中成药**：至宝丹，每服 1 丸（3 克），开水调服。紫雪丹，每服 1.5～3 克，凉开水送服，日 1～2 次，用于昏迷、谵妄、痉挛抽搐者。藿香正气水每服 1～2 瓶，用于中暑轻症。

**预防**　加强产褥期卫生宣传，住房要适当通风换气；夏季分娩衣着、被褥不宜过厚，中暑症状一旦出现，即应及时置产妇于通风处呼吸新鲜空气，多饮淡盐水、西瓜水、绿豆汤，以控制病情发展。

## 5.6　其他产后病证

### 5.6.1　恶露不绝

产后恶露持续 20 天以上仍淋漓不断者，称恶露不绝。由于产后失血耗气，气虚不摄；或瘀血阻滞，湿热蕴结；阴虚内热，肝郁化热；以致冲任不固，热扰冲任。或瘀血内阻，胞衣残留，影响冲任，血不归经而引起恶露不绝。

**辨证论治**

**1.　气虚型**

**临床表现**　产后恶露不止，量多或淋漓不断，色淡红，质稀薄，无臭气。小腹空坠，神倦懒言，面色㿠白，舌淡红苔薄白，脉缓弱。

治法：补气摄血。

方药：益气摄血汤。

太子参 30 克，黄芪 30 克，炒白术 9 克，炒山药 12 克，首乌 12 克，五味子 9 克，杭芍 15 克，煅龙牡各 30 克，坤草 30克，炙甘草 9 克，水煎 200～300 毫升，早晚 2 次温服，每日 1

剂。

加减：伴腰酸痛，膝软无力者，加炒续断 30 克，鹿角胶 12
克（烊化兑服），艾叶炭 9 克。

中成药：人参归脾丸，每次 1 丸，每日 3 次。

**2. 血热型**

**临床表现** 恶露过期不止，量多，色深红，质稠粘或有臭秽
气。面色潮红，口燥咽干，舌红，脉虚细数。

治法：养阴清热止血。

方药：保阴煎（5）加减。

生地 12 克；山药 12 克，杭白芍 12 克，黄芩 9 克，续断 15
克，旱莲草 12 克，丹皮 12 克，甘草 6 克。水煎 200～300 毫
升，早晚分服，每日 1 剂。

加减：胸胁胀痛、心烦、舌苔黄、脉弦数者，宜疏肝解郁、
清热凉血，方用丹栀逍遥散加旱莲草 12 克，女贞子 9 克，茜草
12 克，生地 12 克。水煎 200～300 毫升，分 2 次服，每日 1
剂。

**3. 血瘀型**

**临床表现** 恶露淋漓不爽，量少，色紫黯有块，小腹疼痛拒
按。舌质紫黯或边有紫点，脉弦涩而沉实有力。

治法：活血化瘀止血。

方药：生化汤（61）。

当归 12 克，川芎 9 克，桃仁 9 克，炮姜 6 克，炙甘草 6
克。水煎 200～300 毫升，早晚分服，每日 1 剂。

加减：血量多、腹痛甚者，加益母草 30 克，生炒蒲黄各 12
克，炒灵脂 9 克。

小腹坠痛、倦怠乏力者，加党参 30 克，黄芪 30 克。

恶露臭秽者，加蒲公英 12 克，金银花 12 克，牡丹皮
12 克，连翘 12 克。

中成药：益母草膏，10 毫升，日 3 次，冲服。

生化汤丸，每次1丸，日3次。

## 5.6.2 产后大便难

产后大便艰涩，或数日不解，或排便时干燥疼痛，难以解出者，称为"产后大便难"。因于分娩时失血，营血骤虚，津液亏耗，不能濡润肠道；或阴虚火盛，内灼津液，津少液亏，肠道失于滋润，传导不利所致。

### 辨证论治

**临床表现** 产后大便干燥，数日不解，或解时艰涩难下，无腹胀痛，饮食如常，面色萎黄，皮肤不润，舌淡苔薄白，脉虚而涩。

治法：养血生津，润燥通便。

方药：四物汤（69）加味。

当归12克，川芎9克，生熟地各12克，白芍药9克，桃仁9克，杏仁9克，火麻仁9克，全瓜蒌30克，麦冬12克，黄精12克，桔梗9克。水煎200～300毫升，早晚分服，每日1剂。

加减：气喘自汗，头晕目眩，精神疲倦者，加党参30克，黄芪30克。

口干咽燥，舌红少津，脉细数者加玄参12克，石斛9克。

脘腹胀满者，加枳壳9克，厚朴9克，山楂12克。

**单方验方**

香油、白蜜适量调匀，温开水冲服200毫升，早晨空腹顿服，每日1次至大便转为正常停服。

麻苏粥：苏子9克，芝麻30克，捣碎煮粥饮服。

番泻叶3克，冲水代茶饮。

**预防** 产后适当活动，增加肠蠕动。多食蔬菜、水果、多饮水。

### 5.6.3 产后发热

产褥期内，出现发热为主症，并伴其他症状者，称产后发热。产后发热病因，或产后瘀血停滞，阻碍气机，营卫失调；或产后百脉空虚，腠理不密，卫外不固，外邪侵袭，营卫不和；或阴血暴虚，阳无所依，浮越于外；或邪毒直犯胞中。临床必须辨证论治。

**辨证论治**

**1.外感型**

(1) 外感风寒

**临床表现** 产后恶寒发热，头痛肢体疼痛，无汗，或咳嗽流涕，舌苔薄白，脉浮。

治法：养血祛风，散寒解表。

方药：荆防四物汤 (33) 加减。

荆芥9克，防风9克，白芷12克，前胡9克，羌活9克，当归9克，川芎6克，白芍药9克，干地黄9克，薄荷6克，桔梗9克。水煎200~300毫升，分两次服，每日1剂。

(2) 外感风热

**临床表现**：产后发热，微恶风寒，头痛，咳嗽，口渴，微汗出或无汗，舌尖边红，苔薄白或薄黄，脉浮数。

治法：辛凉解表，疏风清热。

方药：银翘散 (101)。

金银花12克，连翘9克，淡竹叶9克，荆芥9克，牛蒡子9克，薄荷6克，桔梗9克，淡豆豉9克，芦根9克，甘草6克。水煎300毫升，早晚分服，每日1剂。

(3) 邪客少阳

**临床表现** 新产后寒热往来，口苦咽干，舌苔白润，脉弦。

治法：和解表里。

方药：小柴胡汤 (89)。

柴胡 9 克，黄芩 9 克，党参 12 克，甘草 6 克，生姜 3 片，姜半夏 12 克，大枣 5 枚。水煎 200～300 毫升，早晚分服，每日 1 剂。

**2. 血虚型**

**临床表现**　产后失血过多，身有微热，自汗，头晕目眩，心悸少寐，腹痛绵绵，手足麻木，舌淡红，苔薄白，脉虚微数。

治法：益气养血。

方药：益气养血清热方

太子参 15 克，黄芪 15 克，黄精 12 克，阿胶 12 克（烊化），当归 9 克，川芎 6 克，白芍药 12 克，生地 12 克，麦冬 9 克，旱莲草 12 克。水煎 200～300 毫升，早晚分服，每日 1 剂。

加减：午后潮热，两颧红赤、口渴喜冷饮、大便干燥、小便黄赤、舌红苔薄黄而干、脉细数者，加玄参 12 克，知母 6 克，地骨皮 12 克，柏子仁 12 克。

**3. 血瘀型**

**临床表现**　恶露不下或甚少，色紫黯有块，腹痛拒按，口干不欲饮，舌质黯有瘀斑或瘀点，脉弦涩。

治法：活血化瘀。

方药：生化汤 (61) 加味。

当归 15 克，川芎 12 克，桃仁 12 克，炮姜 6 克，炙甘草 9 克，益母草 30 克，丹参 15 克，丹皮 9 克。水煎 200～300ml，早晚分服，每日一剂。

**4. 感染邪毒型：（同产褥感染）**

## 5.6.4　产后身痛

产褥期内，出现肢体酸楚、疼痛、麻木、重着者，称"产后身痛"。由产后血虚，筋脉关节失于濡养；或产后外邪乘虚而入，留着经络、关节、气血运行受阻，瘀滞而引起。

## 辨证论治

### 1. 血虚型

**临床表现** 遍身疼痛，肢体酸楚麻木，头晕心悸，气短懒言，面色萎黄，肌肤不泽，舌淡红，苔少，脉细弱。

治法：补血益气，温经通络以止痛。

方药：黄芪桂枝五物汤（29）加减。

黄芪15克，桂枝9克，白芍药12克，生姜3片，大枣5枚，当归12克，川芎9克，鸡血藤12克，丝瓜络12克，秦艽9克。水煎200～300毫升，早晚分服，每日1剂。

加减：腰痛明显者，加桑寄生15克，续断30克，补骨脂12克。

纳少便溏者，加山药12克，炒扁豆12克，薏苡仁30克。

大便燥结者，加肉苁蓉12克，火麻仁12克。

### 2. 风寒型

**临床表现** 产后周身关节疼痛，屈伸不利，或痛无定处，或疼痛剧烈，犹如锥刺，或肢体肿胀，麻木重着，步履艰难，得热则舒，舌淡苔薄白，脉细缓。

治法：养血祛风，散寒除湿。

方药：独活寄生汤（18）。

独活9克，桑寄生15克，秦艽9克，防风9克，细辛3克，当归12克，白芍药12克，川芎6克，干地黄9克，杜仲12克，牛膝12克，党参15克，茯苓12克，甘草6克，桂心6克。水煎200～300毫升，早晚分服，日1剂。

加减：肢体重着明显者，去甘草，白芍药、干地黄、加苍术9克，茯苓12克，木瓜12克。

### 3. 肾虚型

**临床表现** 产后腰脊酸楚疼痛，膝软乏力，或足跟痛，舌淡红，苔薄白，脉沉细。

治法：补肾壮腰膝。

方药：补肾活络方。

制附子6克，川断30克，杜仲12克，补骨脂15克，熟地12克，山萸肉9克，枸杞子12克，木瓜12克，秦艽15克，细辛3克，炙甘草9克。水煎200～300毫升，早晚温服，日1剂。

加减：腰膝冷痛，带下清冷者，加鹿角霜12克。

**4. 血瘀型**

**临床表现** 产后身痛，四肢关节不利，或伴下腹痛，恶露排出不畅，舌紫黯或有瘀点，脉沉涩。

治法：活血祛瘀，通经止痛。

方药：身痛逐瘀汤（68）。

桃仁9克，红花9克，当归12克，川芎6克，秦艽12克，羌活9克，没药9克，灵脂9克，香附12克，牛膝15克，地龙9克，甘草6克。水煎200～300毫升，早晚分服，每日1剂。

**预防** 产后充分休息，增强营养，使正气恢复；避免风寒，以防外邪侵袭，暑热季节勿过贪寒凉，以防寒湿外侵；产后2～3日，无手术创伤者，应离床适当活动，以防瘀血阻络。

## 5.6.5 缺乳

产后乳汁甚少或全无，称为"缺乳"。又称"乳汁不足"或"乳汁不行"。乳汁由血所化，赖气以运行，气血源于水谷精微。多因气血虚弱，化源不足，则无乳可下，或肝郁气滞，脉络壅塞，乳不得下而引起。临床以乳房柔软为虚，乳房胀硬而痛为实。

### 辨证论治

**1. 气血虚型**

**临床表现** 产后乳汁少，甚或全无，乳汁清稀，乳房柔软无胀感，面色少华，神疲纳少，舌淡少苔，脉虚细。

治法：益气养血，佐以通乳。

方药：通乳丹（76）。

党参 15 克，黄芪 15 克，当归 9 克，麦冬 12 克，木通 6 克（或通草 6 克），桔梗 9 克，猪蹄蹄一只。用猪蹄煮汤代水煎药 200～300 毫升，早晚分服，每日 1 剂。

加减：产妇体虚明显者，改党参为人参 3 克，浓煎兑服。

纳少便溏者，加茯苓 12 克，山药 12 克，白扁豆 15 克。

## 2. 肝郁气滞型

**临床表现** 产后乳汁分泌甚少或全无，胸胁胀闷，乳房胀硬，或扪及结节，精神抑郁，或有微热，纳差，舌苔薄黄，脉弦细或数。

治法：疏肝解郁，通络下乳。

方药：下乳涌泉散（92）。

当归 12 克，川芎 9 克，生地 12 克，白芍药 12 克，柴胡 9 克，青皮 9 克，天花粉 12 克，王不留行 9 克，炮山甲 15 克，漏芦 9 克，桔梗 9 克，甘草 6 克，通草 6 克，白芷 12 克。水煎 200～300 毫升，早晚分服，每日 1 剂。

加减：胸闷纳呆明显者，去生地、天花粉、加陈皮 9 克，佛手 9 克。

乳胀有硬结者，去生地、甘草，加夏枯草 12 克，连翘 12 克，橘络 12 克，香附 12 克。

身有微热或乳房有热感者，加蒲公英 9 克，白蒺藜 12 克，黄芩 9 克。

**中成药**：下乳涌泉散，每袋煎水 300 毫升，日服 2 次，每日 1 袋。

**其他疗法**

针刺：以膻中、乳根为主穴，少泽、天宗、合谷为配穴（用法见针灸手册)。

饮食疗法：气血虚弱者，用鸡血藤 30 克，红枣 10 枚，桑寄生 12 克。水煎 300 毫升代茶饮。生芝麻 30 克，嚼服。

外治法：用橘皮适量，煎水热敷乳房。配合用木梳向乳头方向疏理乳房，可促气血流畅，乳汁得通。

**预防**

保持乳头清洁，及时治疗皲裂。(用植物油涂局部)。

按时哺乳 (产后 12 小时即可开始哺乳，每 3～4 小时一次，每次 15～20 分钟)。每次哺乳要将乳汁吸空。

保持心情舒畅。

多进高营养、高热量的流质饮食，勿食煎炸辛辣之物，以保乳汁充足通畅。

## 附

1. 回乳：炒麦芽 100 克，生山楂 60 克，水煎 200 毫升，温服，每日 1 剂。配合芒硝外敷 (芒硝 500 克分装两个布袋，敷两乳，用宽布包扎固定)。

2. 乳痈初起，症见恶寒发热，乳房肿胀触痛者。双花 12 克，连翘 9 克，牛蒡子 12 克，全瓜蒌 15 克，天花粉 12 克，黄芩 9 克，青皮 9 克，陈皮 9 克，生栀子 6 克，皂刺 9 克，柴胡 9 克，甘草 6 克，水煎至 200 毫升，低温服，每日 1 剂。

若未成脓者，用仙人掌去刺、捣烂敷患处。已成脓应即时切开排脓。

3. 乳汁自出：不经婴儿吮吸而自然流出者，称为"产后乳汁自出"。亦称"漏乳"、"乳汁自涌"。气虚者，乳汁清稀、量少，乳房柔软不胀。治法：补气固摄。服：太子参 15 克，黄芪 15 克，炒山药 12 克，芡实 12 克，莲子肉 12 克，山萸肉 9 克，五味子 9 克，云苓 12 克，炙甘草 6 克。水煎 200 毫升，温服，每日 1 剂。

肝郁乳汁自出者，乳汁浓，乳房胀满，**心烦易怒**，舌红苔薄黄，脉弦数。治法：平肝清热。服：柴胡9克，黄芩9克，郁金9克，丹皮12克，栀子9克，夏枯草12克，生牡蛎30克，玄参12克，淡竹叶9克，赤芍15克，木通6克，水煎200毫升。待凉服，每日一剂。

## 5.6.6 产后排尿异常

新产后小便不通，或尿意频数，甚而小便失禁者，统称产后排尿异常。多因素体虚弱，产后更虚，气虚膀胱失约，或肾气不固，膀胱气化失职，或手术损伤引起。

### 辨证论治

**1. 气虚型**

**临床表现** 产后小便不通，小腹胀急，或小便频数或失禁，少气懒言，四肢无力，面色少华，舌质淡，苔少，脉缓弱。

治法：益气通利。

方药：益气通脬饮。

太子参30克，黄芪30克，白术9克，山药12克，木香9克，枳壳12克，桔梗9克，茯苓12克，通草6克，车前子9克。水煎200～300毫升，早晚分服，每日1剂。

加减：小便频数失禁者，加益智仁9克，金樱子9克，五味子9克。

**2. 肾虚型**

**临床表现** 产后小便不通，小腹胀满而痛，或小便频数，甚则遗尿，面色晦黯，腰膝酸软，舌淡苔润，脉沉细而迟。

治法：补肾温阳，化气行水。

方药：肾气丸 (66)。

干地黄12克，山药12克，山茱萸9克，茯苓12克，牡丹皮9克，泽泻9克，肉桂6克，附子9克。水煎200～300毫升，早晚分服，每日1剂。

加减：尿频或失禁者，加桑螵蛸12克，复盆子12克，补骨脂15克，生龙骨30克，煅牡蛎30克。

### 3. 产伤

**临床表现** 产后小便不能约束而自遗，或排尿淋漓挟有血丝，舌苔正常，脉缓。

治法：补气固脬。

方药：黄芪当归散（28）加味。

黄芪30克，当归12克，人参15克，白术15克，白芍15克，甘草9克，生姜6克，大枣3枚，猪尿脬1个，白芨12克，水煎200～300毫升，日1剂。

服药期间卧床休息，若久漏不愈，已成尿瘘者，应仔细检查，以手术修补。

**其他疗法**

针灸疗法：取关元、气海、三阴交、阴陵泉、水道各穴（选用），针刺或艾灸。

引尿法：用温热水熏洗外阴，或用温开水冲洗尿道口周围，以诱导排尿。

热敷法：于下腹部放置热水袋，可促使膀胱收缩而排出尿液。

（国培）

# 6 其他妇科疾病

## 6.1 子宫肌瘤

本病是女性生殖系统较常见的良性肿瘤之一。以月经量多，经期延长，下腹坠胀为特点。有的可无任何症状，仅在查体发现。属中医"症积"的范畴，多与正气虚弱，气血失调，气机阻滞，瘀血内停，或痰湿内阻，积之日久，日益增大而形成。

### 辨证论治

**1. 气滞型**

**临床表现** 下腹症块，推之可移，痛无定处，伴小腹胀满不舒。舌苔薄润，脉沉弦。妇科检查：宫体增大，质硬，表面凸凹不平。

治法：行气导滞，佐以活血消症。

方药：香棱丸（91）。

木香 9 克，丁香 6 克，三棱 9 克，枳壳 12 克，青皮 9 克，小茴香 6 克，莪术 9 克，炒川楝 12 克。水煎 200～300 毫升，早晚分服，每日 1 剂。

加减：月经后期量少，可加当归 12 克，川芎 9 克。

下腹痛甚，块下痛减者，加益母草 30 克，生蒲黄 12 克，炒灵脂 9 克。

**2. 血瘀型**

**临床表现** 下腹症块坚硬，固定不移，疼痛拒按，面色晦黯或见褐斑，肌肤不润，口干不欲饮。月经量多或延后，或漏下不止，色紫挟块，行经腹痛，块下痛减，舌质紫黯，边有瘀点，脉沉涩。妇科检查同气滞型。

治法：活血祛瘀，软坚散结。

方药：活瘀散结方。

桂枝9克，桃仁9克，当归12克，川芎9克，赤芍药12克，枳壳15克，川牛膝15克，丹参30克，三棱9克，莪术12克，夏枯草12克，生牡蛎30克。水煎至200~300毫升，早晚分服，每日1剂。平日服用。

加减：于月经期血量多挟块、伴腹痛者，去夏枯草、生牡蛎、加生蒲黄12克，炒灵脂9克。

血崩不止者，去三棱、莪术，加太子参15克，三七粉（冲服）3克。

月经延后或闭止不行而腹痛者，加血竭（冲服）3克，泽兰12克。

3. 痰湿型

**临床表现** 下腹症块，质不甚坚硬，经期或后延量少，或闭止不行，带下量较多，色白质粘腻，形寒畏冷，胸脘痞闷，舌黯苔白腻，脉细濡或沉滑。

治法：理气化痰，破瘀消症。

方药：开郁二陈汤（36）。

青皮9克，陈皮9克，香附12克，川芎6克，木香9克，槟榔12克，制半夏12克，苍术12克，甘草6克，生姜三片，茯苓12克，莪术12克。水煎至200~300毫升，早晚分服，日1剂。

加减：月经量少，或经闭者，加丹参30克，川牛膝15克。

胸闷恶心纳呆者，加鸡内金12克，神曲30克，焦山楂30克，去莪术。

带下色黄、质稠、味臭者，加苦参30克，龙胆草12克，去半夏。

中成药：七制香附丸，每次1丸，日3次，适用于气滞血瘀型。

大黄䗪虫丸，每次 1 丸，日 3 次，适用于正盛体壮之血瘀型。

## 6.2  子宫内膜异位症

子宫内膜组织出现在子宫腔以外时，称为"子宫内膜异位症"。以继发性、进行性痛经，月经失调及不孕为特点，属于中医的"痛经"、"崩漏"、"症瘕"、"不孕症"的范围。是由气血运行不畅而导致冲任瘀阻，胞宫功能失调引起。

### 辨证论治

本病以气滞血瘀型多见。

**临床表现**　经前 1～2 天开始腹痛，行经第一天剧痛。并逐年进行性加剧。腹痛。腰骶痛并放射至会阴、肛门、或大腿部。月经量多，或经期延长，淋漓不断。常有不孕史。舌质紫黯，苔薄白或薄黄，脉沉弦或涩。

妇科检查，可见阴道后穹窿或宫颈有紫兰色结节，子宫后倾，粘连固定，活动受限。子宫后壁、子宫直肠陷凹处，宫骶韧带可触及黄豆及蚕豆大小的结节，质硬、触痛明显。附件区可触及不活动性囊性包块，有轻压痛。

治法：活血化瘀为主。

方药：膈下逐瘀汤 (25)。

当归 12 克，炒五灵脂 9 克，川芎 9 克，赤芍 12 克，桃仁 9 克，红花 9 克，枳壳 12 克，延胡索 9 克，牡丹皮 12 克，香附 12 克，乌药 12 克，甘草 6 克。水煎至 200～300 毫升，早晚分服，每日 1 剂。

加减：神疲乏力，纳差者，去五灵脂，加党参 30 克，黄芪 30 克。

下腹冷痛喜热者，去丹皮、赤芍，加小茴香 9 克，吴茱萸 9 克。

伴输卵管不通而不孕者，加透骨草 12 克，炮山甲 15 克，皂刺 9 克。

**其他疗法**

中药灌肠法：丹参 30 克，川芎 9 克，三棱 9 克，莪术 9 克，制乳香 12 克，没药 12 克，红花 9 克，血竭 3 克。浓煎 150～200 毫升，待温度降至 37 度左右时于晚上睡觉前保留灌肠。

**预防** 矫正宫颈管狭窄、子宫过度后屈，以免因经血瘀滞而引起经血倒流。

月经期避免不必要的盆腔检查。

避免手术操作时引起的子宫内膜种植。

# 6.3 不孕症

女子婚后夫妇同居两年以上，配偶生殖功能正常，未避孕而不受孕者，称原发性不孕。中医称"无子"、"全不产"。如曾有过生育或流产后，未避孕又两年以上未再受孕者，称继发不孕，中医古称为"断绪"。

属先天性生理缺陷者，非药物所能治疗，不为本节讨论内容。如古人所谓"五不女"（螺、纹、鼓、角、脉）。肾主生殖，不孕与肾的关系最密切。临床以先天肾气不足，精血亏虚的肾虚不孕最多见。另外，肝郁气滞、疏泄失常，气血不调，冲任不足；及脾虚湿盛，阻滞胞宫，寒凝血滞等。亦可导致不孕。

## 辨证论治

**1. 肾虚型**

（1）肾阳虚型

**临床表现** 婚后久未受孕，月经后期量少，色淡或月经稀发甚而经闭。面色晦黯，腰酸腿软，性欲淡漠，带下清冷淋漓或滑脱而下，或带下甚少而阴部干涩，小腹冷感，大便溏薄，小便清长，夜间尤甚，舌质淡，苔薄白，脉沉细或沉迟。

妇科检查往往子宫发育不良。

治法：温阳益肾，养血调冲。

方药：益肾养血调冲方。

仙灵脾 12 克，紫石英 30 克，巴戟天 9 克，续断 15 克，鹿角霜 12 克，川椒 1.5 克，枸杞子 12 克，当归 12 克，川芎 9 克，白芍药 12 克，熟地 9 克，木香 9 克。水煎至 200～300 毫升，分 2 次温服，每日 1 剂（经期停服）。

加减：气短乏力，小腹下坠者，加党参 30 克，黄芪 30 克。

带下冷滑不禁者，加芡实 12 克，金樱子 9 克。

小便清长，夜间频数者，加益智仁 9 克，桑螵蛸 12 克，煅龙骨 30 克。

(2) 阴虚型

**临床表现** 婚后久不孕，月经先期，量少，色红无块，形体消瘦，腰腿酸软，心悸失眠，五心烦热，口干，午后低热，舌红苔少，脉细数。

治法：滋阴养血，清热调经。

方药：六味地黄汤（41）加减。

生地 15 克，山茱萸 9 克，山药 12 克，牡丹皮 12 克，泽泻 9 克，地骨皮 9 克，当归 9 克，白芍药 15 克，旱莲草 24 克，女贞子 9 克，红花 9 克。续断 30 克。水煎至 200～300 毫升，分 2 次温服，每日 1 剂。

加减：口干，舌苔少津者，加玄参 12 克，知母 6 克，麦冬 9 克。

心烦少寐者，加柏子仁 9 克，五味子 9 克，炒枣仁 30 克。

中成药：六味地黄丸，每次 1 丸，每日 2 次。

**2. 肝郁型**

**临床表现**　婚后多年不孕，月经周期先后不定，经前经期腹痛，经行不畅，血少色黯，挟块，经前胸胁乳房胀痛，精神抑郁，烦躁易怒，舌黯红苔薄白，脉弦。

治法：舒肝解郁，养血调经。

方药：舒肝调经汤。

柴胡9克，郁金9克，川楝子12克，香附12克，当归9克，川芎6克，白芍药9克，生地12克，桑椹子12克，枳壳12克，益母草15克。水煎200～300毫升，分2次服，每日1剂。

加减：经前乳胀痛有硬块者，加夏枯草12克，橘核9克，路路通9克，生牡蛎30克。

经少难下，腹痛甚者，加莪术12克，延胡索9克，生蒲黄15克，去生地、桑椹子。

舌红苔黄，脉弦数者，加丹皮12克，栀子9克，玄参12克，去桑椹子。

中成药：逍遥丸，每次6～9克，每日2次。

七制香附丸，每次1丸，每日2次。

**3. 痰湿型**

**临床表现**　婚后久未受孕，形体肥胖，月经延期，血少甚或闭经，带下量多，质粘稠，面色㿠白，头晕心悸，胸闷泛恶，舌苔白腻，脉滑。

治法：燥湿豁痰，化瘀开窍。

方药：燥湿豁痰方。

炒苍术9克，炒白术9克，天竺黄9克，姜半夏12克，橘络9克，生蒲黄12克，莪术9克，石菖蒲9克，制胆星9克，枳壳9克，姜竹茹9克，茯苓12克。水煎至200～300毫升，分2次温服，每日1剂。

加减：气短、带下量多者，加党参15克，黄芪15克，炒白芍 15 克。

月经后期量少者，加仙灵脾 12 克，续断 30 克，当归 12 克。

**4. 血瘀型**

**临床表现**　婚后久不孕，月经后期，量少，色紫黑，有血块，伴腹痛、拒按，块下痛减，舌紫黯或舌边有瘀点，脉弦涩。妇科检查多有盆腔炎症。

治法：活血化瘀。

方药：桃红四物汤 (75) 加减。

桃仁 9 克，红花 9 克，当归 12 克，川芎 9 克，赤芍 15 克，白芍药 15 克，莪术 12 克，延胡索 6 克，乌药 12 克，香附 12 克，丹参 30 克，水煎至 200~300 毫升，分 2 次温服，每日 1 剂。

加减：腹痛喜暖者，加小茴香 9 克，艾叶 9 克，

输卵管不通者，加皂刺 9 克，透骨草 12 克，炮山甲 15 克。

盆腔炎块致下腹时常作痛者，加鸡血藤 15 克，连翘 12 克，三棱 9 克。

**5. 气血虚弱型**

**临床表现**　婚久不孕，月经后期，血少，色淡，质稀薄或闭经，面色萎黄，神疲乏力，纳谷不佳，头晕，心悸，两目干涩，舌淡苔薄白，脉细弱。妇科检查多有子宫发育不良。

治法：补气养血调经。

方药：毓麟珠 (98) 加减。

党参 15 克，黄芪 15 克，炒白术 9 克，茯苓 9 克，当归 9 克，川芎 9 克，熟地 12 克，白芍药 12 克，阿胶 12 克 (烊化)，菟丝子 12 克，川椒 1.5 克，仙灵脾 12 克。水煎至 200~300 毫升，分两次温服，每日 1 剂。

加减：带下过少，阴部干涩，性欲低下者，加紫河车 30

克，鹿角胶 12 克。

行经下腹隐痛不舒者，加鸡血藤 12 克，益母草 15 克。

中成药　十全大补丸，每次 1 丸，每日 2 次。

**其他疗法**

川芎嗪注射液 4 毫升，加注射用水至 10 毫升，缓慢注入宫腔。于经血干净 3～5 天至排卵前期使用，隔日 1 次，3～4 次为 1 疗程。用于输卵管阻塞者。

盆腔炎症、输卵管不通所致不孕，可配合丹参注射液 10 毫升加入 5～10% 葡萄糖注射液 500 毫升中作静脉滴注，每日 1 次，10 日为一疗程。

中药煎液作保留灌肠：丹参 30 克，红花 12 克，桂枝 9 克，透骨草 15 克，鸡血藤 15 克，制乳香 9 克，制没药 9 克。浓煎至 100 毫升，每晚睡前灌肠，10 日为一疗程，经期停用。适用各类瘀阻疼痛症。

# 6.4　阴挺

妇女子宫下脱，或阴道壁膨出，前者为子宫脱垂，后者为阴道壁膨出。中医统称为"阴挺"。又称"阴脱"、"阴菌"、"产肠不收"等。临床以子宫从正常位置沿阴道下降，子宫颈外口达坐骨棘水平以下，甚至子宫全部脱出于阴道口作为诊断子宫脱垂的标准。主要病机是由于产伤未及时修补，产后过早参加重体力劳动，气虚下陷，肾虚不固而致胞络损伤，不能提摄子宫而引起。多因分娩时临盆过早、难产、产程过长，产时用力太过，或产后过早劳动，操劳过重，久咳，便秘，或素日体虚，房事不节，多产等引起本症发生。

## 辨证论治

### 1. 气虚型

**临床表现**  子宫下移或脱出阴道口外，劳累则加剧，小腹下坠，四肢无力，少气懒言，面色少华，小便频数，带下量多，质稀色白，舌淡苔薄，脉虚细。

治法：益气升提。

方药：补中益气汤（7）（方见第 5.6.1 恶露不绝）。

加减：腰酸、带多清稀者，加续断 30 克，金樱子 12 克，芡实 9 克。

### 2. 肾虚型

**临床表现**  子宫下脱，腰酸腿软，小便频数，夜间尤甚，头晕耳鸣，舌淡红，脉沉弱。

治法：补肾固脱。

方药：大补元煎（13）加减。

熟地 12 克，山药 12 克，山茱萸 12 克，茯苓 9 克，枸杞子 12 克，杜仲 12 克，续断 15 克，金樱子 12 克，鹿角胶 12 克（烊化服），芡实 9 克，黄芪 15 克。水煎 200～300 毫升，分 2 次温服，每日 1 剂。

### 3. 湿热型

**临床表现**  子宫脱出阴道口外，脱出部分红肿溃烂，黄水淋漓，带下量多，色黄或挟脓血，秽臭，伴口渴发热，小便黄赤，局部灼痛，舌红苔黄腻，脉数。

治法：清利湿热。

方药：龙胆泻肝汤（38）。

龙胆草 9 克，栀子 9 克，黄芩 9 克，车前子 9 克（包），木通 6 克，泽泻 9 克，生地 9 克，当归 12 克，柴胡 9 克，甘草 6 克。水煎 200～300 毫升，分 2 次温服，每日 1 剂。

加减：寒战高热，腹痛尿频灼痛者，加石苇 15 克，蒲公英

15 克，金银花 15 克，延胡索 9 克。

**其他疗法**

单方：棉花根 60 克，枳壳 30 克。水煎 200 毫升温服，每日 1 剂。或金樱子根 60 克，水煎 200 毫升温服，每日 1 剂。

针刺疗法：主穴维胞（关元旁开 6 寸），子宫、三阴交。配穴长强、百会、阴陵泉，每周针刺 2～3 次，2～3 周为 1 疗程。

外治法：五倍子 15 克，枳壳 30 克，诃子肉 9 克，黄柏 15 克，木通 9 克，水煎 1000 毫升，加入冰片 1.5 克，薰洗，每次 10～15 分钟，每日 1～2 次，日 1 剂。

子宫托：适用于一度、二度脱垂，无感染者，需在医师指导下使用。

手术治疗：上述各法无效者，可选用适当手术。

# 6.5 阴吹

妇女阴道时时出气，或气出有声，如矢气者，称为阴吹。若无其他不适感，则不作病论。本病多因肠胃津液枯燥，腑气不通，或因中气不足，或因水饮停聚中焦，以致谷气不通而引起。现代医学认为多由分娩时损伤阴道而致组织松弛引起。

## 辨证论治

**1. 肠燥型**

（1）热结肠胃

**临床表现** 阴中时时排出气体，气出声粗响亮，大便燥结难解，口干渴喜冷饮，舌红苔黄燥，脉数。

治法：清热润燥，理气导滞。

方药：玉女煎（99）。

生石膏 30 克，知母 9 克，熟地 12 克，麦冬 12 克，牛膝 15 克。水煎 200～300 毫升，每 2 次温服，每日 1 剂。

加减：热盛气结肠燥明显者，可加生地12克，全瓜蒌30克，柏子仁9克，鲜石斛9克，杏仁9克，陈皮9克。

(2) 阴虚津枯肠燥

**临床表现** 阴吹时作，形体干瘦，面色枯萎，皮肤干燥，咽干口燥，或五心烦热，午后潮热，大便燥结，小便量少色黄，舌红苔少不润，脉细略数。

治法：养阴生津，润燥通便。

方药：五仁丸 (84)。

杏仁9克，桃仁9克，柏子仁9克，郁李仁12克，松子仁12克，水煎200～300毫升，分2次温服，每日1剂。

加减：津亏无腹胀气滞者，去郁李仁，加全瓜蒌30克，黄精12克，生地12克。

**2. 气虚型**

**临床表现** 阴中排气，声音低沉，伴面色㿠白，气短乏力，心悸，语声低微，小腹空坠，小便频数，大便秘或溏薄，白带清稀量多，舌淡红苔薄白，脉虚缓无力。

治法：益气补中。

方药：补中益气汤 (7) (方见5.6恶露不绝)。

加减：便秘者加肉苁蓉12克，熟地12克。

**3. 水饮停聚型**

**临床表现** 阴中出气，形体肥胖，面色浮白，脘闷纳呆，呕吐痰涎，心悸少寐，头重目眩，大便燥结或粘腻。舌质淡胖，苔白腻，脉弦滑或弦迟。

治法：利湿豁痰，佐以健脾。

方药：橘半桂苓枳姜汤 (31)。

陈皮9克，姜半夏12克，桂枝9克，茯苓12克，枳实9克，生姜三片。水煎200～300毫升，分2次温服，每日1剂。

加减：大便燥结难解者，去生姜，加全瓜蒌30克，芒硝3克。

**4. 肝郁气滞型**

**临床表现** 阴中出气，或续或断，神情抑郁，烦躁易怒，胸胁少腹胀痛；嗳气食少，时欲叹息，大便时干，伴月经先后无定期，经量时多时少，舌苔薄白，脉弦或弦涩。

治法：疏肝理气解郁。

方药：四逆散 (65)。

柴胡9克，白芍药12克，枳实12克，甘草6克。水煎200～300毫升，分2次服，每日1剂。

加减：腹胀、便燥者，加瓜蒌仁30克，桃仁9克，郁李仁12克。

（国培）

# THE ENGLISH–CHINESE ENCYCLO–PEDIA OF PRACTICAL TCM

## (Booklist)

# 英汉实用中医药大全

## （书目）

| VOLUME | TITLE | 书名 |
|---|---|---|
| 1 | ESSENTIALS OF TCM | 中医学基础 |
| 2 | THE CHINESE MATERIA MEDICA | 中药学 |
| 3 | PHARMACOLOGY OF TRADITION-AL CHINESE MEDICAL FORMULAE | 方剂学 |
| 4 | SIMPLE AND PROVEN PRESCRIPTION | 单验方 |
| 5 | COMMONLY USED CHINESE PATENTMEDICINES | 常用中成药 |
| 6 | THERAPY OF ACUPUNCTURE AND MOXIBUSTION | 针灸疗法 |
| 7 | *TUINA* THERAPY | 推拿疗法 |
| 8 | MEDICAL *QIGONG* | 医学气功 |
| 9 | MAINTAINING YOUR HEALTH | 自我保健 |
| 10 | INTERNAL MEDICINE | 内科学 |
| 11 | SURGERY | 外科学 |
| 12 | GYNECOLOGY | 妇科学 |
| 13 | PEDIATRICS | 儿科学 |
| 14 | ORTHOPEDICS | 骨伤科学 |
| 15 | PROCTOLOGY | 肛门直肠病学 |
| 16 | DERMATOLOGY | 皮肤病学 |
| 17 | OPHTHALMOLOGY | 眼科学 |
| 18 | OTORHINOLARYNGOLOGY | 耳鼻喉科学 |
| 19 | EMERGENTOLOGY | 急症学 |
| 20 | NURSING | 护理 |
| 21 | CLINICAL DIALOGUE | 临床会话 |

（京）112号

The English – Chinese
Encyclopedia of Practical TCM
Cheif Editor Xu Xiangcai
12
GYNECOLOGY
Chief Editors Xuan Jiasheng
Li Zhulan
英汉实用中医药大全
主编　徐象才
12
妇　科　学
主编　李竹兰
宣家声

\*

高等教育出版社出版
高等教育出版社照排中心照排
新华书店总店北京科技发行所发行
国防工业出版社印刷厂印刷

\*

开本 850×1168　1／32　印张 15　字数 380 000
1990 年 8 月第 1 版　　1997 年 7 月第 2 次印刷
印数 5 261—9 270
ISBN7－04－002059－9／R·2
定价　15.60 元